GW01184634

I NEVER KNEW THAT

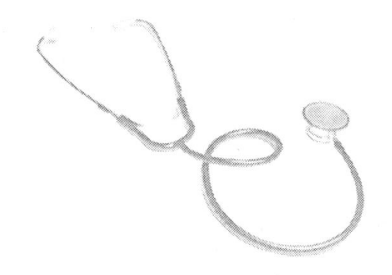

DR. SHANE MISEER

(MBBS. LRCP. MRCS)

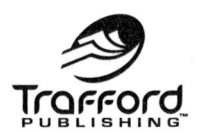

Trafford
PUBLISHING

Order this book online at www.trafford.com/07-0597
or email orders@trafford.com

Most Trafford titles are also available at major online book retailers.

Note for Librarians: A cataloguing record for this book is available from Library
and Archives Canada at www.collectionscanada.ca/amicus/index – e.html

Printed in Victoria, BC, Canada.

ISBN: 978-1-4251-2195-2

*We at Trafford believe that it is the responsibility of us all, as both individuals
and corporations, to make choices that are environmentally and socially sound.
You, in turn, are supporting this responsible conduct each time you purchase a
Trafford book, or make use of our publishing services. To find out how you are
helping, please visit www.trafford.com/responsiblepublishing.html*

*Our mission is to efficiently provide the world's finest, most comprehensive
book publishing service, enabling every author to experience success.
To find out how to publish your book, your way, and have it available
worldwide, visit us online at www.trafford.com/10510*

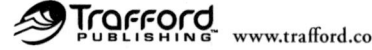 www.trafford.com

North America & international
toll – free: 1 888 232 4444 (USA & Canada)
phone: 250 383 6864 ♦ fax: 250 383 6804 ♦ email: info@trafford.com

The United Kingdom & Europe
phone: +44 (0)1865 487 395 ♦ local rate: 0845 230 9601
facsimile: +44 (0)1865 481 507 ♦ email: info.uk@trafford.com

10 9 8 7 6 5 4 3

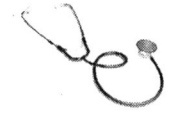

FOREWORD

I was never going to be around forever to take care of my patients. That painful point became clearer as the time approached for me to retire from my practice. Loyal patients and friends would accusingly stab me with "Who will I call when I need a doctor?" Who indeed!

From my years in hospital practice I learned that when the consultant's mother was admitted to hospital she automatically received special attention. I have tried to treat all my patients as though they were my consultant's parents, never taking them for granted, paying attention to what was being confided in me and putting my patient's safety and health first and foremost. Cause no harm – that was the law.

One day my eldest son handed me a book with a note "Dad, read this". I knew then that my time had come to sever the umbilical cord and allow new life to take its course. That little book was "Who Moved My Cheese" (Dr. Spencer Johnson); it made leaving my patients and the comforting cocoon I had woven around me less traumatic.

What could I leave them?

In "I Never Knew That" I have tried to give something back so that leaving, as we all must one day, did not create a complete void with nothing to show for the wonderful relationships my practice had known. Clearly it is not intended to be a textbook of medicine and much of what I have written is my own views. I strongly advise you to consult your own doctor on matters pertaining to your own health and to use "I Never Knew That" as a guide towards that goal.

I Never Knew That

A subject that received scant attention throughout my medical career was Nutrition. Things like: what role does Zinc play in our lives? And how much of it does an adult need to maintain the integrity of the sex organs? And why do school children appear to be getting shorter and shorter? And why are there more and more Infertility Clinics? And why oysters are called 'aphrodisiacs'?

Medicine without Nutrition is like a car without petrol. I was blissfully unaware that I had very little petrol and my learned colleagues did not fare any better.

I suspect the closed mindset towards 'Alternative Medicine' stems from ignorance on the subject of nutrition and the erroneous idea that Alternative Medicine is linked to 'Homeopathic Medicine'. There are over two thousand research articles on Omega 3 Fatty Acids but how many doctors take it as a supplement? And how many prescribe it to pregnant mothers?

When it was reported that Vitamin E did not help in lung cancer were we informed which company had supplied the vitamin that was used in the study? Vitamin E is actually made up of 8 fractions – companies cut costs by using only one of the fractions and this is often a synthetic one to boot. Could this be the reason the vitamin did nothing? Some of the better companies include 4 of the fractions. I am of aware of one that includes all 8 – just as nature intended in a peanut. The letters *dl* before tocopherol (Vitamin E) stand for dex*tro-laevo* – light directed at synthetic Vitamin E molecules enters from the *right* and *left* respectively. Natural Vitamin E allows this light to enter only from the *right* – called *d*-tocopherol. The law permits the public to be kept in the dark about this difference. The cynic, quick to use the 'natural food' instead of a supplement, should know that it would take 4 1/2 *cups* of peanuts to obtain just one day's requirement of Vitamin E!

I have been privileged to perform my own autopsy on GNLD International – a company that introduced me to the subject of Nutrition. I learned from them that the research for the chemotherapy used worldwide in the treatment of cancer hails from their Scientific Advisory Board and that they include the whole orange including the *whites* of the fruit in their Vitamin C slow-release tablet. Their product was the only solvent that could degrease the penguins of oil from tanker spillages and this same product that could clean an engine could be accidentally drunk by a child without harmful side-effects. The list is long.

In recommending their products in my book the company bears no responsibility whatsoever for either the use of their products for the conditions listed or any claims made on behalf of the products. They have no vested interests in this book and their products are only available through appointed agents. I nurture a fervent hope that this policy will change.

Until then the products may be obtained via their website at www.gnld.com or email gnlduk@hotmail.com for more information.

I wish to thank all my patients whose illnesses taught me to better understand medicine and to accept a sincere apology for the times when it failed them. The lesson learnt that very little can be cured and much that could have been prevented.

I dedicate this book to all my patients, my family and friends who never tired of asking "When will it be ready?" And a special thank you to my daughter Sandhya for the proof-reading and my colleagues and dear friend – Professor Charles Swanepoel – who gave me their unstinting support and encouragement. To their good health -

Shane Miseer

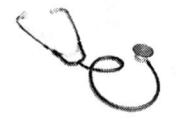

CONTENTS

1.	ABORTION OR MISCARRIAGE	1
2.	ABSCESS/ BOIL	7
3.	ACUTE PANIC ATTACK	13
4.	ALCOHOL	16
5.	ALZHEIMER'S DISEASE	24
6.	ANTIBIOTICS	30
7.	APPENDICITIS	33
8.	ARTHRITIS	38
9.	ASTHMA	44
10.	ATTENTION DEFICIT HYPERACTIVITY DISORDER	56
11.	BEDWETTING	61
12.	BREAST FEEDING	64
13.	CHEST PAIN	70
14.	CHILDREN	76
15.	CONDOMS	87
16.	DEATH	92
17.	DEPRESSION	97
18.	DIABETES MELLITUS	103
19.	DIARRHOEA	113
20.	DIFFICULTY SWALLOWING (DYSPHAGIA)	121
21.	DRINKING WATER	123
22.	ECZEMA	127

23.	EGGS	129
24.	EXERCISE	131
25.	GOING FOR AN OPERATION	139
26.	GOUT	144
27.	HEAD INJURIES	147
28.	HEADACHE	151
29.	HEART ATTACK	155
30.	HEARTBURN	164
31.	HERNIA	167
32.	HYPERTENSION	170
33.	IN–LAWS	175
34.	INFERTILITY	179
35.	IRREGULAR PERIODS	186
36.	LOWER ABDOMINAL PAIN	188
37.	LOWER BACK PAIN	190
38.	MARRIAGE	202
39.	MIDDLE ABDOMINAL PAIN	214
40.	MUSCLE CRAMPS	216
41.	NECK PAIN	218
42.	OSTEOPOROSIS	221
43.	PALPITATIONS	227
44.	PERIODS	231
45.	PILES (HAEMORRHOIDS)	235
46.	PNEUMONIA	239
47.	PREGNANCY	244
48.	SEXUALLY TRANSMITTED DISEASES	259
49.	SEXUAL ABUSE	263
50.	SINUSITIS	268
51.	SORE THROAT	272
52.	SOUNDING OFF	276
53.	STRESS	282
54.	SWELLING OF THE FEET	290
55.	THE ANKLE JOINT	293

56.	THE BABY	297
57.	THE BLADDER	304
58.	THE EAR	317
59.	THE EYE	324
60.	THE HANDS	333
61.	THE HIP JOINT	340
62.	THE IMMUNE SYSTEM	345
63.	THE MEDICINE CABINET	354
64.	THE MENOPAUSE	358
65.	THE MISSED PERIOD	363
66.	THE ORAL CONTRACEPTIVE	365
67.	THE PAP SMEAR	369
68.	THE PROSTATE GLAND	373
69.	THE SHOULDER JOINT	377
70.	THE TESTICLES	380
71.	THE THYROID GLAND	385
72.	THE PENIS	390
73.	THE THERMOMETER / FEVER	396
74.	UPPER ABDOMINAL PAIN	403
75.	VAGINAL DISCHARGES	410
76.	WARTS	413
77.	WEIGHT MANAGEMENT	415
78.	WRIST JOINT	438

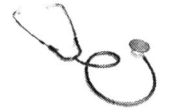

ABORTION OR MISCARRIAGE

When a pregnancy is terminated naturally (called a miscarriage) or deliberately(abortion) before the foetus is 20 weeks old it is not considered viable i.e. it will not easily survive outside the mother's womb. If it is terminated for any reason after the 20th week it is called *premature birth.*

Periods (menstrual flow) are not routinely examined for products of conception and many pregnancies are 'terminated' by the body for unknown reasons and no one is the wiser. The unsuspecting female may note a slightly heavier flow or a bit more pain than usual and think nothing further of it.

Any person who has three or more miscarriages should have investigations to try and ascertain a cause as some of these may be treatable. Circumstances permitting, it is difficult to contain the joy of the parents when it is first confirmed that the partner is pregnant. It may however be prudent to take the pregnancy one day at a time. Announcing the news to all and sundry, rushing out to furnish the 'baby's room and practicing breathing exercises in anticipation of labour that is a whole nine months away will all come to a crashing end if nature has other plans. It may make readjustment to a 'non-pregnant' state more difficult and the emotional recovery phase needlessly painful and prolonged.

The subject of pregnancy and induced abortions are often clouded by emotion and religious sentiments – perhaps more than nature intended. To become pregnant out of ignorance of effective contraceptive measures and then have to bear the consequences of the unplanned pregnancy forever afterwards is often so unnecessary. The unplanned baby will grow up with or without the parents; the state or foster parents can see to this – but what of the parents of the child? Often these are teenagers in school or young adults recently started college or a promising career. There are many reasons why the youngsters may drop out of school or college. Life will never be the same ever again!

Here is a small check list for what is in store for the parents of the baby:

- Be prepared for over 4000 nappy changes until the baby is 3 years old and these may be soiled with urine or faeces or both at any time of the day or night
- Make that 8000 if the pregnancy turns out to be twins
- Forget about parties, movies, night clubs or evenings alone unless one can find a reliable babysitter – and do not even consider one's parents for this role
- The cost of baby feeds and clothes – and one size will not fit forever
- The cost of a nursery if one is working or studying
- Rushing to the doctor/chemist/clinic and often at night. Try finding an all–night chemist or doctor in a hurry. Never mind the anguish over the baby's illness – "Has it got meningitis?" "Could it be his appendix?" And one has to be at work the following morning!
- The first time the baby starts crying and will not stop and then progresses to wild screaming with its legs doubled up and face contorted in pain will make one hit the panic button. The sheer helplessness of being unable to do anything to relieve the suffering or communicate with the little infant as it looks up into your face for help will test the patience and courage of the bravest. The harder and faster one rocks the baby to try to calm it the harder and louder it will scream. One's anxieties and fears will be picked up by the infant as surely as it could read one's mind.

Does the 14 year old school girl with the physical maturity to bear children have the mental and emotional maturity to cope with a baby when she should have been concentrating on getting better grades in school and which dress to wear to the dance? It can take exactly one minute of unprotected sex to change it all – thirty seconds to have a boyfriend ejaculate sperm into an unsuspecting vagina. It may not be possible to control the urge or need to have sex but using a condom responsibly can prevent a pregnancy. Failing that - one has recourse to the 'morning-after' pill to prevent an unwanted pregnancy - bearing in mind that nausea and vomiting are unpleasant side effects of this drug.

Much is made about the psycho–physical aspects of abortion. The body could not give a hoot. It has the theoretical potential to produce twins or even triplets every 9 months for 40 years! Of course, an 'unwanted' pregnancy can certainly be made to become 'wanted'. The teenager with the problem is often frightened out of her wits by the very idea of the predicament into which she got herself. A root–canal treatment at the dentist can only be experienced first hand. Stories of pregnancies from mothers and friends and the media will not completely prepare the young mum–to–be for what is in store. The pregnancy test kit is bought clandestinely in a chemist far removed from home. The entire chemist will, seemingly, know one has had sex. The test is done alone behind closed doors with the heart pounding in one's mouth – "Please God let it be negative and I'll never have sex again". The would–be–father has no inkling of the drama unfolding in the bathroom and that their future hangs on a colour change! 'Blue' and the following will fly: –

- She told me she was on the pill
- How was I to know she was not taking it regularly?
- Why did she not take the necessary precautions?
- I didn't know the condom would break if I used Vaseline?
- We had sex only once – how could she become pregnant if we did it only one time?
- It was only foreplay!
- I never thought I could make her pregnant!

- She told me she could not become pregnant if we had sex during her period
- We did not have a condom and took the chance

Then she must face her parents who may not have been aware their precious 'baby' was having sex at home while they were at work or away for the weekend. How often has it been the teenager is made to follow the dictates of her parents regardless of how the pregnancy and an unwanted baby may change her life forever? Laws have been changed to allow women the right to decide if they wish to have a pregnancy terminated provided it has not advanced beyond 14 weeks. After this period the procedure becomes more difficult to perform and places the mother at risk.

Ending a pregnancy can be done either

- Medically – using drugs or
- Surgically – Suction termination or evacuation done under a general anaesthetic.

There may be some bleeding after the procedure but often not much more than would be expected from a menstrual period. The sanitary pads should show less and less staining with blood over a 24 hour period. If this is not the case medical advice should be sought. There may be some lower abdominal pain but this is controllable with analgesics and should show signs of abating within 24 to 36 hours. The periods may take a month or two after the termination to return to normal. A fever or unwell feeling 3 to 5 days (sometimes even longer) after the termination of pregnancy needs a medical opinion. It is no longer considered necessary to observe a waiting period after a natural abortion and personal choice and nature are allowed to decide about future pregnancies. It may help shorten the 'mourning' period after an abortion.

For at least two months before falling pregnant again it is advisable for both partners to take the following supplements:

- *Omega3* (2 capsules daily)

- *Formula 4 plus* (tablet and capsule) daily
- *Zinc tablets* (1 daily)
- *Calmag tablets* (3 daily)
- *Vitamin E* – 200 I.U. (1 capsule daily)

This is to improve the nutritional status of both prospective parents *before* conception takes place (again) and to improve the quality of the sperm and ovum (egg). Pregnancy should hardly be a 'hit or miss' affair. One will reap as well as one sows – produce the best sperm and egg to do the job. The mother should continue with the supplements *throughout* the pregnancy and *afterwards* for the duration of the breast-feeding period. These supplements will have no deleterious side effects on the baby. Health authorities have only recently been extolling the benefits of Omega 3 for the development of the brain and retina in the foetus and the infant.

After an abortion there are no major physical side effects that should cause concern provided the procedure is performed in a hospital setting by competent and caring staff and no complications arise. There should be a support system to meet the emotional needs of the patient and, where applicable, the male partner. Conception should take place normally thereafter, not that this should be a consideration if the pregnancy was unplanned and unwanted.

After an assault or rape antiviral drugs for HIV and Hepatitis vaccination should be administered immediately and counselling arranged for the victim. If a pregnancy results from this crime the unfortunate victim is entitled to a therapeutic abortion. This is also legal when the mother's life is endangered by the pregnancy or the foetus is found to carry a genetic abnormality such as Down's syndrome. It is often maintained that life is precious and to be preserved at 'any cost' and there are many people with Down's syndrome living with loving parents. It should also not be ignored that as human beings we have the gift of free will. Just as we have been taught to respect life it should hardly be 'at any cost'. Nature has long been a proponent of survival of the fittest and in its great wisdom allows the infirm and deformed to die at birth. The human spirit and the physical body are more resilient than we give it credit. Given time and understanding they will recover from the immediate pain of the loss but it could be criminal to allow to term what nature would have denied and forever after subject the deformed and the parents of the deformed to a life time of suffering under the guise of 'preserving life at all costs'. Mankind has still to grasp that life should have some dignity more than simply the beating of a heart without much quality of life. Once the pregnancy has been allowed to progress to term (maturity) what choice would the parents have *but* to cherish it till death? Death is a part of life, a part of living – man does have control over life and destiny. The electric chair, the genocides, the racial murders, the family murders, the hijackings and gang killings, international wars, religious wars, the road traffic deaths, terrorist murders, euthanasia – are all well known to mankind – but an unwanted pregnancy is wished survival!

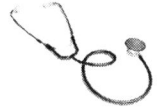

ABSCESS/ BOIL

The skin is the body's largest organ. Normal skin has bacteria (germs) on it. If the numbers become more than the skin can handle or if the immune system becomes compromised because of

- diabetes
- a protracted illness
- poor nutrition
- chronic alcohol abuse or
- stress

the natural defences of the organ are compromised and a 'pimple' can develop. A pimple is a smaller version of an abscess. Sweat glands in the skin open on the surface via pores. Bacteria commonly gain entry through these pores or, if the skin has been damaged, by an abrasion (cracked skin on heels) or thorn prick. If the infection should spread this little pimple gets bigger and turns into an *abscess*.

If the area *around* a pimple starts to spread and becomes red chances are that an abscess is developing. At this time use of an antibiotic may prevent the abscess from progressing to a stage when 'incision and drainage' is the only option i.e. requiring minor surgery. This would mean a local or general anaesthetic depending on its size and where it is situated. Once pus has formed within the abscess antibiotics cannot be relied upon to solve the problem.

Pain from an abscess occurs because the infection and accompanying inflammation lead to the formation of pus and swelling. As the pus accumulates and stretches the surrounding tissue the pain gradually increases in intensity and, once it becomes constant, severe and throbbing, implies that the abscess has reached the point of no return; surgery will then become necessary. Before this stage is reached pain may be present only on applying pressure – this would be the time to take an antibiotic.

If one cannot get to a doctor and pus has started to ooze out from a point on the abscess, (only as an *emergency* measure to relieve the pain), one can squeeze out as much pus as is possible. This will be very painful while it is being done but it can bring much relief by removing some of the pressure generated by the pus. Place the index fingers and swabs/clean tissues on either side of the abscess and apply gentle but continuous pressure to squeeze out of it as much pus as possible. It is advisable to use clean/sterile gloves; a new pair of kitchen gloves may do in an emergency. Be aware that pus is infectious and therefore contagious and all soiled material should be placed in a plastic bag before disposal. Wash the hands thoroughly before and afterwards. Note that this is an emergency measure to relieve pain and a doctor should be seen as soon as possible. Invariably, the opening of the abscess is not wide enough and once it seals itself pus may build up again and one is back to the original problem.

An abscess in the armpit (axilla) deserves special attention. A simple boil can become a 'recurrent' problem - aided and abetted by bacteria that collect in the natural habitat of sweat in this area. The result may be an abscess that could end up being treated in theatre under a general anaesthetic. Correct treatment the first time, with the opening made wide enough and pus drained surgically, may avoid a recurrence.

The armpit is an awkward area because the arm naturally hangs by the side and will put pressure on the abscess and result in more discomfort. Walking about with the affected arm on the hip will help avoid the pressure, as would sleeping with a pillow between the arm and the side. Boils in the armpit can become a nightmare and may persist for months and sometimes years. Sulphur–producing bacteria in the armpit are responsible for producing the 'odour' that seems to plague our sanitised lives. If there is a tendency to boils in the armpit, roll–on type of deodorants should be avoided as bacteria may lurk on the container itself. For the same reason roll–on deodorants/antiperspirants should not be shared with others.

Applying ointments to help 'draw out pus' is a waste of money; left alone nature will force the pus to follow the path of least resistance and push its way out to the surface. It does help to *rest* the affected part as the body is trying to limit the spread of infection and movement will defeat this. A boil must first become 'ripe' i.e. the pus must have formed and be about to burst – before it is ready for incision (lancing).

As a preventative measure regular use of a medicated soap may help reduce the bacterial load on the skin and the frequency of skin infections. Showering at night and paying special attention to the armpits to remove deodorants and antiperspirants used during the day may also help prevent or reduce infection. Avoiding the use of these substances at night allows the pores of the sweat glands to open again. However, the area should be washed again in the morning before application because perspiration occurs during the night and antiperspirants should not be applied once sweat has formed. Most of these products contain aluminium which is used to seal off the pores thereby preventing sweat from being secreted. Bacteria multiply in the sweat and produce the all too familiar odour.

It is safer to use products that do not contain aluminium or those made from natural ingredients that do not contain this metal. Aluminium is absorbed into the body and has long been suspected of playing a role in causing Alzheimer's disease (dementia).

A boil in or around the anus (back passage) should ideally be treated in hospital as its size may be deceptive. What appears as a small abscess on the outside could well hide a half a litre of pus within the rectum. Lesions in this area should be treated under general anaesthetic if one is to avoid future problems. The site is notorious for developing a chronically discharging bead of pus, noticed as a discharge on the underwear or during toiletry. The pocket of pus lies deep within the tissue around the rectum and will intermittently find its way out to the surface just when one imagines one has seen the last of it! This communication (called a 'fistula') between the deeper tissues around the rectum and the skin will always require an operation. It is not usually painful and by virtue of its embarrassing site may go untreated for months and sometimes years. A boil that occurs more than once at the same site often implies that the original abscess was not properly treated. The sufferer may be content to continue stuffing toilet paper in the underwear to absorb the discharge rather than seek advice! Perianal abscesses (around the anus) have sometimes been mistaken for haemorrhoids (piles). The telephonic advice from the busy doctor's surgery to use "the suppository" prescribed previously for piles has the potential for missing an abscess around the back passage as the symptoms (pain and bleeding) may mimic each other.

The skin of the ear canal also deserves special attention. It is very tight; a little pimple can cause excruciating pain because there is little room for the skin to stretch unlike, for example, the skin over the back of the hand. If tugging on the earlobe produces pain this is often a clue that the infection is in the ear canal i.e. the outer ear and not in the eardrum (inner ear) – the latter will not be painful with this manoeuvre. If it is not in the eardrum the problem is less serious though not less painful. A simple incision under a local anaesthetic (spray) will bring instant relief. Alternatively an ointment containing an antibiotic plus steroid may be stuffed into the ear canal – the steroid helps to reduce the unwelcome swelling.

Bacteria (staphylococci) that commonly cause boils in or around the nose are highly contagious and very easily spread to other parts of the body simply by touching the part. These infections will invariably require an appropriate antibiotic taken early rather than late. An antibiotic ointment may be necessary to eradicate bacteria from the nostrils if a person becomes a 'carrier' i.e. the germs are present within the nostrils but are not causing that person any symptoms though he or she can spread it to others. The innocent act of touching the nostril and then shaking somebody's hand has the potential for spreading the bacteria. For the same reason one should avoid coughing into the cupped right hand and contaminating unaffected areas and objects and other persons. Cough into the left hand instead. Shaking hands is a custom well loved by bacteria and viruses for their ease of transmission!

In undermining the immune system the following factors may play a role in infections targeting the skin

- Poor nutrition
- Stress
- Diabetes (too much sugar in the blood – bacteria thrive on it)
- Chronic alcohol or other substance abuse
- The presence of HIV/AIDS

It is noteworthy that 1 can of one's favourite sweetened soft drink may contain up to five tablespoons of sugar. Taken on a daily basis this adds up to more than a staggering 17 kilogrammes of sugar per year! One can per day! Furthermore, it has been shown that a normal white cell (the body's natural defence against infections) can destroy up to 12 to 13 bacteria at any given time within about 45 minutes. Take 6 teaspoons of sugar (in a soft drink/fruit juice) and 45 minutes later this number is reduced from 13 to about 6 bacteria! Eating pastry or a piece of pie reduces the number destroyed by the white cell to a stunning 3 bacteria within 45 minutes! It is hardly surprising that in diabetes, where there is an excess of sugar in the blood, there is a higher incidence of tuberculosis, bladder and skin infections than in the general population. To add to the dilemma the artificial sweetener – aspartame – has been associated with damage to liver cells.

Junk food also impairs one's immune function; the chips, cool drinks, sweets, cakes, biscuits and 'fruit juices' which swell today's shopping baskets are contributing to many diseases our parents and grandparents escaped. Vitamin C – in a slow–release form, zinc supplements and improving the nutritional state may restore the balance in our diet.

Constant exposure to stress depletes the body's stores of *Vitamins A, B, C, and E.* The body cannot *make* vitamins nor can they be *stored* for future use. Therefore, they must be taken in the food or as supplements on a *daily* basis. An orange eaten today will confer no benefit the following day or even six hours later because Vitamin C is used up within hours of ingestion.

Nutrition from most foods has been leeched out through faulty agricultural practices (fertilisers, poor crop rotation) , lengthy storage and refrigeration, canning , processing, freezing, addition of colourants, preservatives and other additives, refining (white flour, white sugar) and cooking. The preparation of a gourmet dish guarantees only food – not always the nutrition the body requires from it.

Does any cook throw away the potatoes and save the water in which the vegetable was boiled? No! Yet the simple act of boiling depletes the innocent vegetable of its natural nutrients. Sugar cane, like all natural foods, is rich in vitamins and nutrients but when it is refined into pristine 'white sugar' only the glucose remains – the rest of that which nature intended is lost in the processing. And the manufacturers will have us believe the bleached crystal is good for us!

By giving the immune system a helping hand to replace what modern day living and sophisticated manufacturing techniques steal from our food a person can reduce the incidence of infection. This can be achieved by taking

- *Vitamin C – slow release* – 1 tablet daily
- *Formula IV Plus* – 1 sachet daily (this contains 15 mg. of Zinc which the body uses to combat infection)
- *Carotenoid Complex* – 1 or more capsules daily
- *Omega 3* – 2 to 3 capsules daily and
- *Vitamin E 200 I.U.* – 1 capsule daily.

The most sophisticated diet on earth cannot supply these requirements. One would have to eat 3 to 4 cups of peanuts a day to obtain one dose of vitamin E! So much for the advice to *eat healthily!*

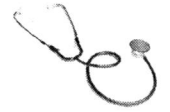

ACUTE PANIC ATTACK

As dramatic as the name of this condition may sound it cannot 'harm' the sufferer in any *physical way*; the person goes into a state of sudden panic for no apparent reason. He or she may actually believe or feel the outcome can be death itself.

Acute panic disorder shares many features with Generalized Anxiety Disorder except for *one important difference* – it is not a chronic condition but happens suddenly and without warning, lasting a few minutes but can also linger for a few hours. The person could be doing his or her everyday chores and, seemingly out of the blue, becomes extremely distressed with difficulty breathing and a sensation of choking. There may be dizziness, shakiness and palpitations – with the heart trying to leap out of the chest – sweating, a dry mouth and an urge to empty bladder and bowel simultaneously.

The attacks may come on without warning and this becomes another source of concern as the fear and embarrassment of such a 'humiliating' display of irrational 'panic' occurring uncontrollably in a *public place or social gathering* may lead to a genuine reluctance and dread of being seen in public.

These are the fears the sufferer may be faced with:

- Fear of the unknown
- Not being in control
- Dying from the attack
- Occurring when the person is alone, in a moving vehicle or crowded lift

- Not being able to function or be able to hold a job and earn a living
- Being labelled as 'hysterical'
- Having a serious mental disorder that doctors cannot fathom or treat effectively
- Permanent brain damage
- Having a heart attack or stroke
- That the children will inherit the disorder from the victim.

The fear may become irrational.

Family and next of kin may not know what to do or expect in the early days of the attacks and it is not unheard of for them to believe that the attack is faked and that the affected person must simply "Pull" him or herself together and "Get on with life". Family support and understanding of the nature of the illness will play an important role in the management of acute panic attacks. There is often an element of guilt on the part of the victim that not everybody believes it is a genuine affliction. Concerned relatives may have had to rush the victim to an emergency unit, often in the middle of the night and on more than one occasion. And, after all is said and done, the busy casualty officer dismisses the 'emergency' with a glib instruction to the duty nurse for a "Shot of valium" and an early discharge!

The underlying cause of these attacks is a chemical imbalance resulting in decreased levels of serotonin – a chemical messenger in the brain (neurotransmitter).The factors precipitating these panic attacks may vary from one person to another. Often there is an underlying reason that invariably and inevitably requires the expertise of a clinical psychologist or psychiatrist to uncover. Over time and with expert guidance the victim may affect a 'cure' or reduce the number and severity of the attacks. The precipitating event may have occurred many years before the condition manifests itself and often the link between the two is not considered, maybe long forgotten or is suppressed within the subconscious. A traumatic childhood experience, such as separation from a loved one due to death or divorce or a sexual assault may form the basis of the panic attacks.

A sexual abuse committed at a young age may lie buried or suppressed within the subconscious and certain associations much later in life may trigger an acute panic attack but the causative factor may not be realised at the time. And if the victim, now an adult, were to make the connection years later to whom would he or she reveal it? And who would believe the claim after all those years? Why had they not spoken up earlier? Would it not be easier for all concerned to forget about the incident? What if the perpetrators had threatened the victims in order to seal their lips? What if the matter went to court and nobody believed them? And what if the perpetrator has long since died? These "What ifs" may bury the origins of the disorder deep within the subconscious!

The parents of the victim may sweep the problem under the carpet hoping, that by maintaining a "Nothing happened" approach, the problem will eventually go away. This does not happen and more often, and in ways that are not always understood, the problem lies buried but not forgotten. The insult will colour the sufferer's life until understanding and release (closure) are found. A person who suffers acute panic attacks should be seen early by a competent professional – not months or years later when all else fails. Spouses and relatives need to understand that without help the attacks may never disappear and the intervals between attacks are simply waiting for the next one to occur.

In the treatment of acute panic attacks drugs are available that help to replace the missing chemical in the brain and one should not be afraid to have them prescribed.

Phaeochromocytoma (pronounced "fee–o–kromo–sight–oma") is a rare condition that has many of the symptoms of acute panic attacks. It is caused by a tumour in the adrenal gland – the small Napoleon's cap–shaped organs that lie one on top of each kidney. Tests can be done to confirm the diagnosis for this treatable condition. However, to do this first requires the condition to be considered. Several years often pass between consulting one psychiatrist and another until the penny falls.

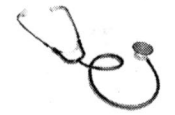

ALCOHOL

lcohol is a drug and if it was discovered today would probably not be passed by the Medicines Control Board as safe for public consumption. Like any other drug the body and the liver, in particular, view alcohol and paracetamol in the same way – as *poisons*.

There is no part of the human body that alcohol cannot affect – from the oesophagus (gullet or food pipe) and stomach, liver and pancreas, heart and blood cells to the nerves of the limbs and the part of the brain that controls coordination and the ability to walk, to the penis and the foetus. It is a *depressant* and not a stimulant, as is often believed. It depresses the part of the brain that controls one's inhibitions allowing the person to do things he or she would not ordinarily do e.g. table-top dancing in a restaurant.

How much it will take to produce an effect will depend on a number of factors: –

- The person (newcomer or seasoned drinker)
- The type of alcohol (fizzy ones get absorbed faster e.g. Champagne – because the gas i.e. carbon dioxide in the drink disperses the alcohol quicker, exposing more of the stomach to the drug). Mixing any alcohol with a fizzy beverage will have the same effect. In medicine this principal is used to get better and faster absorption of certain drugs (effervescence)

- Iced drinks will take longer to get absorbed; while hot drinks are absorbed much faster because the heat improves circulation to the stomach – Beware the 'hot toddy'!
- The quantity imbibed – the same amount of alcohol taken over a longer period than if it was gulped down allows for slower absorption and gives the liver more time to break down the alcohol.

The effects of alcohol can only be felt once it enters the blood stream. If one has been 'forced' to take more than one feels comfortable with for whatever reason – showing off to friends/ peer pressure/ hosts with heavy pouring hands/ sheer greed/ not knowing how to say "No thank you"/ experimenting in unchartered waters/ drinking too fast/ free drinks – one can sabotage the absorption by slipping away discreetly to a toilet or other appropriate outlet (flower bed) to deliberately vomit out the contents of the stomach - even if it means sacrificing the juicy steak one had before the debauchery. If one has decided to go this route one can 'assist' the vomiting by first taking at least half a litre of water - preferably warm. This gives the stomach a 'bulking effect' to help in ejecting the contents and also reduces the harm one can do (precipitate bleeding) at the junction of the foodpipe (oesophagus) with the stomach. On a lesser note, the more content/bulk to the vomitus the less 'noise' one is likely to make while vomiting – dry retching is noisier and more uncomfortable! Flushing the toilet to coincide with the act of vomiting may also mask the noise.

Once alcohol has *entered the blood* it is much like traffic on the motorway – there is no way out! The liver can only break down alcohol at a *fixed rate* no matter how much enters the blood. Only the *rate of absorption* from the stomach can be manipulated i.e. how quickly the alcohol enters the blood stream. A fatty meal or snack (nuts/cheese), taken before or with alcohol can delay this absorption.

Taking Vitamin B complex supplements may help the liver perform its functions better and - with a poison on its hands - all the help it can get will be welcome. Using non–carbonated mixers or shaking off the carbon dioxide from fizzy mixers, diluting the alcohol as much as possible and taking longer over a drink will also help slow down the rate of absorption (and avoid the call for a refill!). The usual push to "Drink up mate!" can be parried with "What's the rush?"

Habitually taking neat or undiluted alcohol can cause cancer of the throat and the risk is greater if cigarette smoke is added. In the stomach alcohol can cause an inflammation of the lining of the stomach (gastritis) and predispose to stomach ulcers. Its prolonged abuse can damage the pancreas and lead to diabetes (a type particularly difficult to control – called Brittle Diabetes). Alcohol can lower the blood sugar and cause one to blackout or induce an alcoholic fit: this can lead to falls and consequent injuries and, if the head is involved, will cause symptoms difficult to separate from the effects of alcohol. Many an alcoholic has been held overnight for drunkenness in a police cell only to be found the following morning dead from a brain haemorrhage - caused by an unsuspected head injury.

Alcohol is a *direct toxin* (poison) to the liver and the heart. Continued exposure may cause cirrhosis of the liver and enlargement of the heart and eventual failure of these organs. The incidence of cancer of the liver is higher when it is affected by cirrhosis. Alcohol also affects the nerves of the body (neuritis) producing the tremor or 'shakes' and numbness of the hands and feet. Because there is a lack of sensation in the extremities minor injuries go unnoticed – resulting in painless ulcers.

Alcohol can also affect the part of the brain that controls *coordination and balance*, especially in the legs. This makes walking progressively difficult and eventually the victim may end up in a wheelchair. The *strength* in the legs may be normal (unlike a stroke victim) but the person cannot make his feet go where it should (loss of coordination). The balance mechanism is impaired making walking unaided, at first, difficult and later, as the condition deteriorates and the alcohol abuse continues, impossible. Every drink thereafter will make the chances of recovery more remote. Discontinuing the poison and taking supplements of Vitamin B Complex, Thiamine and better nutrition may reverse the damage if it is caught in time.

An important deterrent to the carnage from drunken driving is performing a breathalyser test or blood sampling in every road traffic accident (like checking the driver's licence and registration) as a routine and not only when drunkenness is suspected.

Pathologists should develop an accurate fingerprick test for blood levels of alcohol - as for diabetics. This would make on the spot checks possible without the need for the services of a district surgeon. If the blood level of alcohol is found to be above the accepted level the driver's licence should be suspended with immediate effect. A firearm discharged into an innocent pedestrian killing the latter or maiming him permanently is viewed as totally unacceptable to the next of kin, the public, the perpetrator, the victim (if he or she is still alive), the police, the magistrate/judge. The perpetrator, if he is seen to be waving said firearm, may be regarded as a terrorist and be shot on the spot. But a drunken driver, who kills a pedestrian or motorist, and at times an entire family, is hardly seen in the same light. Can killing with a gun be different from killing with a front fender? Drunken-driving is described as 'an accident' – the media does not report the incident as a 'homicide'. The moment a person who has taken alcohol sits in the driver's seat and turns on the ignition he or she is being irresponsible – there is nothing 'accidental' about the tragedy that may follow the decision to drive under the influence of alcohol.

Every pub or hotel regularly has its fire extinguishers checked by the Fire Department. Wherever alcohol is served breathalyser testing should be mandatory before taking to the road. Drunks who walk home should be equally culpable. The hotel's responsibility to its clients should extend beyond ensuring the fire extinguishers are working – there may never be a fire in the life of the hotel but deaths from drunken driving are daily scourges.

While drinking and driving is taboo so should *drinking in pregnancy*. If it can be proven (?) by the baby that its mother took alcohol while the baby was a foetus this should be grounds for instituting compensation claims against the mother! Drinking in pregnancy (like smoking) should be labelled 'child abuse' because alcohol can affect development of the foetal brain and show itself by later relegating the unfortunate child to being at the back of the class in its academic potential. These babies are also growth retarded and the faces show changes that can be identified as part of the Foetal Alcohol

Syndrome. Thalidomide earned itself a name in the banned category of substances but alcohol (and smoking) hardly appears to qualify!

The weekend drinker is under the impression that this "Is not so bad" and believes that he or she avoids the harmful effects of alcohol by being a teetotaler on weekdays. This is not true. The weekend binge bombards the liver with excess alcohol in a shorter space of time and becomes more toxic than the same quantity spread over seven days. The definition of an alcoholic is any person, regardless of age, sex, occupation, social status or religion, who needs alcohol *in order to function normally.*

Functional Alcoholics do not consider themselves as 'alcoholics' because they

- Do not get drunk
- Do not drink before breakfast
- Do not suffer from tremors (shakes)
- Do not absent themselves from work
- Do not suffer from withdrawal symptoms
- Can go for long periods without a drink
- Only take alcohol as part of their 'job requirements' at office lunches, client meetings in restaurants and seminars.

Friends, relatives, spouses, work colleagues and employers may be too embarrassed or afraid to confront the person and thereby aid and abet the abuse.

Women have only relatively 'recently' been introduced to alcohol and their genetic make-ups have yet to acclimatise to the ravages of this poison – unlike their male counterparts! This makes women more susceptible to cirrhosis of the liver. Professional women in the 'thirty-something' age, striving to keep pace or stay ahead of their male associates, are finding out what men have been accustomed to doing for generations – quietly becoming alcoholics! Women have still to learn that, like nicotine, alcohol is another drug they can well do without. The stresses that women have created for themselves in competing with both men and women in the work place have not made alcohol an unwelcome crutch.

The alcohol industry has not been slow to capitalise on the preferences of the fairer sex. Many of today's alcohols are cleverly disguised with pleasant tasting fruit juices and soft drinks – no longer the gut burning raw taste of whiskey, brandy, gin, vodka or rum! The *type of alcohol* that is taken makes no difference to the liver or the damage that it causes. After it is absorbed from the stomach it is converted in the liver into glucose and aldehyde. It is the latter that poisons the liver. The glucose provides an 'empty' calorie and though its nutritional benefit is minimal it will lead to obesity; alcohol is the 'unseen' calorie. The body becomes 'tolerant' of the effects of alcohol and, with time, more and more must be consumed to achieve the same effect. Today's glass of wine will soon become two and then three and very soon the whole bottle can be consumed and, in promoting the macho image (men and women), the brag becomes "I can hold my liquor". Translated simply this means the person is becoming tolerant (immune) to the toxin in terms of drunkenness but the physical damage to the organs will escalate.

Men have been drinking alcohol for so long that their genes are being modified by the toxin and are carrying a special code that can detect future alcoholics. Technology may one day be able to remove the offensive gene and hopefully prevent alcoholism in the offspring. This possibility could extend itself to other inherited conditions like diabetes, Alzheimer's disease and Huntington's chorea.

In chronic alcoholism, as the disease progresses, and long before it begins to affect the brain, the spouse needs be aware that there is little way that the affected partner will ever be able to recover from the addiction unless admission is sought into a hospital or institution for 'drying out' and rehabilitation. Withdrawal of the drug (as for any substance abuse) is the first priority. Refusal to enter such an organised programme should be taken as a definite sign that there is little future in such a relationship. The alcoholic cannot easily be relied upon to do this voluntarily because *insight* into his (or her) illness may be lost – he or she simply *cannot see the harmful effects* of the drug on the person and those around.

The next priority is psychotherapy in which inner struggles and neurotic disturbances that may have been the basis of the ensuing addiction can be dealt with. These services are not always available and private care is expensive. *Social acceptance* of alcohol as a recreational drink has been a major stumbling block in getting early help when the abuse first gets a grip on a family. The wife is often too embarrassed to disclose to family members or friends that such abuse exists, persists and steadily progresses – with resultant deterioration in marital relationships. It is almost a given that a relationship is dysfunctional if alcohol abuse is involved.

The drunken husband who arrives late at night and demands food and sex is unlikely to find much support or sympathy and the spouse (unless she has been attending sessions at Al-Anon or receiving professional assistance herself) cannot cope with the abuse and invariably presses buttons that bring on further verbal, physical and often sexual abuse. This can only lead to a widening of the rift between the partners. Children often witness the abuse and, sadly, also suffer the consequences.

Some alcoholics may develop paranoid *delusions* and accuse their spouses of infidelity. Alcohol often makes them impotent and, to hide behind the shame of their lost manhoods, blame the wives – who refuse to have sex with their husbands because they are drunk. Citing his impotence as a reason for not having sex, when he himself is ignorant of the true cause of his erectile dysfunction, will add more fuel to the fire. Jealousy is the commonest and most dangerous feature of alcoholic paranoia and may even provoke the partner to murder the spouse. The alcoholic makes infidelity the scapegoat for the loss of his manhood as this is easier to accept than blaming the drug as the underlying cause. The wife who thinks and hopes that last night 'may be the last time', and promises are made by the addict to this effect, is often continuing in a relationship that will add up to just so many wasted months and then years. The addict *must agree* to voluntarily get professional help otherwise the relationship is doomed. Alcoholism is like any illness/ addiction – it requires treatment: one cannot treat diabetes with denial, empty promises, hope and prayers alone!

Delirium tremens occurs in alcoholics who have been deprived of alcohol for whatever reason (admission into hospital for an unrelated condition and the addiction is not brought to the attention of medical personnel). It presents with severe shakiness, sweating, rapid heartbeats, restlessness, agitation, sleeplessness and confusion. This condition has a high mortality rate and must be treated in hospital as a medical *emergency.*

While one glass of red wine (no more) has been shown to be beneficial to the heart it is the skin of the red grape that really has the benefit and one helping of these grapes (about 8 to 10) per day should avoid the need or excuse for alcohol. The benefit in the grape is an antioxidant called hercetin.

Until the brewers, publicans and politicians who sanction its revenue-generating existence are not made accountable for the cost in terms of illness, lost lives, broken homes and relationships, the carnage from drinking and driving and all the other facets into which alcohol has seeped, this bottled drug will continue to rob us of the George Bests of the world.

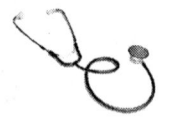

ALZHEIMER'S DISEASE

This is a disease of advancing years – the hereditary types may appear earlier. The longer one lives the higher the chances of getting it. The disease is caused by a degeneration of nerve cells in brain tissue that eventually form 'plaques' (or 'scabs') that can be detected on a brain scan. There is no easy test that can confirm the disease short of a biopsy of the brain.

Picture each nerve cell as a kite with a tail. Join a string of kites together one behind the other all the way from the brain to the toe and one has the structure of a single nerve. In Alzheimer's disease the 'tails' within the brain gradually become entangled with each other. This forms the 'plaque' that is visible on brain scans. It is a slow process characterised in its early stages by gradually increasing *forgetfulness for recent events*. While this is true not every forgotten key and mislaid wallet implies that this disease is in progress. The memory loss happens gradually and progressively over a period of many months i.e. it steadily gets worse. Today's forgotten key and wallet in time will include forgetting what was taken at breakfast and later - the pot on the stove. This is a serious omission from the memory bank and potentially dangerous. It should be a strong warning that this affliction may be present. Ignorance about the disease and perceived social stigmata attached to it often make next of kin have difficulty accepting the diagnosis or that it could happen to *their* loved one.

As the condition progresses more and more difficulties are experienced. Clothing is put on incorrectly – back to front, more than one garment is worn and socks do not match. "Am I going to the hairdresser today?" "Uncle Jack is coming to tea", "May I have my lunch now?" – may be repeated again and again.

Carers or relatives may ignore that the reasoning powers of the mind are not functioning normally and the unwary will respond normally – "No, mother, this is not your week at the hairdresser. I have just told you that for the tenth time!" Levels of frustration will increase, needlessly. The brain is not functioning normally and, therefore, cannot understand the explanation that has been offered. A close parallel would be trying to show a two-year-old how computers work! The memory bank of learned information is non-existent in the two-year-old and has been forgotten in the person with Alzheimer's disease. This can be quite traumatic for loved ones that watch the gradual, almost unbelievable, deterioration of their parent and often go into a phase of denial. It is difficult to come to terms with the lifetime memories of a wonderful person who is now painting the walls with excrement from the toilet bowl!

Sleeping difficulties can keep everybody awake with loud shouting and sometimes singing and restless pacing of the floor. And all through this the memory for events that occurred in their earlier years remains remarkably clear – childhood friends and birthdays and their weddings are recalled with such clarity that next of kin who are not familiar with the characteristics of the disease will, understandably, not readily believe that their loved one has a problem. The adage 'First in last out' applies admirably to the failing memory. To complicate matters and confuse next of kin and friends - in the early stages it can be very difficult even for professionals to differentiate Alzheimer's disease from the normal ageing process. There may well be times when thought processes are functioning normally giving the semblance of normality, thereby creating a doubt that the condition actually exists. Asking questions that require a simple "Yes" or "No" for answer may also convey the picture of normality unless a more detailed answer is expected and the reply waited for! Asking "How was your day?" should not be followed immediately with "Were you okay?" The former would require a more structured reply – difficult for an Alzheimer's patient whose thought processes may not be normal. Answering "Yes" to the latter question could fool the unwary or continue the denial that the condition exists. It is very important that the person electing to care for such a patient should be aware of the special circumstances of this disease. Often it is an inexperienced next of kin or spouse. This has the potential for creating more than one patient in the house in a very short time and making management of the patient difficult - much to the detriment of the hapless victim. Bearing testimony to this are the exasperated cries of "Mother! Why are you wetting yourself on the lounge carpet?" Medical opinion should be sought early because there maybe other potentially treatable causes for the dementia – e.g. an underfunctioning thyroid gland (hypothyroidism) or a forgotten (often minor) head injury that may have happened several weeks or months previously resulting in a bleed within the skull (subdural haematoma) which may be surgically treatable. By causing pressure upon the brain tissue such a bleed may mimic Alzheimer's disease. A brain tumour could also masquerade as Alzheimer's disease.

There is currently no cure for this affliction but there are drugs that may slow the rate of deterioration. Measures that can help delay or avert it rely on keeping the mind active from an early age e.g. playing chess, Scrabble, draughts, card games (bridge), reading, solving crossword puzzles and attending social functions and get-togethers. Isolation in a home, where next of kin have to work and the victim is left alone out of necessity or is plonked in front of the television, as so often happens in an institutionalised setting, may lead to an earlier deterioration. Loneliness is the curse of the elderly! Does it play a more important role in the onset of this disease than is given its due? Have the fragmentation of the family unit and the demise of the extended family system given birth to another disease of the twenty first century?

If the person is kept occupied with simple tasks like peeling potatoes (with a potato-peeler!) helping in the garden and arranging laundry these will go a long way to staving off the eventual deterioration. Restlessness, agitation and sleeplessness can, and should, be controlled with medication to allow caregivers the respite of adequate sleep and rest so that the care of their charges does not ultimately suffer. It also ensures that the patient is not having the addition of sleep deprivation to make his or her load from the disease heavier.

The smaller independent family unit – often a couple and one or two children (a product of our times and a far cry from the 'extended family' system) will set the stage for institutionalised care and place an expensive burden on society. It should be the responsibility of every individual to *prevent* disease before it happens because there is very little that conventional medicine is able to *cure*. Conventional medicine is too busy treating disease to pay more attention to its prevention even though small measures are in progress .The downside is that if disease prevention is successful, and this should be the goal – the medical profession and drug manufacturers may have to seek alternate livelihoods.

Omega 3 fatty acids are obtained from fish oil and have been shown to have anti-inflammatory properties and, because Alzheimer's disease has its pathology based on inflammatory changes in the nerve cells (neurones), these fatty acids may help to prevent or slow down the relentless degeneration of brain cells. There are other benefits to taking Omega 3. It also helps in arthritis, depression, cardiovascular disease and the changes that take place with age. Antioxidants have been shown to be responsible for many of the changes that take place in almost every disease process as well as the cell's ultimate degeneration when it dies. Vitamin E is a powerful antioxidant and together with Omega 3 should be given to assist in preventing or slowing down disease and, in particular, this form of dementia. These are not drugs and because they are made from natural foods (grain and fish respectively) there are no serious side effects.

On a practical note, bicarbonate of soda sprinkled liberally on urine-soaked clothing and bedding can eliminate the smell of ammonia and, for sheer cost saving and effectiveness, has few equals. In Alzheimer's disease expect bladder (and bowel) control to be less than perfect .Caregivers should acquaint themselves with the disease (books in the local library, the Internet) to better understand the condition and thereby improve the overall management of the patient. In addition, there are Alzheimer's support groups whose services may be enlisted.

Access to and the use of electrical equipment or gas appliances has the potential for serious injury to life and property. Forgetfulness can result in pots boiling over on the stove and starting a fire and doors being left unlocked inviting intruders. Wandering from home is well known and unbelievable distances may be covered – begging the need to have 'Medic Alert' bracelets detailing contact names and numbers. These could save the carers much anxiety, the police wasted time and effort – and reduce the risk of road accidents and muggings. Bathtubs have the potential for drowning or flooding and should always be supervised. A plastic chair in a shower has the following advantages: –

- Much safer than having to step out of the bathtub and run the risk of slipping
- Easier to manage
- Makes it easier to dry the patient while still seated in the chair
- Leaves both hands free and
- Saves water!

It is often difficult for teenagers to live and cope with a grandparent who has Alzheimer's disease. It maybe embarrassing for them to have friends over and have the whole house reeking of urine, as is bound to happen when incontinence sets in. Better understanding of the condition and its complications can only make for improved relationships, given that teenagers may well have their own problems without having to cope with an adult that swears and curses without reason. There is a stigma attached to labelling the elderly parent or grandparent as being 'mentally insane'. How do teenagers 'introduce' the strangely-behaving grandparent to their friends? Furthermore, siblings of the patient run the risk of the condition being hereditary, with its attendant baggage of anxiety and depression. Open discussions with their medical practitioners are necessary.

Weight loss is often part of the condition for a number of reasons. The person may simply forget to eat or be hungry! Nevertheless, beware the abuse that can be meted out to these unfortunate patients. The carer may discard the food intended for the patient and nobody will be the wiser. Similarly, because the patient is unable to complain, verbal, physical, sexual and emotional abuses are possible and must be guarded against. The size of the fee does not necessarily determine the quality of care. Children and the elderly are at potential risk from such evils.

The caregiver should understand that of almost all the conditions he or she could be faced with the care of the demented patient must be the most challenging. Next of kin who attempt to share such a responsibility should be warned they could end up becoming physical and mental wrecks themselves. Weekend respites and deserved holidays should be the order of the day and planned in advance in collaboration with family and institution. Often one family member (usually the most gullible or the unmarried son or daughter) is taken advantage of and responsibility is not shared. The adage has oft been stated: The integrity of a society is gauged by how it takes care of its elderly.

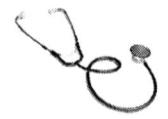

ANTIBIOTICS

These are one of the most frequently prescribed groups of drugs. What long-term effect they will turn out to have on the human body (and those of our domesticated animals) only time will tell. For the present, mankind is grateful for their availability because a short 100 years ago infection became the biggest killer. These little miracles of science have been responsible for changing the face of disease.

They are usually prescribed as a course and should always be completed even though the symptoms of the illness may have begun to improve soon after starting treatment. Failure to do so encourages the appearance of drug resistance. Bacteria (and viruses) have become adept at adapting their cell structures to protect themselves against the 'killer' drugs - illustrating the powerful instinct for survival that all living things have

Resistance to antibiotics is a major problem in the treatment of tuberculosis. TB patients do not complete the six month course because they feel so much better after a month or so and then drop out. This has led to the emergence of dangerous new breeds (strains) of TB germs that often do not respond to conventional drugs. This *drug resistant tuberculosis*' is turning a potentially treatable infection into a killer – and only because the infection is not hit hard and long enough for the medication to effectively kill the bacteria – instead of just 'stunning' them for a short period. This 'resistance' occurs with antibiotics but not with medication for conditions like diabetes, hypertension etc. This is because the target is a living organism that can adapt - or die!

In the presence of HIV AIDS the incidence of TB has increased and the tuberculosis bacteria have an opportunity to get a stranglehold.

Drugs are often taken after a meal unless otherwise stated. Antibiotics like tetracycline and erythromycin should be taken an hour *before* a meal or two hours after. Some of them may cause side effects and these should be mentioned to the prescribing doctor as soon as possible. If the latter cannot be reached the nearest hospital – emergency unit or the poisons information centre should be contacted. These telephone numbers should always be kept accessible for emergencies.

If one is allergic to any medication this must be mentioned to the doctor. A 'Medic-Alert' bracelet should be worn at all times stating the relevant information – "It will speak for you when you cannot!" When consulting medical personnel (doctor, dentist, radiologist) all medication currently being used should be disclosed – the oral contraceptive pill, laxatives, antacids, herbal remedies and other alternative medicines are often overlooked as 'medication'! Dyes that are injected into a vein e.g. for an intravenous pyelogram (IVP) (during which X-rays are taken of the kidneys and bladder) can also cause allergic reactions.

The discovery of penicillin introduced one of the earliest, effective, injectable forms of antibiotic. That painful discovery holds sway more than half a century later.

Patients are often under the impression that antibiotics given in an injectable form work faster. This probably carries over from an era not so long ago when the medical profession found one more way to reinforce their 'superior' healing powers - the injection! If the truth were known the 'bronchitis' that the patient has been nursing for two or more days *without* treatment will not fare any the worse for waiting another hour, which is how long it would take for the medication to get into the blood! And, while there may be exceptions, the patient who has an illness that is serious enough to warrant an injectable antibiotic should probably be on his or her way to hospital! How often is an injection requested "Because it works faster" part of the quest for instant gratification – or ignorance about antibiotics?

Ideally, if a drug is administered by injection as an outpatient it is safer to be observed at the hospital or surgery for at least 15 to 20 minutes so that if an acute allergic reaction does occur the patient will be close to medical attention. Furthermore, there is no guarantee that if a particular drug has been taken in the past *without* untoward side effects this may not happen in the future!

Some of the more common side effects of antibiotics are nausea, skin rashes and loose stools. Certain antibiotics can change the 'environment' in the vagina and encourage yeasts like thrush to flourish and cause a vaginal itch/discomfort plus a discharge. The use of cultured yoghurt orally may help avoid this. As an emergency measure, when pharmacies are closed and the doctor is away for the weekend, plain, unsweetened yoghurt may be applied directly to the vaginal area to relieve the symptoms of thrush.

Any bleeding spots in the skin, particularly around the buttocks and the legs, and the development of symptoms like fever, shaking chills and headache that were not present before the antibiotic (or any drug) was taken warrants a telephone call to a doctor – preferably the one who prescribed it.

Antibiotics for cystitis (bladder infection) should, as far as possible, not be taken *before* a sterile urine sample has been collected for laboratory examination. If the specimen cannot be sent immediately it should be passed into a sterile container and stored in the refrigerator overnight. A single dose of antibiotic may clear the urine of detectable organisms but will hardly eradicate them. The urine should always be 'cultured' to identify the bacteria and the correct antibiotic for that organism.

It is important to take extra fluids (water and not fruit juice!) to flush the antibiotics out of the kidneys after they have performed their function - wherever they were required. This reduces the risk of harmful effects of the drug on the delicate tissues of the kidneys. This risk is increased during the night when the kidneys naturally 'slow down' the production of urine; better to have sleep disturbed by taking extra water and have to get up to pass urine than risk possible kidney damage.

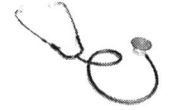

APPENDICITIS

The appendix, as it is known today, is a far cry from the original organ. In herbivores (vegetarian animals) like the cow the appendix is a hollow tube about 15 cm in length and performs a vital function in the digestion of carbohydrates, producing a rich source of yeasts and healthy bacteria. However, in man this function has largely disappeared because of the reduced intake of carbohydrates and his preference for meat. Accordingly, evolution has shrunk down the appendix to the size of a little finger. The rudimentary organ is a stark reminder of how our diet has changed over generations!

The appendix is situated at the bottom end of the caecum, the 'half-way house' between the small intestine (gut) and the large intestine. It has a narrow opening that leads into the cavity of the caecum and if this should become obstructed can cause inflammation and / infection of this appendage. It is the bane of parents' lives every time junior has an abdominal pain "Is it the appendix, doctor?" Appendicectomies have been the bread and butter of surgeons for generations and will continue to be until the 'defunct' organ disappears completely.

The appendix lies in the right lowermost quadrant and can become inflamed in any age group. Although appendicitis is not common before the age of two it becomes increasingly so during childhood and adolescence. Symptoms usually begin with *fever, vomiting and a vague pain in the belly* that may initially begin in the upper part of the middle of the belly and over time (+/-24 hours) move down to the right lower abdomen. Though vomiting is not persistent it is rare to find a child with appendicitis without this symptom. Sleep during an attack would be difficult.

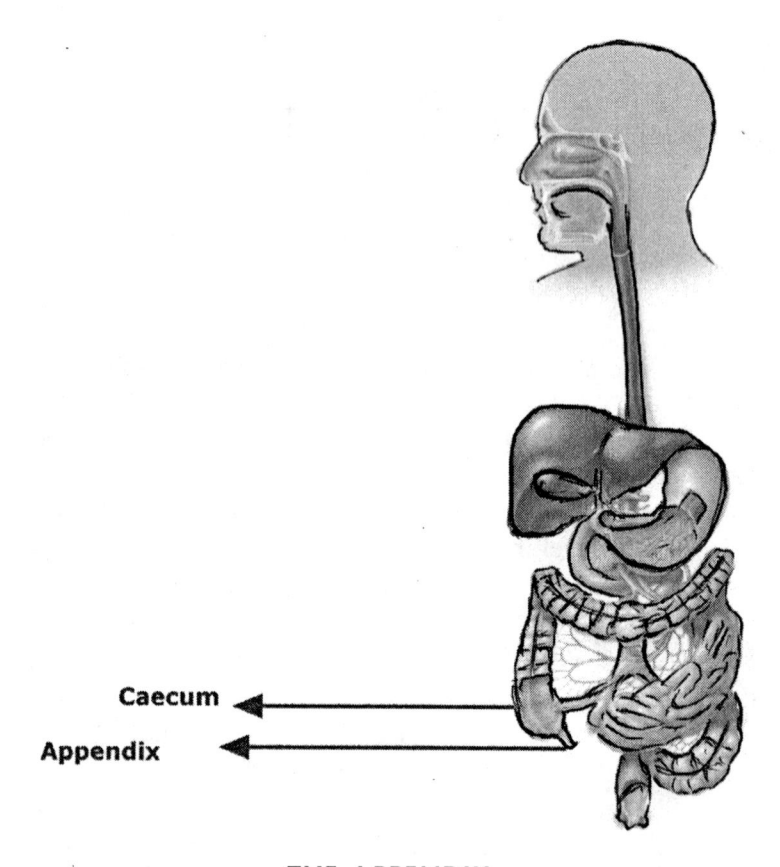

Caecum

Appendix

THE APPENDIX

The pain may be mild at first but becomes steadily and progressively worse and there is a *great reluctance to move*. A child with abdominal pain who is eating and jumping around is very unlikely to have appendicitis. Diarrhoea (watery stools) is not the usual picture of this illness and usually points to gastroenteritis. However, in an infant or child with diarrhoea, vomiting and abdominal pain – appendicitis should be suspected as they may rupture their appendices more easily - placing them in a higher risk category.

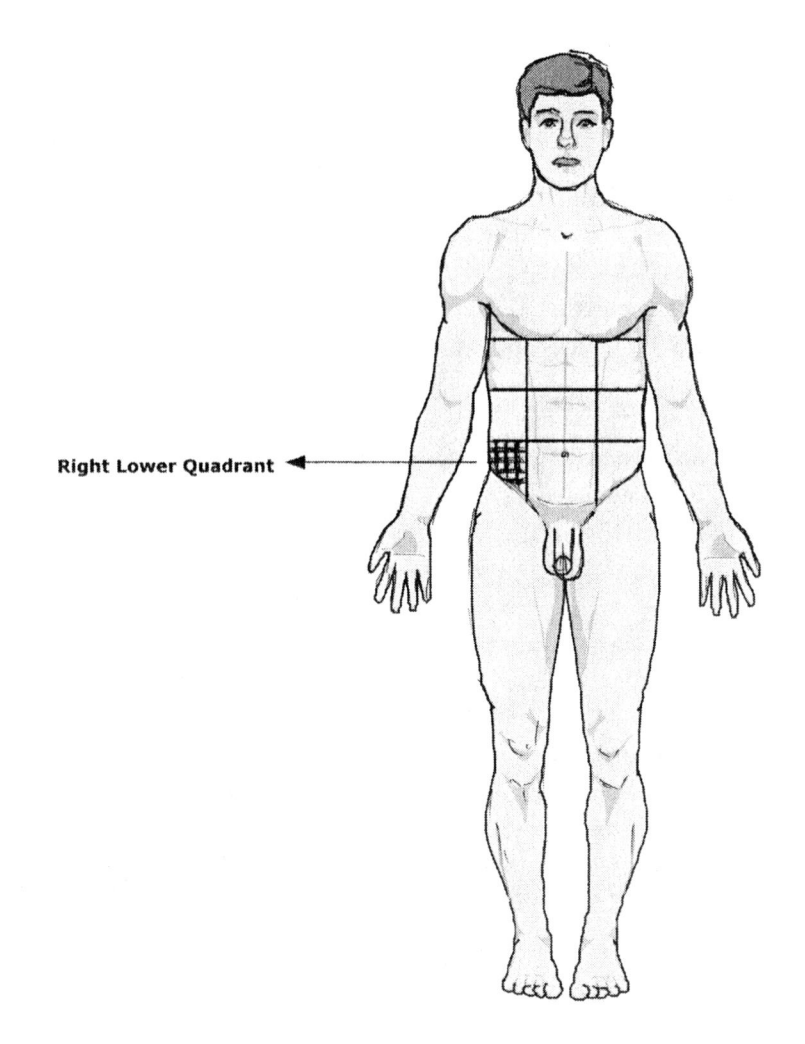

Right Lower Quadrant

THE RIGHT LOWER QUADRANT

Unlike that of typical appendicitis in other age groups, in the elderly fever may be absent and because of obesity, lax abdominal walls or previous abdominal surgery the pain maybe vague or completely absent. *An elderly person* who becomes unwell for any reason or simply goes off food without apparent cause should, unless proven otherwise, be suspected of having either *appendicitis, cystitis (bladder infection), or prostatitis (in a male)*. In this age group cystitis may occur without the usual 'burning sensation' and the frequent passage of small quantities of urine. These diagnoses are easy to miss in the elderly. Gangrene and perforation of the appendix occur more frequently in the aged. Once the appendix has been removed 'appendicitis' need never be considered again as a cause of abdominal pain.

Appendicitis *in pregnancy* will always pose special diagnostic problems because abdominal pain is often experienced during pregnancy and is usually explained away as part of the vagaries of having a uterus that is steadily increasing in size.

Clues to alert one of the possibilities of appendicitis are:

- The pain is different from that experienced before
- There is usually fever and vomiting
- The pain becomes steadily worse
- A normal pregnancy does not cause fever
- The typical site for the pain will not be the same as in a non–pregnant person – it is usually higher up in the belly depending on how big the uterus has become.

Surgery for appendicitis should not pose a threat to the pregnancy unless there is a complication e.g. If the appendix should rupture.

Any person who develops an abdominal pain should be restricted from eating any solids until the nature of the problem is established. Introducing food into the stomach when appendicitis or any other abdominal illness (gastroenteritis, gallstones etc) is brewing will complicate matters further. Animals rely on instinct and will not eat if they are unwell. Give 'rehydration fluid' made up of 8 teaspoons of sugar and ½ teaspoon of salt added to a litre of water. At least 2 – 3 litres (for an adult and proportionately less in a younger patient) is all that should be allowed or be necessary in the first 24 hours until some clues arise to further assist in the diagnosis. Adding the salt to a litre of soft drink (like 'Fanta') maybe more palatable - given that it already contains sugar. Withholding food for 24 hours will not harm the patient provided that rehydration fluid intake is maintained. If the patient should require surgery the presence of food in the stomach may delay the operation or increase the risk of aspirating stomach contents into the lungs during the anaesthetic.

As mentioned elsewhere the *temperature* should always be checked with a thermometer, and more than once, to ascertain its true level and its progress after that. Is it returning to normal, increasing or staying constantly elevated? Not every pain in the belly will be due to appendicitis. When the diagnosis is uncertain the patient can be hospitalised for observation. This may ease the stress on parents who feel very vulnerable when their children are involved. They may live a distance from the hospital, have problems with transport or have had a previous experience with surgical complications. A single parent, and this is invariably the mother, should also deserve special consideration.

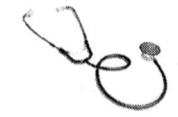

ARTHRITIS

A 'joint' is where two bones meet and arthritis simply means an inflammation of a joint – no other part except the joint.

The term 'arthritis' does not specify the type and it may be due to:

- Gout
- Rheumatoid Arthritis
- Osteoarthritis
- An injury
- Infection

Whenever the term 'arthritis' is used it implies that the joint is *swollen and painful*. Pain without the swelling is called 'arthralgia'. Pain occurring in muscle (called myalgia) is not arthritis. It is important to know or identify the type of arthritis as this may influence treatment. Taking Aunty Mary's 'arthritis tablets' from the Day Hospital may relieve the pain and swelling but treatment may entail more than just taking analgesics and they do have side effects – user beware!

Swelling of a joint that occurs immediately after an injury may be due to bleeding within the joint and the suddenness of the swelling must prompt immediate medical attention. The presence of blood in the joint will act as an 'irritant' and will hamper healing. Such an injury needs an X-ray and if this is normal the joint should be aspirated. Under a local anaesthetic a needle is introduced into the joint (often the knee) and fluid is removed. This will immediately reveal if bleeding has occurred. All joints normally have some fluid for lubrication – if it is inflamed the lining within the joint makes an excess that will stretch the joint capsule and cause swelling and pain.

Removing the fluid (aspiration) will bring immediate pain relief. The excruciating pain of gout, if it occurs in the knee, elbow or shoulder, can often be relieved by aspiration. These joints are easily accessible for needling. If a cartilage has been damaged within the joint the 'anti-inflammatory' tablet found in the medicine cabinet will not rectify the problem and may mask the symptoms and, by delaying, may convert a simple tear of the cartilage into an irreparable one.

Any pain developing in a joint should warn the person to immediately put it to rest i.e. no weight-bearing or active use of the joint. The spine is often ignored as a 'joint'. It is made up of dozens of small joints at each vertebral level (bones of the spine). If the jaw joint (temperomandibular) is inflamed it also needs to be rested i.e. avoiding chewing anything hard, yawning widely or laughing heartily! The habitual chewing of gum may set the scene for developing inflammation / arthritis of the jaw joint, the treatment of which can be frustrating as the jaw cannot be effectively 'rested'. Injury to a joint (or muscle) sustained while exercising or being engaged in a sporting activity should be followed by immediate cessation of any movement of the affected part until, wherever possible, a diagnosis has been established and appropriate treatment instituted.

How often has the injured player continued to play for the sake of the game and made matters worse. The body has no other way of signaling that there is a problem except through the sensation of pain – whether it is a sprained ankle or a heart attack – ignore it at one's peril! A fracture may not result in a 'broken' bone – a thin 'hairline' fracture may not be detected on ordinary X-rays except with a bone or MRI Scan. This is not always undertaken because of the lack of facilities for such investigations and the costs involved. Bone usually heals within six weeks of the injury and in that time the pain should be settling. If it persists longer further investigation is required.

Any *stiffness* occurring in the small joints of the fingers or hands occurring in the morning on arising and gradually disappearing after a period of time (from 10 to 60 minutes – depending on the severity) requires a medical opinion. This symptom could be the start of rheumatoid arthritis and may present at any age – even in children! The efficacy of treatment is measured against the time it takes for the early morning stiffness to disappear - the shorter the interval the milder the inflammation.

A *fever accompanying a painful swollen joint* may be serious as it could be due to an infection within the joint and this will require hospitalisation and potent antibiotics - usually given by injection. In an elderly person or in a joint that already has long standing 'arthritis' the pain and swelling may not be that obvious and the diagnosis is often missed or delayed. Beware!

Arthroscopy is the introduction of a lighted tube (scope) into a joint to view its interior. It is reserved for the bigger joints when the diagnosis is not clear or, as in the knee joint, when a torn cartilage is suspected. This can be repaired or the torn part excised through the scope. This 'keyhole' surgery obviates the need for an open operation – with its longer recovery period and higher incidence of complications like infection.

The drugs used in arthritis have some important side effects that are often ignored in the search for 'immediate' pain relief

- *Gastritis*–causing pain in the region of the stomach (below the lower end of the breast bone) due to inflammation in the lining of the stomach - sometimes progressing to an ulcer
- *Bleeding* from the stomach lining or ulcer. The bleeding may occur without any symptoms to warn the user anything is amiss. Many people do not look at their stools. If the bleeding is heavy it will change the colour of the stool to black; iron from the digested blood in the stomach turns black. Taking iron tablets will similarly discolour the stools. Any such change (in the absence of iron tablet ingestion) must be reported to the doctor. Drugs that may be responsible for bleeding from the gut – warfarin (used to 'thin the blood'), aspirin, dispirin, med lemon with aspirin, any of the more specific arthritis drugs called 'non-steroidal anti-inflammatory drugs [NSAIDs] or Prednisolone (a steroid) should be *discontinued immediately*. Taking an antacid

(or sodium bicarbonate as an 'emergency' measure) will help to relieve the gastric inflammation. A person who has an active ulcer in the stomach or a history of such ulcers in the past must consult a doctor before taking these drugs

- *Kidney damage*: This is another serious side effect of NSAIDs that may occur without symptoms. These drugs may also cause swelling of the feet. The person afflicted with arthritis is usually elderly and in this age group the function of the kidneys tends to become impaired – again without much warning to the person. This places patients in this age group at greater risk of kidney damage.

A recent change in bladder habit causing a person to pass urine more frequently, especially at night, should alert one to kidney involvement. This may also be a warning of early prostate enlargement in men. In either case a doctor should be consulted. The use of these drugs in the elderly should be tempered with more caution. The urine should be examined at intervals and the presence of blood and protein prompting further investigation.

It is tempting in this era of instant gratification to use potent drugs to control joint symptoms where bed rest may have been helpful. Furthermore, it is unacceptable (to the affected joint!) to take a potent anti-inflammatory to simply *relieve pain* and then go off to play a few rounds of golf or slip down to the supermarket. Inflammation will not respond that quickly and more harm is done by having the patient believe that the injection "Worked like a charm!"

NSAIDs should be taken after a meal – a slice of toast and a cup of tea may not be adequate. The fluid intake should be increased to at least 3 litres - taken in quantities throughout the day *and last thing at night*. This is the time when the production and excretion of urine is normally reduced allowing these potentially toxic drugs to accumulate in the delicate tissues of the kidneys. The inconvenience of having to waken during the night is a small price to keep the kidneys from being damaged! *Arthritis may not kill anybody but kidney failure can*!

The elderly are at special risk for several reasons: –

* They are often on *medication* for high blood pressure and almost all of these drugs may cause the blood pressure to drop making the person lightheaded and triggering a stumble or fall when they assume the erect position too quickly

- Dizziness is a side effect of NSAIDs,
- Their *blood pressures* take longer to correct when they stand up suddenly from a seated or lying position. This may make them lightheaded and at further risk of stumbling or falling
- Inadequate *fluid intake* is a common failing in the elderly because they hate going to the toilet so often! Or they simply forget to take extra fluids
- The losses of fluid from diuretics (used in hypertension) that make them pass more urine also tend to cause dehydration

It is little surprise that the elderly person 'stumbles' (and this is all that it takes to do it!), breaks the upper end of the femur (hip bone) and then falls to become one more victim of a fractured hip and the orthopaedic surgeon's bread and butter.

One in four women (they also have more arthritis than men) who break their hips will die from the fractures or complications that arise from them. In the USA alone there are over 220,000 fractures of the hip every year and of these 30,000 die. Is it fair for the very person afflicted with arthritis to suffer even more from the overzealous use of drugs?

Other common side effects of NSAIDs are drowsiness and swelling of the feet. They tend to retain salt in the body and where salt goes water will follow. With this in mind the amount of salt in the food should be reduced – not that anybody should be using much salt anyway! These drugs should be used with caution in patients who have heart failure because of the risk of salt retention and worsening cardiac function. For similar reasons patients with hypertension should be wary of taking NSAIDs for they may elevate their blood pressures.

These drugs and their concomitant use with alcohol (that will cause further dehydration and increase the risk to the kidneys), certain cough mixtures and sleeping tablets taken while driving, working with machinery or on heights should be avoided because of drowsiness. Pregnant and breast-feeding mothers should not be exposed to such medication.

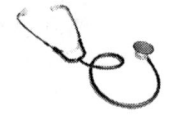

ASTHMA

It is not surprising that reports worldwide quote an increase in the prevalence of this condition. The past hundred years, as mentioned elsewhere, has seen a concerted effort to impair the body's Immune System.

How did this happen? One can trace the decline: –

- Beginning with the introduction of steel rollers in 1890 to process a more refined wheat
- The manufacture of more and more processed foods
- The addition of preservatives
- The phenomenal increase in the consumption of 'highly refined' white sugar and the ready availability and tasty appeal of convenience foods – especially in the recently migrated rural population to urban cultures and 'westernised' eating habits
- Aggressive advertising, especially, in third world countries to encourage more and more of the virginal and more impressionable youth to take up smoking.

The furore over marijuana as a substance of abuse is laughable when tobacco, with its 2000 separately identified carcinogens (cancer producing agents), and alcohol are socially acceptable and the powers that be that regulate the introduction of drugs and their use turn a blind eye to these toxic substances. From the tobacco farmers (the very root of the chain that produces the filthy cigarette) to their retail outlets, the advertising companies, sporting bodies, other parties with vested interests and the Revenue Services - there is money to be made. While this remains the main objective the evil that tobacco is and how it contributes to lung disease (not to mention all the other diseases that stem from this) will keep the incidence of asthma 'on the increase'!

Preventative medicine, if it were to be made truly effective, could sound the death knell of the medical profession, the drug manufacturers and the Medical Aid schemes. Who will have need of their services if people were not ill?

Asthma is a *wheezy chest* condition that occurs *again and again* at intervals. One episode of bronchitis can also produce a wheezy chest but this does not make it asthma at the time – unless it recurs. Not every asthmatic may have a wheeze; *a cough that persists* may masquerade as asthma. Is this the 'wheezy bronchitis' many patients have been so labelled because the profession is tardy in making the diagnosis of 'asthma'?

This reluctance works to the detriment of the patient's health because

- Identifiable causes are overlooked
- The education of the asthmatic is wanting
- The correct medication is often not instituted and
- The many precautions given an asthmatic are missing (avoiding dispirin and NSAIDs, preservatives in foods etc).

It is understandable that the undiagnosed asthmatic who cycles to work or plays soccer will believe that the shortness of breath that the person experiences when active is due to the 'exercise' and being 'unfit'! This is often 'Exercise Induced Asthma' – the correct diagnosis and appropriate treatment will produce the feeling of having an 'extra pair of lungs'!

Many potential asthmatics are afraid to be labelled as such because of the seeming need for chronic medication – particularly the much maligned 'pump'. The ill informed often believe that using the inhaler/pump or the nebuliser will make the user 'addicted' to it for the rest of the person's life. Or that these preparations will weaken the heart if used for any length of time. Nothing could be further from the truth. Taking a tablet or syrup orally exposes the stomach, the liver, brain, kidneys – the entire body from the head down to the toes – to the effects of the drug, whereas using an inhaler puts a minute quantity of the medication exactly where its action is required i.e. in the lungs.

In comparison taking a tablet every day for the rest of the person's life for diabetes or hypertension would appear more acceptable. The fear and reluctance to use inhalers often stems from the historical background of these devices. In the early years of their introduction their accuracy was unreliable and the user sometimes received toxic doses of medication that were fraught with undesirable side effects – targeting the heart and nervous system. These sometimes resulted in fatalities.

The inhalers and the drugs they contain have been made very safe provided they are used in the prescribed way; each 'puff' is accurately measured. The technique may appear simple, and it is, if one important point is remembered – the canister must be depressed (to activate it) *and* the breath taken *simultaneously* through the mouth. The principle is the inhaled air must carry the aerosol medication into the depths of the lungs and not, as is often the case, spraying the medication into the mouth and *then* inhaling – it is not the mouth that needs the treatment but the lungs!

The technique is simple but it has to be demonstrated, otherwise the patient loses out for there is no other way to get the medication into the lungs except by inhalation. Success is user dependent. Furthermore, the patient *must be able to* take a deep enough breath in order to get the inhaled air to carry the aerosol into the lungs. This would be difficult if the chest is tight (bronchospasm). In this situation to rely on the inhaler is begging for trouble. The nebuliser, which is not dependent on technique or the ability to take a deep enough breath, will be far more effective. The medication is carried into the lungs in a jet of air carrying tiny droplets of water mixed with the inhalant medication. In hospital practice the nebuliser has the added advantage of using oxygen to carry the medication – the home nebuliser uses room air. Asthmatics' chests are tight and are therefore getting insufficient oxygen and this will also make them more short of breath. This begs the point that acquiring a home nebuliser carries a risk that the patient or caregiver may feel over confident that, armed with this equipment, this is all that is required and lulls the person into a false and dangerous sense of security.

The advantages of being in hospital are: –

- The benefit of measuring and monitoring the precise level of oxygen in the blood
- Oxygen therapy itself
- Nebulisation – using oxygen instead of room air in the nebuliser
- Chest X-rays to exclude the presence of a lung that has collapsed – this is a small but not uncommon risk in asthmatics – or a lung infection (pneumonia)
- Intravenous medication to relieve the tightness
- Assisted ventilation – if this becomes necessary. A tube (endotrachael) is inserted into the bronchial tube through the mouth and a ventilator does the breathing. The presence of the tube as it passes through the vocal cords into the lungs will prevent the person from speaking. Pen and paper may be used for communication.
- Round-the-clock monitoring of progress.

Home nebulisation should not be seen as the equivalent of treatment in hospital!

Children, and some adults, who cannot master the technique of using the inhaler correctly may attach the inhaler to a plastic device or breathing chamber (spacer) in which the medication from the inhaler is squirted into the chamber and an opening at the opposite end of the bottle allows one to breathe in the contents. In an emergency a 'Styrofoam cup (or plastic soft drink bottle) can be used wherein the mouthpiece of the inhaler is made to fit tightly into a hole cut out at the bottom end of the cup or plastic bottle. The medication is then squirted twice in quick succession into the cup (or bottle) and the person uses the open end of the cup (or bottle) to fit over the mouth and inhales several times as deeply as possible.

In the evaluation of the person whose chest is tight, even if the person is not known to be asthmatic, certain guidelines should always be observed to avoid the disasters that continue to occur. In an infant or young child the presence of difficulty breathing means it is already late and without further delay the child should be rushed to a doctor or nearest hospital. The usual setting is a cough that has become steadily worse i.e. producing more and more phlegm that may be difficult to bring out but can be heard bubbling in the chest or upper throat. The child's breathing is faster than normal (count the number of breaths in one minute using the second hand of a watch – greater than 30 per minute.

Signs of severe breathing difficulties are

- Reluctance to take feeds or fluids
- Increasing restlessness and agitation
- Crying and intolerant of being made to lie down flat – breathing and the resultant agitation become worse in the supine position – the child preferring to sit and hold the head up in order to straighten the air passages - trying to get air into the lungs more easily
- Reluctance to speak/cry as the breath is being saved instead for breathing – the 'quiet' child may well be having a very tight chest and in grave danger of going into respiratory failure and possibly dying. Waiting for the skin colour to change to blue before seeking urgent treatment is really courting disaster!
- Flaring of the nostrils
- Pulling in of the spaces between the ribs as the child breathes

In an older child or adult when the chest is starting to deteriorate the breath rate starts to increase. The normal rate in this age group is between 12 and about 18 per minute. If a fever is present (always check with a thermometer and not the traditional hand on the forehead!) this will also push up the breath rate but here the breathing is *not difficult,* simply faster. At this stage two puffs on the inhaler – Berotec or Ventolin or other similar product – (*not* the steroid inhaler as this is used as a preventative measure and takes much longer to take effect) should easily relieve the tightness – as measured on the *peak flow meter* - before and after the inhaler is used.

If the response is not good enough in terms of the tightness (subjective) or the PFR (peak flow rate – which is an objective measurement) within the space of 10 to 20 minutes and, if a nebuliser is not available, another two puffs of the non-steroidal inhaler is permitted. Failing a response within the next 10 minutes the child must be taken to hospital.

If a nebuliser is available add 1 ml of the medication and 1 to 4 ml of water (preferably warmed – cold water may precipitate further tightness) depending on the age of the patient. For young children who may not tolerate long periods on the nebuliser (they hate the idea of a mask 'obstructing' their breathing even further) use 1 ml of the medication and only 1 ml of water. The quantity of the medication always remains 1 ml whether it is for a child or adult. Be aware that the harder the child cries the deeper it is breathing and the more effective will be the nebulisation.

Every asthmatic should have an emergency supply of prednisolone (5mg.) to be taken in a single starting dose of between 6 to 8 tablets – preferably not on an empty stomach – to reduce the side effect of stomach inflammation (gastritis) and the start of a stomach ulcer. Medication to protect the stomach can be used along with the steroids.

If the decision has been taken (by the doctor) to use a course of steroids the tablets may be taken in two ways – either 6 – 8 tablets daily at once (after the main meal) for 14 days or the same number daily for 7 days and thereafter reducing the number of tablets by one each day for 7 days. The tablets take up to 4 hours to become effective but are the mainstay of treatment of acute asthma as they address the inflammation that occurs in this condition.

The underlying principle in the treatment of an asthmatic whose chest has changed for the worse is to *'over treat'* the condition even if the change is considered to be mild. If one previously used the inhaler once daily – increase it to 4 times daily. Using the peak flow meter should guide the management. Treating an asthmatic without it is akin to monitoring blood pressure without the sphygmomanometer (blood pressure recording machine). It is difficult to predict which particular episode of tightness will land the patient on a ventilator in the intensive care unit! Treat every tight chest with care.

Situations that could kill an asthmatic

- "It is 3 am – I'll wait until daybreak to get to the doctor"
- "It's not that bad!"
- "I've got the nebuliser – I should be okay"
- "My pump ran out"
- "I lost the inhaler"
- "I left it in my other handbag".

The tightness is always underestimated and the airways can quickly become tight enough to kill the patient from sudden respiratory failure – the cessation of breathing. It can take minutes for the chest to close down and the ambulance may not get there in time.

In an asthmatic attack the chest muscles that are used to breathe harder behave like any other muscles that are being exercised to the point of exhaustion - they produce lactic acid and, over time, the acid accumulates - impairing the function of the chest even further. Excess lactic acid is toxic to cells and results in *muscle fatigue*; the asthmatic literally becomes too tired to breathe. Fatalities in asthmatics will continue until they are educated about some problems that occur in this condition that are different from other chronic ones - like diabetes and hypertension. The most important difference, and a factor responsible for many of the deaths in asthma, is the patient *underestimates the severity of the attack* and does not believe that anything serious would happen in a short space of time. The reality is that the chest can 'close' within minutes – tight enough to make breathing impossible and death within a matter of minutes. Asthma is largely a controllable disease but with time the asthmatic becomes blasé about the condition and a cavalier attitude often prevails.

Furthermore, a poorly controlled chronic asthmatic has a higher risk of dying from an acute tight chest because invariably the episodes of bronchospasm mean a trip, often in the middle of the night to the doctor or hospital emergency unit. Do such asthmatics become depressed with the chronicity of their illness and its seeming incurability? And would they gladly trade illnesses with hypertension, for example, where the most that is required of the patient is to take a tablet – unlike in asthmatics where the responsibility often goes beyond this?

In asthma changes can occur more unpredictably, more swiftly and with more serious consequences. Furthermore, changes in the weather may not push up a person's blood pressure but spell disaster for asthmatics.

Any change from the usual behaviour of the chest – a cough that was not present the day before or more tightness than usual – should be the first warning that something may be amiss. This should warrant the following measures

- checking the degree of tightness more often with the peak flow meter
- using the inhaler more often
- taking a starter dose of Prednisolone
- using the nebuliser
- seeing the doctor or
rushing to hospital.

Just as blood glucose monitoring machines are available for diabetics the peak flow meter should be mandatory for every asthmatic. It gives the patient an accurate measurement of the tightness. Using "The way one feels" as a guide could spell disaster.

The tight chest often occurs at night and especially in winter when temperatures tend to fall. Air that is being inhaled through the open mouth is not receiving the benefit of being warmed by the rich blood supply in the lining of the nostrils. This situation occurs when the nostrils are blocked making it easier to breathe through the mouth because of the shorter distance between the mouth and the lungs. Cold air tends to precipitate an attack by making the airway tubes go into spasm. Homes should be heated in winter and especially at night when temperatures are much lower. Drying out of the ambient air can be prevented by placing a bowl of water in the room or hanging up washed, wet clothing to dry (not in front of the heater because of the fire hazard).The *change in weather* and its effect on asthma should highlight why there are empty beds in asthma wards in summer and standing room only in winter.

The Peak Flow Meter is the most accurate means available to the asthmatic at home or in a surgery to measure how tight the chest is at any given moment. It may vary with different times of the day or night and, therefore, in the initial work up of an asthmatic or later to review progress - the peak flow rate should be measured:

- in the morning on waking
- at midday
- in the evening
- on retiring at night
- at about 3 – 4 o'clock in the morning when asthmatics are known to 'dip' – i.e. the peak flow readings (PFRs) become lower

When the patient is asleep he or she may only be awakened if the chest becomes tight enough to arouse the person. If the PFR falls, but not sufficiently to waken the person, breathing will continue with less oxygen getting into the lungs because of the ('mild') degree of bronchospasm. These 'dips' will go undetected if the PFR is not measured. Any degree of failure to get adequate oxygen into the blood – as may also occur in those who snore – is bad news for the heart especially if this happens over prolonged periods.

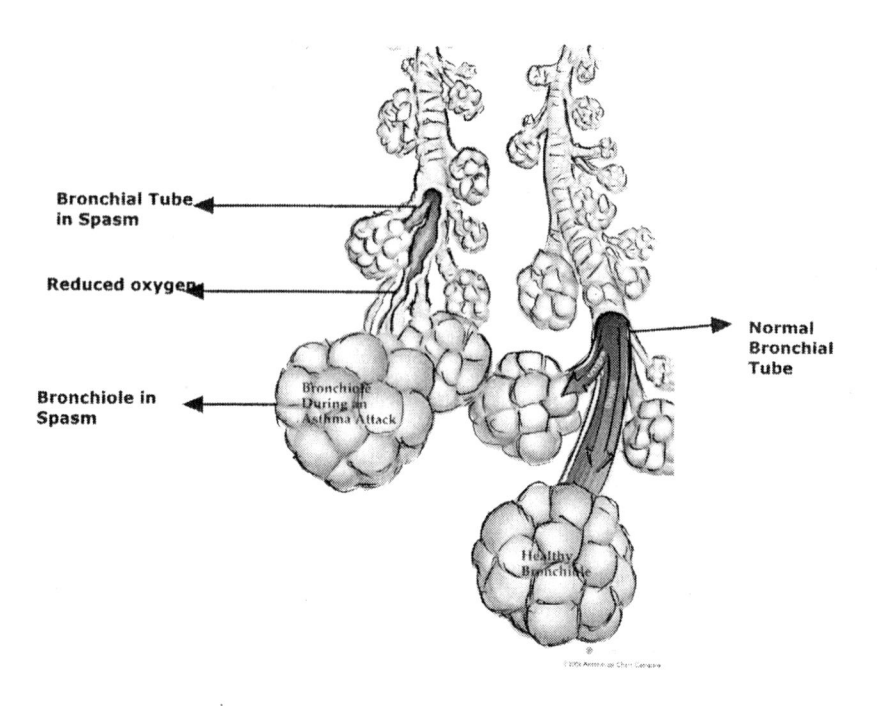

Bronchial Tube in Spasm

Reduced oxygen

Bronchiole in Spasm

Bronchiole During an Asthma Attack

Normal Bronchial Tube

Healthy Bronchiole

UNDERSTANDING ASTHMA

It is useful to have a profile of these readings to get a 'baseline' of normal, to know if the readings change during a period of broncho-spasm and also to detect *early morning dips*. If the latter are present a longer acting preparation can be taken at night to cover for these periods of otherwise undetected tightness. Using the person's height and a special chart the PFR can be calculated. Obviously, this will change with time, as a youngster grows taller.

Exercise (on a static bicycle or simply skipping) can be used to bring out latent or suspected 'exercise induced asthma'. Measure the PFR before and after the period of exercise and then repeat the exercise *after* using the nebuliser or inhaler (correctly!). This will establish the diagnosis of *exercise induced asthma* (the PFR readings will reflect changes accordingly) and also measure the response to treatment. If the diagnosis of exercise induced asthma is confirmed two puffs on the inhaler should be used about 20 minutes *before* any exercise.

Asthmatics with bronchospasm (tight chest) often have difficulty bringing up phlegm because the latter is often dry and sticky. This will irritate the bronchial tubes further. The viscid sputum is hardly surprising considering that the problem is aggravated by the effects of 'dehydration' – a factor often ignored because the problem is not that of 'diarrhoea' for which the importance of fluid intake is well known. Normally the bronchial tubes along with the upper airways (trachea, pharynx and nasal passages) produce up to 3 litres of mucus per day to keep the airways moist. This should give some idea of how much more fluids are necessary in an asthmatic who is too busy concerned about the chest to worry about food and fluids!

Many a person (young and old) is reluctant to use the inhaler and loses out on a very effective form of treatment. The inhaler is 'cumbersome' and has not the same facility as a tablet slipped into a pocket and unobtrusively popped into the mouth when required – sometimes in the middle of a rugby match! The snout of the inhaler may look 'comical' and ungainly when positioned in the mouth; it does not resemble conventional medication and can make the user become self-conscious and nonconformist in a world of cruel, teasing young peers who may view its use and the user as a bit 'freakish' – becoming the receiving end of schoolboy tomfoolery and, perhaps, a missing inhaler!

The underlying pathology in the airway cells is *inflammation*. It is inflammation that makes the tubes go into spasm and only steroids (in tablet, inhaler or injection form) address this problem.

Other drugs – called b agonists (Ventolin/ Berotec) help to open the bronchial tubes and smaller airways but do not address the inflammation. The anti-inflammatory effect of steroids may be enhanced by using *Omega 3* (salmon oil). *Vitamin E* should also be taken for its powerful antioxidant effect.

During inflammation anywhere in the body O2 (oxygen) breaks up and becomes separated into O + O. These are the so called 'free radicals'. Nature does not allow oxygen to separate and each free radical frantically searches for a 'partner' to become O2 again. A free radical is akin to a mate desperately seeking a partner. The more free radicals present at the scene of the inflammation the greater the damage to tissue. Antioxidants, if they are present at the site of inflammation (whether in the bronchial tubes in asthma or the heart muscle in angina) help to mop up the free radicals thereby limiting the damage. Vitamin E and *Vitamin C* are powerful antioxidants.

Vitamin E also helps red cells transport oxygen more effectively – a function that is crucial in an asthmatic.

Should the asthmatic require additional support *Herbal Respiratory* tablets – one twice daily – should be added and, in an attempt to protect the cells of the lungs and airways, *Formula IV Plus* – 1 sachet daily should be taken in conjunction with the Omega 3 capsules.

Conventional medicine has a worrying limitation and many patients end up with bad lung disease from chronic asthma and cigarette abuse and are told that "The hospital cannot do any more" for them. All of the drugs currently used in asthma have side effects; if the oral steroids cause a bleeding ulcer in the stomach this, often life saving medication, may be withdrawn. However, none of the natural alternatives mentioned above have any detrimental side effects. They should be started early in conjunction with normal medication – not in place of it.

Asthma, when it occurs early in childhood, has a better chance of disappearing as the child grows older. Such a patient should never take up smoking because, if the condition should reappear later in life, as it can, one will have the added disadvantage of the damage from the cigarettes to contend with and this could easily lead to 'end stage respiratory (lung) failure'. The victim may end up a respiratory cripple, relying on home oxygen for the remainder of the person's life.

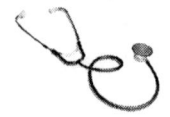

ATTENTION DEFICIT HYPERACTIVITY DISORDER

Attention deficit hyperactivity disorder or ADHD is not terminology that has been used for long even though the condition has been present for generations; has it become more prevalent? Is the condition being recognized and reported better?

Are we doing things to our children to make it easier to develop this condition? Are the answers linked to the frightening statistic that the incidence of Cancer in children has doubled in the past 12 years in Britain? A mere one hundred years ago, which is the batting of an eyelid in terms of the millennium and the evolution of the world, the biggest killer of mankind was *Infection* – today it is *Heart Disease and Cancer.*

What have we done in one hundred short years to achieve this remarkable turnaround in disease patterns and mortality? The underlying causes could also be linked to ADHD

- Food – the way it is grown, processed, stored, cooked and refrigerated
- Television and its barrage of advertised junk food and beverages, the lack of exercise and subsequent obesity from hours spent each day glued to the set
- Transport and its link to the lack of exercise and resultant
- Obesity and emission of lethal fumes from motor vehicles and industry,

- Pollution of our waters by industry and agriculture and the subsequent toxicity to our marine life, fruit and vegetables through insecticides and fertilizers that permeate into our crops, soil and eventually into drinking water
- Damage to the ozone layer that allows harmful irradiation rays of the sun to enter our atmosphere
- Working mothers and the role oral contraceptives have played in their supposed emancipation
- Surrogate 'parents and caregivers' - i.e. the crèche and pre school!

In the animal kingdom offspring are taught instinctively by the parents and the young learn at a pace determined by nature to ensure, primarily, survival. The skills embrace the ability to flee from danger (and to this end man shares the benefits of sudden surges of adrenaline and steroids when faced with stress) and the instinct to find food and to preserve the line of the species (procreation).

In trying to produce the 'super kid' (the child that the parents aspired to be but failed to become) do we over stimulate the child beyond the pace nature intended? So that the entire biological clock has been made to tick faster resulting in an earlier maturation that robs them of the innocence of childhood? Is the grade one child finding his mental development beyond that of his or her peers and the level expected of a child of that age? And is sexual maturity being attained at an earlier age? Statistics do indicate a rise in the incidence of sex crimes committed by younger offenders.

The capacity to procreate outstrips the mental maturity that should have developed pari passu with the gonads resulting in teenagers charged with sex at an age that nature did not intend to happen so early. Are we creating misfits with the removal of the mother and her replacement with the crèche, television or preschool? Are we *creating* the 'inattentive' child?

The present generation of young children have been exposed to foods and drinks such as their parents never had – crisp chips, fruit juices sweetened and 'unsweetened' (the sugar content of almost 6 oranges lurk innocently under the almost criminal advertising of 'no sugar added' in one glass of orange and most other fruit juices) soft drinks, cakes, sweets, ice cream, battered and fried chicken, hamburgers, fish and chips, polony, salamis, liver and fish spreads, Vienna and other sausages and a whole variety of other processed meats, dairy products from cows being primed with hormones and protected with antibiotics to increase productivity to meet the demands of consumers and farmers, margarines, samoosas, pastries and pies, biscuits and cakes!

How often do parents lament, but do little about it "He just won't eat his veggies"? Why would he eat his veggies when he has chips that dad brought home (for himself) and sweets that grandpa bribed him with so that he could get some peace and quiet around the house until the parents arrived from work to fetch the children? How many trolleys are dutifully loaded with the above mentioned junk foods and beverages accompanied by the familiar lament "He just won't eat any fruit!" And "I've tried everything to lose weight but nothing seems to work?"

The young parents of today are the products of the television pioneers. Their children will be more television-wise than the parents since the first advertisements reached the small screen. Today's child is being brainwashed from an earlier age and is an expert on the advertised products and has become even more 'supermarket-wise' than their parents! Advertising on television has changed our buying and eating habits. Thus far we have managed to ban smoking from the small screen – but there is a long way to go yet.

Reading a storybook has a pace dictated by the speed of the reader. Compare this with the lightning speed at which each frame changes on television. The child must keep pace with this speed or miss the sequence of whatever it was viewing at the time. This must, of necessity, challenge the child's brain to assimilate information faster. Is this another explanation for the increased numbers of 'hyperactive' children? Who will grow up to be another impatient and intolerant motorist committing road rage?

One of the biggest culprits of the state of our health must be the intake of sugar. The powers that be rightly pronounce that the sugar is innocent. The point that is missed is its inclusion into so many manufactured foods. Smoking one cigarette a day may not be sufficient to cause much harm but twenty will. One teaspoon of sugar per day may not be detrimental to our health – but is this the consumption of the average child or adult? Therein lies the rub and calls the bluff of those that sanction the use of refined sugar. All carbohydrates that are eaten, regardless of whatever form they are taken, are all converted into 'glucose' – whether it is a piece of cake, slice of bread, rice, pasta or alcohol. The body stores any glucose that is not used by first converting it into fat. This fat, and any other additional fat taken in the diet is stored as fat. However, the body cannot store protein - therefore this has to be taken at each meal.

Whenever sugar is taken the level of glucose in the blood rises and each time insulin is produced to bring the level down again. The amount of insulin produced may not always be that fine tuned and invariably the insulin lowers the blood glucose level to lower than normal. In a child (or adult) this lowered blood sugar will produce symptoms of jitteriness, irritability and restlessness that may translate into lack of attention, boisterousness and disruptive behaviour.

In a preschooler it may result in aggressiveness and a quick pinch or punch aimed at any recipient – peer or adult – the mother apologizing that the child is "Very crabby today" and another sugared pacifier is given, often in desperation, to calm down the child.

In a classroom, with a slightly older subject, the disruption may translate into a lack of attention and disturbance of other pupils leading to academic backwardness and unruly behaviour. This could sow the seed for a future lack of self-esteem from being repeatedly admonished or even punished because he or she has earned a reputation for such behaviour and, in time, this becomes the 'norm' for that child. Such behaviour may also alienate him or her self from the other children in the class; once the label sticks change becomes more difficult. The classes may be too large to allow the teacher to recognize the problem. Having a 'human relations' or 'resources officer' (as is customary in the workplace) would be useful provided referral is requested early. Teachers should be taught to recognize pupils with attention deficit hyperactivity disorder or who are suspected of having it. Not every inattentive or disruptive child may have ADHD

– making it important the child is referred early and the diagnosis confirmed and treated by professionals (psychologists).

Children who leave home without breakfast or adequate nutrition may be setting themselves up to be hypoglycemic (low blood sugar) by 10 o'clock because the normal liver has only sufficient glucose for about four hours from the time of waking. By mid-morning the child is inattentive and may well display symptoms of low sugar. How many schools insist their young protégés have breakfast as ardently as whether they have done their homework? How many teachers themselves have breakfast? And how many educationists understand what should consist of a *nutritious breakfast*? Oats, 'Weetabix' and 'Pronutro' share pride of place.

The following supplements could ensure a sound start in the development of the child on its way to adulthood as it passes through school:

- *Omega 3* – one capsule daily
- *Calmag tablets* (the number determined by the age – less than 8 years 1/day; between 8 and 12 – 2/day and after that 3 daily)
- 1 helping of *Nutrishake* daily
- *Vitasquare* tablets are chewable forms of vitamins along with being a food supplement and could play an important role in the child's growth.

Before Ritalin is recommended to a child with ADHD, given the side effects of this drug, little is lost by using the above supplements. Omega 3 and Calmag have been shown to benefit children with ADHD.

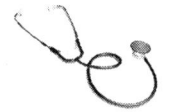

BEDWETTING

The first time and how it is handled then may determine its outcome in the future. When it occurs urine has left the bladder and no amount of shouting or screaming will get it back to where it should have been. But this will turn it into a major issue in the child's mind, making it more difficult to prevent future 'accidents'. The bedwetting is usually discovered some time *after* the 'accident', often the following morning. The child will be unable to correlate the fuss with the actual loss of bladder control that occurred while the child was asleep. As with a pup that has not been house trained the 'wetting' is never deliberate and shouting or, worse still, punishing the pup for soiling your prized carpet will tell the pet nothing – it cannot tell a Van Dyk cross weave from a patch of grass in the garden! It knows only that you are upset and feel the pain you may have inflicted – the offending original deed long since forgotten. The carpet can be cleaned and the bedding can be washed but the memory of the pain from the spanking and the shame will linger on – sometimes for life. The problem is magnified if other members of the family and friends are informed.

Life and sleep, in particular, can easily be transformed into a major undertaking to ensure the bed remains dry – playing detectives and setting up electronic devices to warn the parents that the urine has leaked. An offer of love, understanding and patience could be more important in the management than any other measure. The child needs to understand that the problem is not serious and that there is nothing abnormal about the 'incontinence' or the child – even if it should happen again and again.

Factors that may precipitate or aggravate the condition:

- A urinary tract (bladder) infection
- Worms irritating the bladder
- Psychological problems e.g. a class bully, a cane-wielding teacher, an abusive sibling
- Possible problems of a sexual nature – could there be underlying molestation?
- Taking fluids and fruits with high 'juice' or water content about one and half hours before bedtime
- Coffee taken in the afternoon may continue its diuretic effect (stimulating the excretion of urine) well into the night (coffee has no place in a child's diet).

Does the onset of bedwetting coincide with admission into a new school or different class, a change in teachers, the moving away of a close buddy or the separation of parents? Has there been a falling off in class grades either before or after the bedwetting started.

To keep some perspective on the problem bear in mind that the person responsible for the wet bed is one's own child and that if he or she were diagnosed as having leukemia the bed wetting would become like 'nothing' – there would be no fuss or bother and the mishaps dismissed without so much as a murmur.

'Without' leukemia the same wet bed could become a war between adult and child. The least amount of fuss required to change the clothing and bedding should be the cornerstones of management for a condition known to disappear over time.

In the meanwhile, discreetly protect the bed with plastic liners and have spare sheets and pyjamas at hand. It may also be useful to have a liner for the blanket or a cover over the blanket that can be easily removed and washed. The older child should not be subjected to wearing an absorbent pad – this may save the linen but it would be an additional humiliation and further entrench the embarrassing problem into the impressionable mind.

The general practitioner would be the first port of call if the condition persists beyond a week or so and a few simple investigations may clarify the picture. If this is unsuccessful the advice of a psychologist may be sought after discrete discussions with the teacher and doctor. As a last resort there is medication available that is taken at night to help improve bladder control.

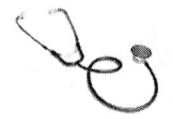

BREAST FEEDING

If there is an area where man' s meddling has been made to revert to that which nature had intended then breast feeding must take pride of place. Sanity has prevailed where the manufacturers of baby formula feeds had got a strangle hold on infant feeding. However, this has been more as a result of pressure from health departments than the goodness of the business sectors' hearts. Nothing man can make will match a mother's milk.

Mothers should also be actively discouraged from using the following reasons not to breast-feed: –

- Insufficient milk
- Had to go back to work
- Didn't want boobs that hung like pendulums
- The idea of a leech sucking me dry
- The gynaecologist advised against it
- My nipples were inverted / painful
- I had a bad/difficult /painful experience the last time
- My husband did not want me too
- I was inexperienced
- It embarrassed me to expose my breasts in public
- I was always too tired to get up at night to feed the baby on demand

Dairy farmers ensure that their 'milk producers' are well fed, receive adequate vitamin supplements, antibiotics and even hormones to improve the quality and quantity of milk. Our mothers should be offered no less! Omega 3 – 2 capsules daily, Vitamin E – 200 I.U. – 1 capsule daily and Calmag at least 3 daily should be continued through the breast feeding stage to be passed on to the baby through the milk. There are many drugs that can be transmitted to the infant through milk and mothers must draw the attention of the doctor or pharmacist before any medication is prescribed.

Omega 3 fish oil has been shown to help in the development of the brain and retina of the eye of the foetus. These continue to develop until long after the baby is born. Breast milk has everything the infant requires until the age of four to six months after which the amounts of iron and the total calorie concentration would become inadequate. At about this time solid feeds or formula feeds should be introduced.

During pregnancy high levels of progesterone keep milk production to a minimum. After the birth the level of this hormone falls and this stimulates milk production. There are two important hormones involved in the production of milk:

- OXYTOCIN   The hormone is made in the brain (in the hypothalamus). Within seconds of the nipples being stimulated – as in suckling – the message is carried by nerves from the nipple to the brain and oxytocin is released into the blood. It is carried to the breast milk glands which are then stimulated to contract resulting in the ejection of milk from the breast.
- Once milk is *removed* from the breast only then will *more* milk be produced and this can continue indefinitely – in some economically deprived communities a three year old could still be breast feeding.
- PROLACTIN   The hormone stimulates the breasts to produce milk and is also responsible for the increased size of the breasts during pregnancy in preparation for its role in lactation. It explains why the breasts of the newborn male or

female infant can sometimes produce milk (called 'witches milk') from their own breasts because of the presence of this hormone carried over from the mother. In pregnancy there is an increase in the level of oestrogen that helps promote the production of prolactin. While prolactin controls the *production* of milk it is not responsible for the *ejection* of milk from the breast. The increase in prolactin levels fills the breast with more milk in readiness for the next feed.

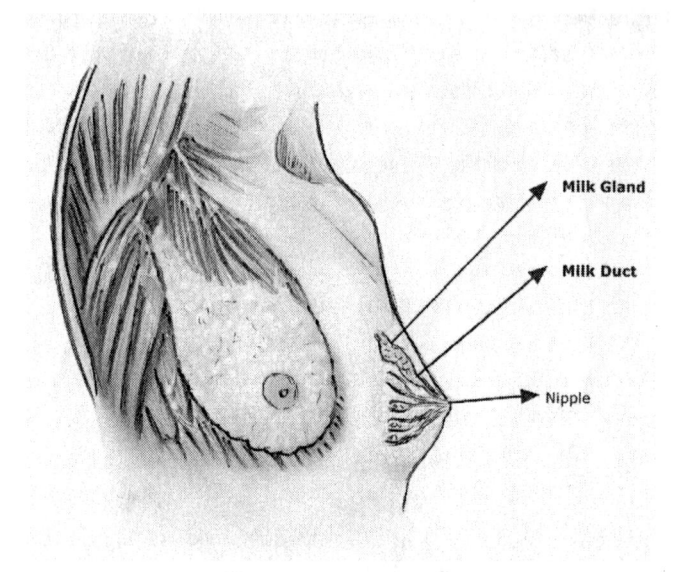

Milk Gland

Milk Duct

Nipple

ANATOMY OF THE BREAST

Suckling on the nipple stimulates the production of more prolactin to maintain the ability of the breasts to lactate. Alternatively, there are drugs available that can suppress the production of the hormone when breast feeding needs to be terminated.

Suckling on the nipples does two things: –

1. Sends messages via nerves to the brain to release prolactin
2. Triggers the release of oxytocin from the brain (Hypothalamus) that stimulates the ejection ('let down') of milk from the breast.

As with any other hormone in the body those involved in the production of milk require adequate vitamins, enzymes and trace elements for their production. Taking Formula *IV Plus* would supply the necessary minerals, proteins, enzymes, sterols and lipids.

The role of water or hydration should not be underestimated. The cells lining the respiratory(air) passages normally produce up to three litres of mucus daily and this does not take into account the extra mucus produced if one has a 'runny nose'! Add to this the fluid required to produce milk and one can gauge the importance of taking adequate water to ensure sufficient milk production. Is it any surprise so many mothers give up in frustration saying they cannot produce enough milk for their infant who is then switched to a 'formula feed'?

The physical contact between mother and infant and the life giving drink that flows into the hungry mouth allaying the pangs of hunger satisfies the first basic instinct in the infant's slow progress through life i.e. the instinct of hunger. This instinct is so powerful and inborn that the touch of the nipple on the cheek will automatically cause the infant to open its mouth and turn toward the offered nipple in readiness to be fed. If a finger touches the infant's cheek it will also instinctively open its mouth in expectation of the nipple.

Babies should be allowed to nurse about twenty minutes or longer on each breast to feel sated and get the benefit of the energy rich *hind milk* that follows the initial flow of colostrum. Feeding on demand avoids the situation where the infant becomes so hungry that the need to feed becomes a battle between the pangs/pain of hunger and the nipples in its attempt to wolf down the milk as fast as possible. This begs sore and battered nipples and the gulping of unnecessary air that will have to be brought up sooner or later or face the consequences of possible colic! Other mammals also feed on demand.

It is tempting to start the young entrant into the rat race in an independent mode and relegate it into a separate room with its own bedding and its other recently acquired worldly possessions. However, it is overlooked that the infant spent nine months of its existence in an environment that was very close to the mother, safe, warm and protected, where food was in constant supply and hunger and thirst were unheard of; where the thermostat did not fluctuate and it never knew pain or a wet or soiled nappy or strange and loud sounds and the tantrums of jealous fathers denied their conjugal pleasures; or overzealous siblings poking, prodding and fussing and showing signs of emotional neglect with the arrival of the new addition.

To husbands that claim sole ownership of their wife's breasts, parts of her anatomy that, until the infant arrived he had privy to, let it be known that the breast may be a secondary sex characteristic and plays not a small measure in the erotica that surrounds sex but their *primary function* is to provide the only source of food nature intended for the newborn. That pang of jealousy on seeing the greedy infant as it attacks the exposed breast with such gusto must be stifled. Perhaps, if the father was allowed to sample the milk, the taste of which he has long since forgotten, it may put the breast issue to rest!

Inverted nipples should not be a reason to withhold breast-feeding because they can be corrected during the pregnancy.

If breast milk is not used up regularly (and allowed to accumulate) the breast/s will become engorged with milk and risk infection – milk is an excellent culture medium in which bacteria can multiply. Any breast-feeding mother who develops pain in the breast must see the doctor *early* as this may prevent the infection from progressing into a full blown abscess that will require 'incision and drainage' in theatre. If caught early a simple course of antibiotics may abort the infection. However, if it should develop into an abscess the milk should be expressed into a feeding bottle, heated to sterilize it and be fed quite safely to the infant.

The transfer of maternal antibodies begins while the foetus is within the uterus and continues to be supplied after the birth through the milk. These antibodies build up immunity and protect the newborn from infections. This first introduction to the outside environment is a crucial time for the infant and it needs all the help it can get.

Research has clearly demonstrated that infants fed on breast milk are less prone to gastroenteritis; this is hardly surprising as this is one product that is 'untouched by human hands'. In today's world

of fast foods and instant gratification it is small wonder that no bud-
ding entrepreneur has come to the rescue with bottled breast milk
for time-bedevilled mothers and for those who, for one reason or
another, cannot or will not breast-feed! Breast-fed babies are prone
to fewer allergies.

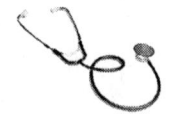

CHEST PAIN

To a layperson there is only one organ in the chest that is of major concern when chest pain occurs: "Is it my heart?" This overriding concern is not unjustified as without the heart there is nothing! However, there may be several causes for chest pain that are not related to this organ. These include the trachea (windpipe), oesophagus (food pipe), pleura (lining covering the lungs), ribs, muscles and skin around the chest and anxiety.

If chest pain occurs the first point to consider is: whether the pain is on the right side of the chest, middle or the left. If the pain arises from the right side this usually excludes the heart as being the cause of the pain. It may be due to the pleura, ribs, muscle or the skin. Pain in the lower part of the chest on the right side may be caused by the liver, gall bladder, right kidney or the last two ribs (which, unlike the ten pairs above, are free floating and not attached to the breastbone in front – as are the others).

The lung per se cannot 'feel' pain but the double layered lining (pleura) that surrounds each lung is very sensitive. The covering or outer lining of *any organ* (kidney, liver, heart brain and gut) is very painful if inflamed or stretched.

Pleurisy is usually the result of a lung infection that has spread from the lung to the pleura and this is often preceded by a cough, phlegm and possibly fever. The most important symptom that draws attention to this diagnosis is the severe pain over the affected side of the chest that occurs during breathing; coughing becomes almost impossible. The person often supports the chest wall with a hand to avoid the pain from stretching the pleura during coughing.

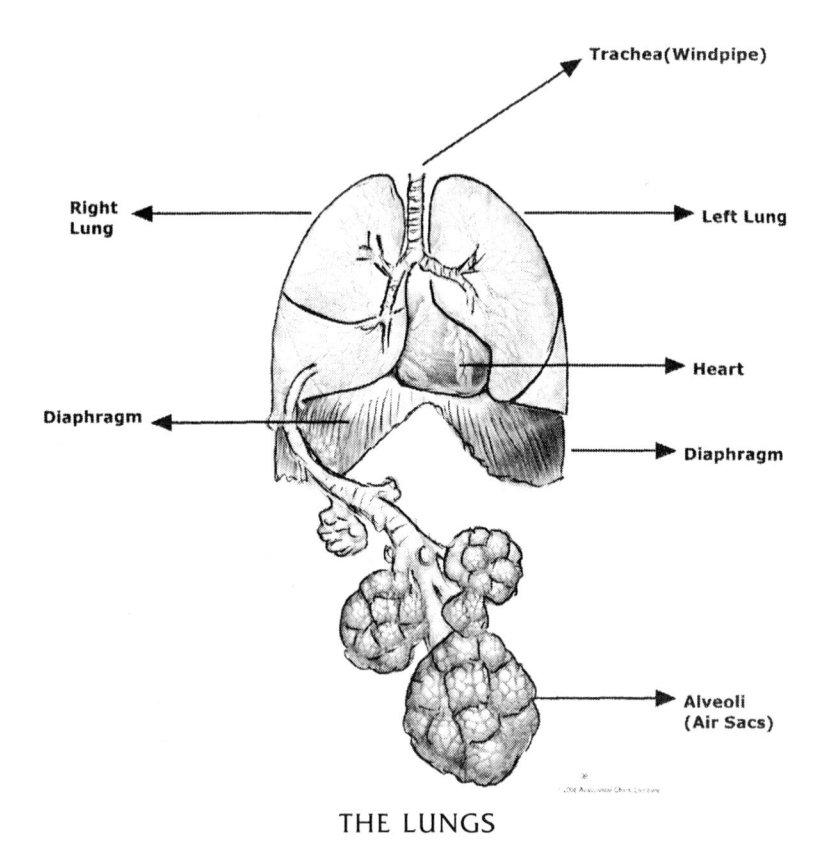

Trachea(Windpipe)

Right Lung

Left Lung

Heart

Diaphragm

Diaphragm

Alveoli (Air Sacs)

THE LUNGS

If the ribs are the source of the pain there is usually a *history of injury* resulting in a fracture of the rib/s. This is accompanied by severe pain that only occurs if a deep breath is taken or coughing is attempted. The pain may be severe enough to make breathing shallow and coughing almost impossible. If the person can cough easily the diagnosis of a fracture is very unlikely. Fractured ribs are no longer treated by bandaging the chest wall as this restricts breathing and if sufficient air does not enter the chest one or more lobes of the lung may collapse or develop pneumonia. Adequate pain relief and deep but controlled breathing, without any explosive movements, is advised.

The main concern with a fractured rib is not that the bone is broken but whether the pleura (lining around the lung) has been punctured by the broken ends. This will cause the lung to collapse and the clue this has occurred is usually the presence of unusual shortness of breath (difficulty breathing). The severity of this shortness of breath depends on how much of the lung has collapsed (shrunk). If outside air is allowed into the space between the two layers of the pleura the lung will collapse resulting in a pneumothorax – pneumo= air.

This is a surgical emergency and is treated by introducing a tube into the chest – it is placed in the space that has been 'created' by the presence of the air within the pleural space (pneumothorax). This tubing is connected to a suction pump that removes the accumulated air from the pleural cavity allowing the lung to re-expand. This means a hospital stay until the opening in the pleura has naturally sealed and the tube can be removed. The tubing is kept in place with a stitch. While this procedure may appear 'gruesome' it is not a major undertaking and can be done at the bedside and under a local anaesthetic.

Shortness of breath occurring after a

- Motor vehicle accident
- Impact injury
- After a bout of severe coughing or
- Sometimes an asthmatic that suddenly deteriorates (given that an asthmatic attack will also cause shortness of breath) requires an urgent chest X-ray. This reinforces the advice that home nebulisation for sudden episodes of tight chests has this potential for fatal outcomes if the management of such attacks becomes cavalier. If the tightness has not responded to an inhaler or nebuliser within about twenty minutes the patient must be referred to a hospital urgently.

Pain from muscles that lie between the ribs (the meat in 'spare ribs'!) and those that cover them and, lower down, pass onto the abdominal wall may also mimic that of a fractured rib – with or without the story of trauma. If the pain is due to inflamed muscles (myositis) it is also worsened by movement of the arms, chest or belly muscles and though there is some relation to breathing or coughing the latter is not as severe as with a fractured rib or pleurisy – the patient may still be able to cough, unlike in a fracture where severe pain will make this almost impossible.

Pain arising from the skin may occur from shingles. When the rash that accompanies this condition is present it consists of several small 'pimple' like lesions much like those seen in acne or chicken-pox. There should be this similarity because shingles is caused by the same virus that causes chickenpox – the latter at a young age. After the infection has cleared the virus may reside (sometimes perma-nently) in some nerves of the skin. In shingles the first day or so may not be accompanied by pain. It is often difficult to make the diagnosis without the telltale rash unless its possibility is considered. That the pain is of a burning nature and there may be some itching may be clues when the rash has not yet appeared.

At the points where each of the upper six to seven ribs meet the breastbone in front of the chest a joint is present. This may become the site of an inflammation producing pain in the chest. A clue to the diagnosis is that pressing over the specific joint produces pain. Lying on the affected side and moving the arm or lifting a weight may also aggravate the pain. A virus (in a condition called Tietze's syndrome) or a simple inflammation (costochondritis) have been implicated and, when the left side is affected, may mimic a heart attack. If the pain occurs over the left chest the possible causes include the heart (angina) or pericarditis (inflammation of the lining around the heart) along with the other causes pertaining to the right side as mentioned above.

The pain from angina (see chapter on Heart attack) is usually related to exercise or some exertion. It is commonly situated in the centre of the chest and may spread across to the left arm, the neck or the jaw. It is often described as tightness or burning – *never* sharp like a needle. The further away from the centre of the chest the pain occurs (past the left nipple) the less likely it is due to angina. Angina usually lasts 10 - 15 minutes and upwards but almost never a few seconds or one - two minutes. It does not normally persist the whole day - allowing the affected person to continue his or her normal activities as though nothing was the matter.

Women and diabetics may not always present classic textbook features of angina. There may not be significant chest pain, the pain may not always be associated with exercise and it may not be severe. The medical profession should have a lower threshold for suspecting heart disease in these two groups. The following should arouse suspicion:

- Unexplained weakness
- Tiredness
- Shortness of breath
- Dizziness and nausea unexpected for the particular female, especially if she is menopausal.

In these situations the risk profile helps in considering the diagnosis of angina or a heart attack viz.

- age
- family history of angina or heart attack
- smoking
- obesity
- lack of exercise
- past history of angina or a heart attack
- hypertension
- diabetes mellitus.

An ECG (electrocardiogram) and blood tests may clarify the diagnosis. Blood tests can measure certain substances that are released into the blood when heart muscle cells are damaged for lack of oxygen - as happens when a coronary artery is blocked. If the blockage is complete and no blood is able to pass to the area that artery was supplying the result is a 'heart attack' (myocardial infarction). If the blockage is *not* complete and blood is able to flow past the obstruction this will result in 'angina'. An echocardiogram may identify the damaged heart wall. This is similar to an ultrasound examination done in pregnancy to examine the foetus, except that here the heart is the focus of attention.

Pain from the oesophagus (foodpipe) e.g. heartburn may cause some confusion in terms of identifying angina. Many a patient experiencing pain from a heart attack (especially a male) will first assume this is 'heartburn (that he may have experienced in the past) and self medicate with an antacid or 'Enos'/'Alka Selzer'. Heartburn occurring for the first time in an older person (35 years and above) must seek professional advice. Receiving an antacid without excluding a heart attack is unacceptable.

If an antacid or other medication has been effective in the past and now no longer relieves the symptoms this requires investigation – beware the repeat prescription for more antacids or other 'stronger' preparations. Also, if there is a change in the character of the familiar heartburn or the pain occurs during or soon after exercise a doctor's opinion should be sought - not another dose of 'Rennies'!

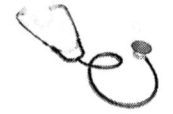

CHILDREN

Given time, and like eating food, man often loses sight of the real reason why we have children: to ensure continuity of the species. Without the instincts of eating and procreation (in that order) Homo sapiens would have been extinct millions of years ago.

The last one hundred years may be used to illustrate how the number of children per family has changed and the factors that helped to determine the number varied from:

- the availability of food
- the influence of diseases and how this dictated mortality rates
- the introduction of the concept of 'Family Planning' and more effective methods of contraception
- education in family size to match the resources of the country at large and the individual family in particular
- the disappearance of the mother from the home environment and the accompanying shift in care-giving from the parent/s to grandparents, nannies, crèches and nursery schools.

Children and infants are being awakened as early as 5 o'clock in the morning in order to be taken to a crèche at the mother's work place or a caregiver, often long distances away from home. The bonding that should have been taking place within the home environment is now being shared with strange people and places. The child now has two 'homes', sometimes three, when the child is taken from the crèche to an intermediate child minder to cope between the hours when the crèche closes and the parent arrives later from work.

How have we altered the child and its development into an adult by the changes that have been made in its formative years? There is a difference between the five year old of today and that of thirty years ago when the latter, more than likely, had one parent present (dad worked) in a 'single home' setting for longer periods during the day. This was a crucial time when the child was first being introduced to his or her new environment – where it had the opportunity to learn and explore in the company of its mother. This is probably how nature intended it because animals do not use caregivers and 'day mothers' to fulfill the functions of the parents.

If this relationship between mother and child is not adequately developed from the time of birth, and continued for a 'reasonable' period (at least until the child enters formal school), the situation is ripe for creating problems for the child later in life and, possibly, into adulthood.

Earlier introduction of the child into a crèche or preschool allows the mother emancipation and a certain equality of the sexes. But are we misguidedly shortening the interaction between mother, child and environment that may be so vital in preparing for more mature schoolgoers rather than more 'academic' ones? Are parents trying too hard to produce the cleverest infant, crèche-attendee, preschooler and pupil and paying less attention to the other parameters that are also important in a child, soon-to-be-teenager and adult?

Sometimes we hasten the rate of development and the level of achievement to match our own expectations, to match or better the competition, to match the demand for the academic because business and industry are more concerned with turn over and what will work better for the company than whether the 'academic' is burning out from stress and building up to an earlier death from hypertension, heart attacks, diabetes and cancer?

Mothers are no longer seeing child minding as an important function when they are trying to balance the need to achieve more with their lives and earn extra income. The state of the economy worldwide has changed from the immediate period after the last world war, when there was a boom in almost every sphere of industry, until about the seventies when the bubble started to shrink and eventually burst in the eighties - when companies started to 'downsize' and retrenchments became the order of the day. The boom was expected to last forever and businesses grew bigger and bigger. We know this to be incorrect.

Overnight the price of oil shot up and petrol almost dried out. Interest rates went up and, almost pari passu with the realization by women that the world that men moved and lived in was not the prerogative of the male sex, women were joining the work force – nay – were even expected to do so! This left the care of the children dependent on the expertise and love, or the lack thereof, of grandparents and strangers. The last 'war effort' did more than produce ammunition and electrical parts; it gave women their first taste of independence and the need for crèches.

Remuneration for work done will never show its worth in any other business as it would in the care of children because the character and personality of the child is being moulded from birth and it takes a special kind of caregiver that will see another person's child as her or his own. This is unrealistic and well nigh impossible when the remuneration of care givers are often pitiful. The caregiver in a crèche may be a minder with no qualifications, a teacher with minimum qualification who cannot find work in a normal school or a caregiver trained and appropriately qualified to give the child the specialised care it needs. This child in the crèche may one day produce a future president, professor, wife batterer, terrorist or hijacker. Who will later interview the caregiver for the details that went into shaping the destiny of the child that produces the adult rapist or successful bank manager?

Grandparents should not easily be given the task of child minding. This alternative to the crèche may seem attractive because

- it is cheaper
- the parents assume the grandparents would be 'offended' at the very thought of remuneration

- the parents also assume that the grandparents are happy to oblige - after all the grandchildren are the apples of their eyes
- the parents would much rather trust the grandparents than a total stranger in the care of their precious child
- the child or children are familiar with their grandparents
- grandparents may subscribe to the notion that they are better qualified.

These children are sometimes caught up in undisclosed turmoils between parents and grandparents. Views on child rearing, eating habits and what foods are best – when they vary markedly between the parents and grandparents – have the potential for conflict. The situation becomes even more complicated when there are differences between maternal and paternal grandparents. These two groups may vie for the attention of their grandchildren by currying affection with gifts and luxuries. The parties involved may be powerless to change or control this knowing full well grandparents are in a position to dictate the terms by virtues of their ages, greater wisdom and experience.

The parents of the children may have totally opposing views on what is best for their offspring. The child is often caught between chips and cookies at grandma's and a stricter 'no luxury nonsense' immediately they are home. This will confuse the child. Furthermore, the luxury items could be used to blackmail the child into better behaviour when they are in the care of the grandparents. The latter may even feel threatened by the 'hyperactive' difficult-to-manage child who has learned the value of a good tantrum.

After an interval of up to twenty years grandparents may feel intimidated by the prospect of child-minding. Grandchildren would have changed in that time and become more demanding, inquisitive and streetwise than the children they had known when they were parents themselves. The widespread media coverage of child abuse also plays a contentious role in the mind of today's caregiver. A smack on the bottom of your own child has never the same implications as one planted on the bottom of another person's baby. Children learn quickly that the smack on the bottom received at home is not forthcoming even when greater liberties are taken at grandma's place. And what does the parent feel who has arrived to collect her precious child - after being painfully separated for up to ten hours - to be informed that her little 'darling' broke grandpa's prized goldfish bowl for which he or she received a smack on the bottom?

Grandparents who have been 'childless' for twenty odd years, having set themselves in their ways and the routines of their retired lives and keeping house the way they have always wanted - now have to cope with the little darling who arrives early on Monday mornings. One day the house is childless and the next there is a ready-made addition – not one that has grown with them over time as their own child did so many years ago.

Then there is the responsibility of the health and safety of the child. This may also cause anxiety as it may be seen as a reflection of the quality and attentiveness of the caregiver should their young charge become ill or, worse still, suffer physical trauma. How do the grandparents inform the parents that some accident has befallen their child - even though it may have been beyond their control? The incident may not have generated the same degree of concern to the parents themselves but could devastate the grandparents.

Furthermore, the latter may be on treatment for ailments common to their age. It is not easy to be in pain from an osteoarthritic joint or be dizzy from the side effects of drugs to be in a fit condition to care for a child – a task that would severely tax the parents themselves or any other caregiver. Age often slows down agility and impairs reflexes that are called upon when young children wish to play and engage in physical activities. Being constantly on the alert to avoid danger can itself exhaust a grandparent.

The caregiver also becomes housebound and where, for many years a certain freedom reigned from minding children of their own and the endless trips to and from school and all the other extracurricular activities that children were subjected to, now all that reappears overnight. How do the grandparents indulge in sexual intercourse that had become the norm during the day – when there is now the patter of little children around the house again? And if the task of minding the child during the day leaves the grandmother physically and mentally exhausted in the evenings where does it leave the grandfather? Entertaining friends, the pursuit of hobbies, the luxury of reading and lying in bed till late - will all suffer or disappear. Grandparents should not be coerced into minding grandchildren.

Children will always be younger than their own parents. This may seem a trite statement but is a point often ignored or forgotten. The life of any individual is measured in decades - not years. The average number is about six to eight, given that some calamity or other does not beset the person before that.

The *first decade* is taken up by the birth, infancy, crèche, preschool and school. The maximum time the parent or parents may ever spend with the offspring in their entire lives is from the time of birth until the child is handed over to the first caregiver – whoever that maybe. The decades that follow are *shared* between caregivers, teachers, lecturers, employers, wives, husbands, in-laws, friends and doctors!

With such a short time at one's disposal and with so many role players involved how does one shape and influence the life that one has introduced into this world? This is another fact that becomes blurred – the child is *brought* into this world, whether by accident or design, and as such has implications for *both* parents whether they remain together or not, whether the parent or parents are alive or not, whether the relationship between the parents remain amicable or not – the cavalier attitude to the responsibility of the offspring is unacceptable.

School curriculae have introduced 'sex education' but this is far short of actually introducing the roles students will play and assume once they leave school and become parents. Some students do not get to leave school before the burden and responsibility of parenthood are thrust upon them. The issues governing marriage, divorce, partner-abuse, child abuse, alimony, child maintenance and contraception are inadequately emphasised at high school level - given that this information every school-leaver will need at some stage in his or her life.

A child cannot be an adult – but how often does it happen that a two year old is expected to have the wisdom of an older child, even that of an adult! "Didn't I tell you not to do that?" – Expecting that once admonished the memory bank will have instant recall the next time the same situation arises. In similar vein: "Don't you know that it is wrong to pull your friend's hair?" and that "It hurts when you do that", that "It is dangerous to get close to the swimming pool", that "Matches can burn your fingers?". The list is long! No! The child "Does not know!" And saying it repeatedly will not change much! And, as an aside, is this how the *inability to listen* gets its first lessons?

The hungry child will not understand, let alone be satisfied, that mum will feed him as soon as she gets home – hunger is not a sensation the brain takes lightly. The same applies to pain: adults interpret pain according to their *own* experiences and perceptions of it. These can only come with time and the child has had limited exposure to pain to be able to respond the way an 'experienced' adult would. And not every adult can tolerate pain! In the management of acute pain (stubbing a toe or squashing a finger) it is often not appreciated that the brain responds to only what is 'troubling' it the most at any one given moment. In the immediate few seconds following the injury *verbal* support from the caregiver will *not* register and the best one can do is to hold /hug the child. A burned part should be immersed immediately under cold water and kept wet for as long as possible until medical help is available. After the initial pain starts to lessen (few minutes) then would be the time to try a diversionary tactic to distract the cerebral input of painful stimuli. Injury produces pain and fear because the unpleasant stimuli may not have been experienced before and comforting the child with a soothing tone will influence the immediate pain and the stored memory of the incident. This would not be the time for apportioning blame for the accident/injury – the why and the wherefore can come later – the injury at hand cannot be undone regardless of who or what caused it! The immediate priority should be pain and damage limitation. The moment of injury is not the time to be shouting and screaming – underlining one's own emotions of anger, guilt, anxiety and "What ifs!" A concerned but calm and collected approach is required and this takes practice in anticipation of the event – like a fire drill.

How often has it been said in the presence of a child: "He never listens to anything that I tell him", "He never does his homework on time", "She hates school", "The teacher says he is not concentrating", "The teacher says she will fail if she does not work harder", "These spots on his face look so ugly"; So-and-so "Is such an obedient child" – "Is always helping her mother do the chores" – "Is doing so well at school" – "Received two book prizes" – "Came first in athletics" – "Takes part in all the games" – "Is always on time" and "Always greets people", "Dresses neatly", "Eats all his food" – the list goes on. All of these emphasize negative qualities in the child in question. How could any of this make him or her feel better, more loved, encouraged or respected or care about making changes to improve?

When praise is lavished in such huge heaps whether the child has just left a loud fart or done very well in some admirable feat – the quality of the recognition ought not be the same. There should be a difference so that praise and reward are given proportionate to the achievement; reward and recognition are important reasons people perform better. The praise must be sincere and befit the deed - not handed out indiscriminately.

Given that most adults assume that the brain of a five year old is in perfect tune with his or her own the adult will assume that the youngster is capable of adult comprehension and deductions. The truth is this is impossible! Such wisdom can only come from years of knowledge and experience! How does one get the child to understand what the adult means at any given moment? Yesterday you smiled and laughed and applauded when the little doll tore out your hair and grabbed at your glasses and everybody thought it was hilarious. What happened today when he tried to do a repeat performance when you had your boss home for dinner and caused the wine to spill onto your nice white shirt? What changed overnight? And why could they not have the same fun again? Why can't adults be more consistent? The child will be confused and may end up being admonished or punished. How does it distinguish between situations? It is not for the child to know this as much as it is for the adult to recognize that the child cannot easily make these distinctions. A similar confusion will occur to a pup that had a great time tearing at an old teddy bear and all had fun with it - and then a smacking when it chewed one's favourite bedroom slippers!

There should be a system in place, developed over time, whereby the child from the age of about three years should be able to recognize that a different set of rules can apply in any given situation: e.g.

- the child has a box of matches and is at risk of starting a fire
- is in the area of a swimming pool and an adult needs to convey quickly and seriously that this is not a game any more and must leave the area immediately
- the child is running up and down the aisles of a supermarket (and unbeknown to some parents this is not an acceptable activity!)

If the child has been accustomed to "Don't do that" dozens of times a day at home how will it respond to "Don't do that" now when the playing field (!) has been changed and the prospect of an audience (other shoppers and children) better than at home?

One alternative that can

- convey a sense of urgency or importance with the minimum of grief for both parent and child
- have a measure of privacy about it
- allow the child to have a say in the decision making
- allow it a way to save face in the presence of company (which is important in building up or preserving self esteem)
– is to establish "The Count of Five".

If the problem is a box of matches the admonition would read "Jonathan put away those matches and that is "1" – the child is immediately aware that a situation exists that is different – "Dad is counting!" Beginning with 1 and at suitable intervals, depending on the urgency of the situation, count up to 2 and then 3 .The child must understand that progress to 4 is becoming a serious transgression as after 4 there is no 5 because 5 equals instant smacking and no further discussions or counting will be entertained. The punishment is then carried out like a 'court sentence' – cool, calm and collected. No raised voices, no talking, no feelings of guilt or remorse and no regard for peer observation of the punishment. The intention is *not* so much to inflict pain (a roll of newspaper makes a loud enough sound!) but the semblance of it. The child learns to avoid the punishment but with a sense of having a say in the matter of whether he or she chooses to be punished or not. Soon the idea of the punishment takes on an imagined severity and over time almost 'never' progresses to beyond the count of 4! It also allows a degree of secrecy whereby only the parties directly involved are aware of the message that events are developing and, if called for, fireworks will out!

The Count of Five should not be used for matters that are not 'crucial' and should not be reduced to a game; the child must get the message quickly that a different set of rules applies at that given moment and the risk of 'punishment' is imminent and will be enforced with no quarter given. In a busy crowd when attention is difficult one may not be in visual contact and the verbal Count of 5 could still be effective. It also saves a lot of unnecessary talking and waste of adrenaline. In a serious situation like "Jonathan get out of the water now and that is 4!" the child should understand immediately that this is not a matter for negotiation and instant obedience is mandatory!

Parents often do not appreciate that the 12 year old who allows his or her room to be 'untidy' has not learned this the day when guests are expected and the state of the room is important for the rest of the house and family. That disregard for orderliness and even cleanliness was learned from somewhere and often the best teachers are the parents themselves.

Parents should have their own joint policy on how things should be done. If one parent has stronger views than the other about generalised orderliness this tug of war will pass itself onto their offspring. If orderliness is the prerogative of the mother (and this is often the case – with father taking a more relaxed attitude – often because he does not clean and tidy as much!) it sends a mixed message to the children. Human nature makes it easier to take the path of least resistance and will go along with the father and then orderliness becomes a 'mum thing' and interested parties 'gang' up on the mother. The child should view the parents as of *one voice* to avoid making it easier for them to take any one parent's side. These decisions should be made in private by the parents and a 'joint statement' presented when the moment is appropriate - and certainly not in the middle of a confrontation. Policies should be seen to be consistent and not easily negotiable. Only rarely should compromise be necessary.

If more than one sibling is involved all discussions should be made in private to allow the one under the spotlight to be able to preserve face and self esteem. This is the same advice given to employers when having to confront employees. In truth this should be applied to any situation of a personal nature where more than the immediate parties concerned are present – bank clerks, post office counter assistants, teachers, shop assistants, hospital admission clerks, doctor's receptionists, doctors on hospital ward rounds, police stations, – there is no need for all and sundry to be privy to personal matters.

Today's child is tomorrow's adult. The end product must reflect upon the formative years. The obese adult, the drug addict, the abusive husband - did not acquire these behaviour patterns overnight.

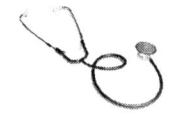

CONDOMS

Condoms did not command as much attention until the spectre of HIV/AIDS reared its ugly head. Where it was once kept under the counter and almost impossible to buy without having to adopt a cloak and dagger approach, today's young school children are having the virtues of this 'French Letter' or FL, as it was known in times gone by, rammed down their throats – along with the 3 R's. In the fight against contracting the HI Virus the mainstay of prevention has been the condom – odd how this piece of latex did not receive as much publicity in the prevention of the other sexually transmitted diseases!

As a contraceptive it is not as effective as the Pill - in that the risk of failure is higher – from rupturing or slippage during intercourse or leakage if not withdrawn carefully soon after ejaculation. Once the penis becomes tumescent (soft) sperm may leak out from the sides; the little bulge at the tip of the condom is designed to accommodate the sperm after ejaculation. Check that it is present before intercourse.

The penis must be ensheathed *before any contact* is made with the vagina as the penis may well contain sperm even though ejaculation has not physically occurred and this may end up as an unwanted pregnancy. It helps to have the condom 'strategically' placed and 'ready for use' instead of having to retreat to the bathroom or the chemist to find one. It is not advisable to have intercourse with the legs of the female partner in the 'closed' position as this will make it easier to tear the condom or cause accidental slippage. Furthermore, the condom may be *'left behind'* within the vagina during intercourse or when extrication of the penis is attempted after intercourse.

While 'one size is supposed to fit all' – individual marked variations in penis size may need to be accommodated. If the organ is unusually small slippage may be a problem and if the organ is exceptionally large then breakage during intercourse is possible. An added precaution as a contraceptive is the use of a spermicidal (kills sperm) cream that is applied within the vagina and the sheathed penis *before* intercourse - to cover for possible 'accidents' with the condom. Over-vigorous intercourse may also damage the condom.

It is often stated that wearing the condom takes away much of the 'feeling' of the penis within the vagina. It is not often appreciated by those who hold this view that if foreplay has been *effective* and arousal of the female partner well executed the vaginal walls become engorged and dilated (to accommodate the erect penis) and the penis will *not* be housed in a 'tight' vagina. Furthermore, it may be an added advantage to be able to prolong intercourse for mutual benefit and this is hardly possible if the penis is oversensitive and therefore more likely to ejaculate sooner when later may be better. The reduced sensitivity induced by the condom in such situations then becomes a blessing. Women will be more appreciative of a less sensitive penis than one that ejaculates prematurely. If premature ejaculation is still a problem wearing two condoms to make the penis even less sensitive may go a longer way to relieving the problem.

Oral intercourse can also transmit STDs and these can be prevented with the use of condoms, making certain that sharp teeth or dentures do not puncture them. It would help if the latter were removed in advance. Condoms also avoid the 'unpleasantness (for some) of having sperm deposited in the mouth. The human bite is reputed to be 'more risky' than a dog bite in terms of its bacterial load. Another good reason for wearing a condom during oral intercourse!

Having intercourse with or without a condom can be a painful experience for the female partner if the vagina is not properly primed with adequate foreplay or a suitable lubricant is not used. Condoms often need some additional lubrication and manufacturers that advertise that they are 'lubricated' have often been found wanting. However, any petroleum or oil based lubrication will damage the condom (Vaseline, vegetable oils). The safest are those that are water based. If saliva is to be used as an emergency lubrication it should preferably be the female partner supplying it as STDs can be transmitted from the mouth of the male.

Anal intercourse should never be performed without a condom; the bottom line is that there should be no contact between the unsheathed penis and the anal area because of the risk of contracting STDs, hepatitis and infection with E.coli. The latter reside normally within the rectum but are responsible for the majority of bladder infections to which women are more prone than their partners. It is physically impossible to 'sterilise' the penis after anal exposure if a condom has not been used. Once the condom has made contact with the anal area (not necessarily penetration of the anus) it is 'contaminated' with bacteria and must never be introduced into the vagina, and after it is removed the hands may be similarly 'contaminated' and will require washing with soap and hot water as though one were scrubbing up for an operation.

After vaginal intercourse the hands should be washed after removing the used condom as it has been exposed to sperm (and may result in an unwanted pregnancy if the fingers make contact with the vagina) and vaginal infections - if these were present.

If either partner has an STD touching each other's private parts will contaminate the fingers and defeat the purpose of the condom when it is being slipped on. This further helps in the spread of infection. In the prevention of STDs, short of abstaining from sex, condoms have become the mainstay. It should be put on before any contact is made with the vagina – inside or out. It should be introduced onto the erect penis like a 'Mexican hat' – made to sit on the head of the penis. A circle is made with the left index finger and thumb and this circle is placed on top of the condom encircling the top of the 'hat' – the tip pointing beyond and above the ring made by the fingers.

The 'top of the hat' must be preserved as such to take up the sperm after ejaculation. If this air bubble contained within the tip is not maintained there is a risk of tearing the condom during intercourse. With the top so maintained the rest of the 'shaft/tube' of the condom is rolled downwards (with the aid of the ring of fingers) down to the base of the penis until it is completely covered.

Manufacturers of condoms should ensure that their products are trustworthy. Expecting the user to look for defects is unacceptable. Short of blowing it up – minute tears will not be detected. A rolled out condom is difficult to introduce onto the erect penis and paves the way for damage. Fingernails may also damage the delicate latex. Ladies beware! The individually wrapped condoms are also difficult to open and risk damage to the latex from teeth and nail. Manufacturers assume that their product is opened in bright daylight and not under cover of darkness when the services of a condom are most likely to be required.

After ejaculation the penis is removed from the vagina with the same ring of fingers encircling the condom at the base of the penis until the entire organ, along with the condom and its contents, is out of the vagina. This should be done soon after ejaculation and *before* the penis begins to shrink down in size. The condom should be held securely so that its contents are not allowed to spill out during extrication. The penis along with the condom is then 'placed' within a plastic packet (if one is available) and through the packet (now being used as a glove) the condom is removed. The penis is extricated from the packet and the latter is then knotted to seal it and the packet (containing the used condom) discarded into a bin. This precaution is important because the condom and its contents are infective if either partner has an STD. If a packet is not handy the hands should be thoroughly washed with soap and water for the reasons described above. Contact with the penis after ejaculation should be avoided by both partners if pregnancy and STDs are to be prevented.

Manufacturers of condoms address the presentation of the product in well-sealed containers but make no provision for their efficient disposal after they have been used. Furthermore, from the pollution point of view future condoms should be made biodegradable; plumbers, beaches, parks and other public places and municipalities would consider this a special blessing. Children may be exposed to these used condoms and are at risk for contracting infections. Used condoms should not be disposed of into toilet pans as they float and do not flush easily; nor should they be discarded from parked cars under cover of darkness.

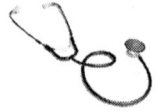

DEATH

There are only two situations in a person's life when he or she will be utterly and completely alone: when one writes an examination and when one is about to die!

Death can occur anytime onwards from the moment the sperm unites with the egg when a male and female have intercourse. *When it will happen depends on a number of factors.* Within the mother's womb, and for a time after it is born, the individual has no control over its own life. When the child starts to crawl it may unwittingly die if it should

- Accidentally crawl into an unguarded swimming pool
- Be killed by a murderous parent who drinks and drives or drives recklessly en route to a holiday destination
- Accidentally swallows a handful of paracetamol (Panadol) tablets
- Be infected with the HI Virus
- Be starved or abused to death
- Succumb to an illness.

From there onwards the individual has the power and the means to kill itself. This may take place as an accidental or deliberate poisoning, a fatal duel on a deserted freeway, a gunshot wound accidental or deliberate or a self-induced death like heart disease and cancer or an unavoidable illness. Illness once used to be due to infections – whether mankind, the vagaries of nature or the will of God engineered this was not always clear. A mere one hundred years ago *'infection'* was the prime cause of death; today – a short hundred birthdays later it is *Heart Disease and Cancer* that kill people. Man has become an expert at self destruction: whether it is the food he eats, the water he drinks, the planet he is destroying or his fellow men that he is hell bent in killing one way or the other – he has become his own worst nightmare. The animal kingdom must sigh and shake its head in despair because with him he will take them whether by poaching, pollution, practicing his science or from the sheer pleasure of killing.

Death is so final. Why is it that our Maker did not choose to inform us how long our sojourn on earth was meant to be? That He has not must demand that we live each day as though it were our last. Instead we go through life as though we will be here forever and that is why we do not to live in harmony with our grandparents, parents, partners, children, in-laws, relatives, friends and neighbours - whether next door, in the next street or the next country.

Working with the terminally ill should be made mandatory for every person to give the ignorant some insight into how life can be altered and how precious it can become when there is a risk of losing it.

Nothing is guaranteed in life. Doctors who preach to patients about the dangers of smoking or overindulging may develop the same diseases themselves. At the most one can *reduce the risks* of dying from disease and disastrous activities – nobody can do more than that because each person has a shelf life that started ticking from the moment of conception. Life is short. The teenager or young adult will not understand this because he or she has not been around long enough to know that time is not unlimited. The unfortunate youngster who develops leukemia or cancer will learn this lesson very quickly – but to what avail? The older adult, who one expects will understand this better, is not advantaged by it. He or she is still coming to terms with what and how much to eat or with deciding when to stop smoking, abusing alcohol or drugs, murdering innocent people or abusing the spouse. Where is the *wisdom of age* when obesity is fast becoming the biggest killer worldwide? The emphasis has shifted to instant gratification: the "I want it all and I want it now" generation.

Partners who live together for a lifetime should understand that the rule is: one will die before the other if the relationship survives long enough. Is it then worthwhile getting together in the first place, knowing full well that their fate is destined to leave one of them behind? The answer is a resounding "Yes" because our genetic coding ensured that this should happen to continue the species. Perhaps the decision to stay in a monogamous relationship can be challenged and therein lies the rub - if man was not monogamous the question of dealing with the death of a partner would not be such an issue!

Death cannot be controlled - just like the weather and taxes can't be. Is there a point to losing sleep and energy over it? Are the children that are the product of marriage another reason for justifying the original relationship? The law of preservation of the species must make the answer affirmative. Indeed, not every relationship may have been a happy one. Animals care not whether their partners are fat, thin, ugly, or beautiful. They mate to preserve the species. We have changed the rules.

The pain from losing a loved one is *normal* – it should be anticipated. Unfortunately the mind finds it too tedious to make the effort to recall the enormity of death *before* it happens. Death and its ramifications will not disappear quickly. This pain will take much longer to heal and the road to recovery is blurred and the brain is too numb to think about the next day - let alone three months hence. Then there is the finality of death that also makes it so 'unacceptable' at the time.

When a person dies well-wishers who comfort the grieving member closest to the one who has died can never feel what the bereaving person is experiencing because five minutes before he or she got to the house the most pressing problem may have been "Who will pick up the children if the funeral is at three o' clock?" The visitor often becomes caught up in the emotion passed on by the bereaved family. However, the grieving person is in no state to listen to *anything* that is being said. Nothing will register and none of the "Please accept my deepest sympathies" has any meaning for the unfortunate person. A handshake or a warm hug may be much more valuable because these do not appeal to the brain (mental) as do physical contact between two people. Injuring a funny bone responds so much better to vigorous rubbing of the part - imagine trying to soothe this pain with a long speech!

The child that has hurt itself will respond much better to a hug than a long discourse about how it should be more careful in the future and that the injury is the result of not listening when told not to climb up the tree in the first place. This is in keeping with the fact that a newborn infant that is never touched by human hands will perish; the power of physical contact is immeasurable and necessary for life itself. When death occurs there is a need for physical contact between those who are living – it reminds them of the existence of people. A hand held in the dark or in the delivery room is more reassuring and comforting than words. Touch is mightier than the spoken word.

One of the most devastating aspects of the death of a spouse is the bedroom. Little is gained by maintaining this room the way it had been. Rearranging it could make it easier to live each day with a positive view to get on with life. Animals do not grieve the way this emotion is known to human beings; society has changed the rules – we mourn the loss of a loved one. Pain on remembering the departed spouse cannot be a pleasurable feeling. What is gained by doing everything in one's power to maintain the pain level? Is it only decorum that dictates the degree and length and depth of the mourning? That a widow may not be seen smiling too soon or appearing to recover too soon? That a certain length of time should elapse before it is becoming for the widow or widower to begin living again? That mourning for a prolonged period or not seeing another person of the opposite sex for years all points to a spouse that loved the late partner all the more? That if it was less than that determined by society, relatives, or friends it should earn their disfavour and disdain?

Going away for a period after the death is like a plaster of Paris cast on a fractured leg; the leg may well heal without the cast but it would take much longer and the end result may not be as satisfactory. To go away allows healing without having to fight the loss continuously and an opportunity to reflect and gain some perspective upon the matter. Sitting in the front row of the cinema gives a blurred overview of the story – one needs to sit in the back row to see it in clearer focus and appreciate the finer details. It does help to talk about the events leading up to the death to almost anybody who shows any interest in listening; the more times it is discussed the lighter the burden will become. The person who does not do this may well be in denial – the road to recovery made more difficult. It is normal, nay, necessary, to cry as much as possible until the tears literally run dry; the tears help to wash out the heaviness from the chest. The person who is supposed to do the listening should do just that - listen!

Cremation should be made compulsory. Apart form the dire shortage of burial space it is macabre that a person who once shared a life and a bed together is now, after death, subjected to a perpetual 'hell' of lying in a coffin and rotting – with maggots crawling out the mouth where once song erupted and the vagina, where once love nestled, is now covered in decay. How could one subject a loved one to such a 'life hereafter'? Cremation is clean and final and helps wipe the slate clean and allows the spouse left behind to get on with his or her life. It avoids visiting a graveside where one knows (but tries to avoid the thought), as a perpetual reminder, that six feet under lies a wooden box with rotting flesh and bone.

Customs will vary with each culture. The Parsees of India allow their departed to lie naked on the roof of a temple to allow the crows to feed upon the flesh until only the bones remain. These then fall through a grid wide enough to allow the bones to fall into an acid bath that then dissolves them.

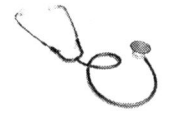

DEPRESSION

This condition is not commonly viewed as an illness but masquerades as a state of mind and successfully escapes attention and, often, proper referral and treatment. Asthmatics suffer the same pitfall – those concerned preferring to have the child labelled as 'wheezy bronchitis' or 'chesty' rather than recognising the true nature of the ailment and allowing for appropriate therapy.

The stigma attached to a disorder even remotely implicating the brain may be strong enough to make the person reluctant to be referred to a psychiatrist. The same patient would have no compunction about seeing an orthopaedic surgeon to deal with a fractured ankle. Add to this a reluctance to use medication to make the brain function better and one is faced with: "It's not so bad. I'll pull myself together"; "I'm sure it's nothing"; "I'll see how I cope and if I can't I'll let you know". It is *expected* that the fractured ankle would be X-rayed and the appropriate plaster of Paris cast applied. Failure to do so could constitute 'negligence' but depression often gets handled differently.

Many theories have been postulated as to the causes of depression. Several factors may play a role. The prevalence of this condition is so high that it has been labeled "The common cold of mental illness". Some of these factors are stress and inadequate levels of neurotransmitters (chemical carriers of nerve impulses) in the brain – namely serotonin and noradrenaline. The picture is not that precise. Not every stressful situation ends in depression and not every depressed person responds positively to treatment with antidepressants. It has also not been established whether the deficiency of the neurotransmitters is a cause or effect of depression.

Underlying the predilection for depression must be the mental disposition shaped in childhood that taught coping mechanisms for crises, making it easier for one person faced with a crisis to deal with it differently from another faced with the same problem. The ability to deal with problems - whether it is the loss of a loved one, retrenchment or coping with a dreaded disease - cannot be developed overnight.

The underlying cause of the depression may not always be obvious to the person who is so affected even though there is often a notable factor. The brain cannot 'see' itself – it needs the condition and its related matters spelled out for it either in writing or through an independent verbal approach such as would be provided by a psychologist. Writing thoughts down on paper allows the brain to have an objective view of itself and the problems that it faces. Having a swollen ankle joint from an injury is a physical ailment and a hand can be literally placed on the problem. How does one do this when the person may not even be aware that the underlying problem is depression? As simple as this exercise is few depressives ever do it and do therapists encourage putting things down on paper?

On the face of it there are not dozens of causes that precipitate depression; invariably it can be linked to one or more of the following:

- Money
- Work
- Sex
- Relationships
- Health
- Religion

Of all of the above the most important factor must be *Health*. Without it none of the others will function and yet this is most often the one that receives the least amount of attention. A cup of coffee for breakfast, a sausage-roll and soft drink for lunch and the proverbial 'cooked' meal for supper and so the wheels of nutrition grind on (or slow down!).

The motorcar gets serviced regularly. Petrol is recognized as being necessary for the car to function and any breakdown receives immediate attention from trained professionals. But the human body is treated with much less respect. So much for the body being created in the image of God!

The stresses of the day and work deplete the body of three essential vitamins: Vitamins B, C, and E. If these are not present in the food or taken as a supplement they are not available to the body. The adrenal gland that is responsible for the production of adrenaline and steroids is compromised in its function. The body produces these hormones in response to stress. It is little surprise that in spite of a full night's sleep the tiredness may persist the following morning The *Formula IV Plus* supplement alone may change this because it supplies essential vitamins, plant sterols, lipids, proteins and minerals.

Human beings are on this planet for only two essential reasons: food and sex (reproduction). Take away the *food* and what is left? A domestic worker may be employed to cook, clean and keep house but does not ordinarily provide sex. This often requires a stable relationship between two people. Depression will depress the libido and complicate matters further. How many family murders have unfulfilled sexual needs as the unknown factor explaining the comment that the couple in question appeared 'near perfect'. If bedrooms could speak the mystery could be unravelled. Sex is the desire of every male but how, when and how much he gets receives scant attention. It is easier to predict and receive the next meal.

The ability to handle *money* may be taken for granted. How many families run into financial ruin because of mismanagement of hard earned incomes? One is required by law to have a valid driver's licence to be able to drive a vehicle competently, but in the handling of a matter as vital as money no such training is demanded or provided. Should this skill be taught more often in school? Banks and similar institutions are only too willing to give such advice; after all it is a subject closest to their hearts.

The role that work plays in people's lives is only appreciated when it is threatened or terminated. The average person may stay with a company for three to four decades, though this loyalty to businesses is changing. Upon retirement or retrenchment the sudden severance of this umbilical cord, that served for so many years as the life blood of the individual and his or her dependents, may lead to depression. This termination is another milestone in man's journey from the cradle to the grave. Retirement may signify the end of a person's usefulness and a step closer to death. If lifetime achievements are not realized at this late stage life itself could become a failure, with broken dreams and unrealized ambitions and, seemingly overnight, appears too late to do much about it.

How one copes with retirement will depend on factors such as:

- Job satisfaction
- Realization of ambitions
- Financial security
- Family support system – the spouse in particular
- Whether the retiree sought refuge in the workplace and only came home to eat and sleep and perchance to dream and have perfunctory sex - because all that may change with retirement.

Now he lies in bed until late in the morning whereas the wife, for all the years when he left for work before sunrise and only returned at sunset, will now be unable to finish her household chores to free her for the rest of the morning. And how does she cope with her chores if husband wants a nice cup of tea every thirty minutes? And now he may have his things lying all over her neat and tidy bathroom. Three meals a day become the new order whereas when he worked she made his sandwiches the night before and only cooked supper as the main meal; she herself settling for a cup of tea and snacks for lunch. And when will she find time to get to the patchwork group on Wednesdays with husband in the house literally behind her back every five minutes, constantly checking on her? How does she cope with sex in the middle of the day when the ironing lady almost caught them in a compromising situation the other morning? And how come they never had all this sex before and who was paying attention to her needs then? And now he has his other retired friends over in the afternoons and they play cards until late and she has to make tea and sandwiches for them.

The pendulum may also swing such that the retired husband's moods may change to being more and more irritable. The smallest differences may blow up into major arguments. Alcohol may find new uses or abuses for the retired husband. Sleep disturbances, worry about whether the pension money will last, concern over health matters, real and imagined, and preoccupation with death may contribute to the problem of depression. Depression does not always have an identifiable cause and this could make its recognition more elusive. One then relies on the symptoms that are associated with depression to alert the next of kin and to seek appropriate help.

These symptoms include:-

- A change in sleeping habits
- Waking in the early hours of the morning
- Changes in appetite with weight loss or weight gain,
- Sexual difficulties – impotence and loss of libido
- Irritability and being short-tempered
- Being easily upset and crying sometimes for no apparent reason
- Loss of interest or pleasure in everyday activities
- Loss of self esteem
- Feelings of guilt and anger because the person recognizes in him or herself a changed personality
- Difficulties at school or in the work place where these had not been present before
- Drop in performance
- The appearance of physical symptoms such as loss of energy, palpitations, constipation, abdominal and chest pains.

There may be thoughts of death or suicide and their existence may be completely unsuspected and only sudden tragedy highlighting the seriousness of the underlying disorder.

Infants are not born depressed. Life's experiences and nutrition play an important role. The incidence of depression in school children is set to increase as more and more pressure to excel is added to their already loaded plates. The elderly pay a double price when this condition affects them because many of the symptoms of depression are passed off as being a natural part of ageing. How many depressed elderly stroke victims languish in granny flats and old age homes – their states of mind fobbed off as being part of the disease whereas an antidepressant or treatment for a possibly underfunctioning thyroid gland could change their lives?

Therapy should include an interview with the partner, attention to nutrition, adequate sleep, exercise and the use of appropriate medication. Not all persons may be keen to receive drugs to improve their minds.

Supplements should include Vitamin C (slow release) 1 tablet daily, Omega 3 – at least 3 capsules daily, Vitamin E 200 I.U. – 1 capsule daily, Formula IV Plus - 1 sachet daily, Herbal Rest and Relax - 1 tablet twice daily and the Herbal Mind Enhancement – 1 tablet twice daily. These are not drugs and, therefore, have no side effects and may help address the nutritional needs of the body at the same time as attempting to relieve depression.

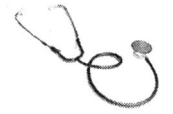

DIABETES MELLITUS

In diabetes the glucose level in the blood is higher than normal. Glucose is derived from food that has been eaten and absorbed into the blood but cannot be taken into the cells where they are required for energy because:

- there is *no insulin at all* (as in the Insulin Dependent Diabetic or type 1 diabetes) or
- the amount of insulin available is *not enough* to get all the glucose into the cells (Non Insulin Dependent Diabetes or Type 2 diabetes).

Without insulin glucose from the blood cannot cross the cell wall (membrane) to enter the cell. Insulin acts as the *carrier* for glucose – like a 'taxi' - carrying glucose from the blood stream into the cells.

Insulin Dependent Diabetes or Juvenile Diabetes occurs in a person under the age of 40 years and usually in childhood or adolescence. When it does the patient becomes ill fairly quickly – over a period of a few days – because there is no insulin and the cells cannot function without glucose. In an older person who develops Maturity Onset Diabetes there is still some insulin present and he or she may get away for fairly long periods – weeks or months – without the condition being detected.

Thirst is not an abnormal sensation and the undiagnosed diabetic does not think anything is amiss until this becomes excessive and abnormal amounts of fluid are being taken to keep the balance between the large amounts of fluid being passed out as (sweetened!)

urine and the amount required to quench an ever-increasing thirst. The problem is aggravated if the fluid taken is in the form of sweetened cool drinks and fruit juices; this is really adding fuel to the fire! The glucose being wasted in the urine and that present in the blood are unavailable to the cells and will lead to weight loss in spite of the good appetite. The extra glucose present in the blood is passed into the urine – the more glucose in the blood the more water is excreted – hence the 'buckets' of urine. The more urine that is produced and passed out the greater the thirst to keep up with the fluids that are being lost; this is an attempt by the body to prevent dehydration.

If for some reason such a person falls behind in the intake of fluids (becomes ill for some reason and does not take much water) dehydration will quickly set in. The body will not tolerate this for very long. As long as the balance between passing out extra urine and taking in extra fluid to make up the deficit is maintained the condition may not easily come to attention. However, *weight loss* and a feeling of tiredness in the presence of a good or *normal appetite* should raise the suspicion that all is not well.

Normal urine does not contain any glucose, protein, blood, pus cells or bile. The presence of any of these may indicate serious disease and requires further investigation. If glucose is present the next step is to have the blood tested immediately to determine whether the amount present at that moment is higher than normal. Normal blood sugar varies from 4 to 6 mmol (per liter of blood). If the blood test reads 11 mmol/L or more at any given moment the diagnosis of diabetes is then confirmed and no further tests may be necessary. If the level is *below* 11mmol/L then a glucose tolerance test (GTT) is necessary: Blood and urine are tested before any breakfast is taken after fasting overnight. 100 ml of glucose powder mixed in water is then taken and the person being tested should rest i.e. without exercising and burning off the sugar. This is the principle of the treatment of diabetes – eating a meal and exercising afterwards to burn off the calories i.e. juggling how much is eaten and how much is worked off. Exactly two hours after the ingestion of the glucose drink urine and blood are again tested for their glucose levels. The rationale for this is that within two hours the glucose should have been absorbed from the gut and insulin, secreted by the pancreas in response to the glucose load, should have cleared the glucose from the blood stream into the cells. If insulin secretion was adequate, the glucose level in blood should have returned to normal even if the fasting level was abnormal i.e. between 6 and under 11mmol/L. (if it was 11mmol/L or above – the GTT as mentioned above was unnecessary). The GTT can be done at home if somebody has a glucose testing machine (glucometer) or at the chemist if the above simple instructions are observed.

If glucose is found in the urine but the level is normal in the blood (taken at the same time) this is not diabetes but indicates that the kidneys have a low 'threshold' for glucose i.e. the kidneys (acting as tea-strainers) have 'bigger holes' than normal and therefore the glucose slips through. The basis for the diagnosis of diabetes is that the *'blood glucose'* level must be abnormally high – not necessarily that the urine has glucose. Relying on the urine alone for the diagnosis is inaccurate. In pregnancy it is not uncommon to have glucose in the urine (called renal glycosuria – glucose in the urine with the kidneys being the cause) provided the blood level is normal.

However, if the urine shows the presence of glucose and blood levels are normal - there is a strong likelihood of the mother developing diabetes later in life. Knowing this should make the person reduce the risk factors that make it easier to develop diabetes viz., *avoid obesity*. Blood glucose levels do not remain constant and, at best, measuring it at that moment is a guide. The best times to check them are after an overnight fast i.e. first thing in the morning or 2 hours after a meal. The latter reading gives a more accurate picture of the ability of the body to deal with glucose or the effectiveness of treatment in controlling diabetes.

Foods that have a high Glycaemic Index (GI) are those that cause the blood glucose levels to be high e.g. – bananas, grapes, beetroot, potatoes; whereas the opposite is true of foods like lentils, legumes and pasta that have a low GI. All carbohydrates, in no matter what form they are taken (chocolates, bread, pastry, fruit juices, sweetened cool drinks, any type of alcohol), are eventually converted into glucose after digestion by the body.

The average can of sweetened cool drink contains up to 10 teaspoons of sugar and taking one can a day adds up to a staggering 17 kilograms of sugar consumed within a year. How many school children, with the blessing of their tuck shop managers, consume 2 cans of cool drinks per day – i.e. almost 34 kilograms of sugar per year!

Each time a cool drink or fruit juice is taken the blood stream is suddenly flooded with glucose and the pancreas is stimulated to produce insulin to carry the glucose into the cells of the body and out of the blood stream - thereby bringing the sugar levels back to normal. In doing this the glucose level often goes down lower than normal and *hypoglycemia* occurs and this creates the urge to have another snack to bring the glucose levels up again. This see-saw effect throughout the day manipulates the glucose levels between high and low and each time the pancreas produces insulin to suit the whims and fancies of every snack, cool drink, fruit juice (sweetened or not) and whatever else takes the fancy that has a high GI.

The young insulin dependent diabetic has no insulin and to date there is no practical way of taking insulin except by injection form because the stomach acid (hydrochloric acid) destroys it if taken orally. In the older diabetic who in non-insulin dependent modifying the diet and exercising can help to control the glucose levels. *Failing this* one has to resort to oral hypoglycaemic agents i.e., drugs that lower the levels of glucose.

The diabetic who has not achieved adequate weight loss as part of the treatment has missed the main cornerstone in the treatment of a condition that has some serious consequences if the glucose is not adequately controlled. Many a diabetic is going to lose a leg or two to gangrene, suffer a heart attack or stroke or risk kidney failure and blindness from uncontrolled diabetes.

Never let it be said or thought for one moment that weight loss is impossible or that, once lost, it cannot be maintained. The body can never increase or maintain weight without something that is being introduced into the mouth, which is the only opening the body has through which food and drink can enter! Anything besides water and most vegetables (except beetroots and potatoes) contains calories that will add to the weight or maintain it. Artificial sweeteners (aspartame) have been shown to cause damage to the cells of the liver and are not recommended. Many so-called 'diet' cool drinks also contain these sweeteners. Cutting down on the total calorie intake will avoid pushing the blood sugar level up and reduce the need for the body to produce extra insulin or get it by injection. Herein lies the secret in the continual battle between blood sugar and insulin secretion: reduce the total intake of calories or use it up by exercising.

Good quality fibre containing soluble (oats) and insoluble fibres (bran) in sufficient quantity (about 35 gm per day), taken 45 minutes before a meal in tablet or powder form will provide a 'bulking' effect within the stomach, reducing the "I could eat a horse!"- type of hunger. It would also act as a sponge in the gut that 'holds' onto ingested food for longer thereby preventing sugar from flooding into the blood and pushing up blood glucose levels - which is the problem for diabetics with no insulin or insufficient amounts.

Fibre helps to keep the levels of cholesterol down by combining with fat in the gut. It has also been shown to help prevent cancer of the gut. The biggest drawback the 'rural' resident who has moved to urban areas is the virtual disappearance of fibre in the diet and the occurrence of diseases almost unheard of in this population group – angina, hypertension and diabetes. For this they must thank the *fast food businesses* that are allowed to sow their seeds of disease on an unsophisticated and unsuspecting people – all in the interest of profit.

The complications that arise from elevated blood glucose levels may be compared very simplistically to mixing sugar in water and watch the consistency (thickness) of the water change. Picture this thickened fluid (diabetic blood) coursing through the arteries and veins and, worse still, through tiny capillaries that are so small one would need a microscope to see them (a spider's web would be too thick!). It is not surprising that capillaries become blocked up. In the early stages this will not cause any major upset but as the blood continues to remain thick (uncontrolled diabetes) more and more of these capillaries will disappear and then progress to bigger vessels and reduce, and subsequently cut off, any further blood supply to the part. This sets the stage for *gangrene.*

Gangrene can occur from any cause that compromises the blood supply to any part of the body, viz., diabetes, hypertension, smoking and a clot within the vessel. It goes without saying that no body part can survive without blood (oxygen and nutrition). The consequences of a river that is being dammed up are easily understood. A blockage to the blood supply in a heart attack is akin to the onset of *'gangrene' of the heart* except that, unlike the toe or foot that are not vital for the normal functioning of the body and may be sacrificed by amputation, a blockage in a coronary artery may bring the function of the heart to a standstill. A flat car tyre does not have the same consequences as a blown gasket in the engine!

The kidneys also depend on very fine capillaries to carry blood to the urine-forming apparatus. Failure of these organs will occur insidiously and, in the early stages, there may be no symptoms. The presence of protein in the urine is usually the first clue that this is happening, making it mandatory to test for it regularly. It is equally important to test the urine for the presence of protein and glucose.

Ketones in the urine of a known diabetic indicate that glucose is not being transferred from the blood into the cells and the latter are using fat for fuel in order to function normally. Ketones are by-products of fat metabolism. The problem with this form of energy supply is the brain cells under normal circumstances only use glucose as a source of energy and ketones in an uncontrolled diabetic are toxic. Ketones(in the urine) + High sugars (in the blood) = Admission into hospital.

The diabetic diet is the diet for everyone, not only diabetics. The meal should be made up in pyramid fashion with the bottom 1/3 made up of carbohydrates, the middle 1/3 of proteins and the uppermost and smallest third – of fats.

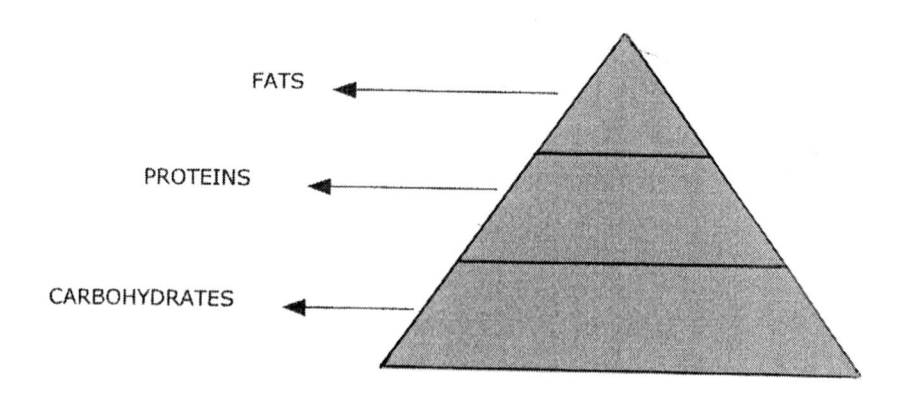

THE FOOD PYRAMID

The body can use animal fat as an immediate source of fuel. If one eats a fatty lamb chop and 90 minutes later engages in physical exercise the fat is used up - but watch a soap opera on television and the fat gets into the arterial walls to lay the foundation for a future heart attack. Carbohydrates should consist of foods with a low glycaemic index and not be simple sugars e.g. potatoes or bread but rather pasta or lentils because these take longer to be broken down and digested, avoiding the sudden flood of glucose into the blood stream. As long as glucose is introduced from the gut into the blood at a rate that prevents sudden surges, the body, with its limited reserves of insulin as occurs in a non-insulin dependent diabetic, can cope with the dietary glucose.

Fructose, (as different from glucose) on the other hand, does not stimulate the release of insulin but is also used by the body as fuel and is therefore a preferred source of food. It has a low glycaemic index and therefore excellent for diabetics.

Exercising twice a day (after breakfast and after lunch) when the bigger meals of the day ought to have been taken will help to burn off the calories. Those that are stored as fats are the extra calories – 'extra' because they are more than were required by the body.

The best late night snack is a helping of oats; one helping is half a cup and with time the tongue or brain can be 'reeducated' to be able to eat it, and many other foods and drinks, without sugar. If a child is taught from an early age to add salt to tea it will learn this taste to be the norm.

Refined sugar is one of the scourges that are surreptitiously responsible for ill health - regardless of what the manufacturers say to the contrary. There are glaring reminders of a recent past that had us believe, and this persists in spite of the efforts of health departments, that cigarette smoking is 'not that bad'. The blatant advertising that associates young people having a good time with cigarettes sticking out of there gullible mouths may just as well have 'mandrax' advertised in a similar manner. But of course that will receive immediate censure – but sugar? Who will associate sugar with an amputated leg or blindness later in life? How many school children buy cool drinks and fruit juices from the tuck shop with the full blessing of parents and school authorities? And as mentioned earlier, who cares to consider that one can (of these seemingly innocent and well-advertised drinks) per day adds up to about 17 kg of sugar for the year and two cans=34kg! Diabetes may appear long after the school principal has retired and the nefarious tuck shop forgotten.

It has yet to filter through to diabetics that the treatment of this condition in the majority of patient begins with weight loss. Where there is a family history of diabetes the only preventative measure for the offspring is to avoid obesity. If a family history of diabetes is absent obesity will still remain an independent risk for developing the condition - along with a host of other diseases.

There is a perception that diabetics may never take sugar in any form be it a cough mixture, a piece of cake or chocolate. This ignores some basic points: if a person is at a birthday party and eats a piece of cake – so what? The blood glucose will go up and this is to be expected. However, it is not the one piece of cake that pushes up the blood glucose that is responsible for all the evils of 'cake' or 'sugar' in diabetes. The body is quite capable of surviving the one episode of elevated blood glucose. What is more important is whether cake is being eaten every day or on most days. The problems arise when the discipline is missing in everyday living, not the occasional 'birthday treat'. Having the odd indulgence can always be balanced with a walk afterwards, adjusting one's next intake of food or temporarily increasing the dose insulin.

Zinc plays an important role in the manufacture of insulin by specialised cells in the pancreas, and the use of Formula IV Plus (1 sachet daily) will supplement 15 mg of zinc and, at the same time, protect the integrity of these and other cell walls in the body by supplying sterols and lipids. Omega 3 (3 capsules daily) and Vitamin E – 200 I.U. units (1 capsule daily) may help to prevent the impairment of blood circulation by thinning down blood - making its passage easier through microscopic capillaries.

Many diabetics will develop high blood pressure at some stage. Levels of cholesterol and triglycerides are also elevated. Given that diabetes, raised cholesterol and high blood pressure are all targeting the circulation it is not surprising that heart attacks, brain attacks (strokes), kidney failure, blindness and gangrene are all common complications of diabetes. To add smoking to this profile is really courting disaster. Nicotine will add one more to the list of causes of compromised circulation. This also reinforces the need to take Omega 3, Vitamin E and exercise.

To this supplementation should be added Fibre tablets – two to three taken with a full glass of water 45 minutes before a meal. The fibre swells with the absorption of water to many times the size of the tablet and gives the gut a bulking effect. This helps to:

- Slow down the absorption of glucose from the small intestine
- Lower the absorption of cholesterol and bile acids (that are rich in cholesterol) from the small intestine (also reduces the risk of developing gall stones)
- Reduce the incidence of heart disease by up to 40 % depending on the amount of fibre taken daily (need 25 - 35 gm of fibre/day)
- Prevent cancer of the large intestine
- make one feel full and less hungry if weight loss is planned

Replacing one or two meals with two scoops of 'Nutrishake' each time will provide excellent nutrition containing all 22 amino acids necessary for protein to be correctly metabolised. Furthermore, it contains fructose, which has a lower glycaemic index than glucose, avoiding the stimulation of higher levels of insulin that glucose does. Currently there are not many meal substitutes that would contain all 22 amino acids.

Cataracts and macular degeneration of the eye are two devastating complications of diabetes and these may be prevented or their progression slowed down by taking *Carotenoid Complex* - between one and three capsules daily. New spectacles will do nothing for these two conditions and visiting the optician for stronger glasses is wasted time and money.

Carotenoid Complex also boosts the immune system and helps to prevent infections to which diabetics are so commonly prone. It also prevents LDL (low density lipoproteins – one of the bad fats in the blood) from being attacked by oxygen - thereby making it less likely to adhere to the arterial walls. This reduces the development of atherosclerosis which narrows arteries and increases the ageing process of cells; the insulin secreting cells of the pancreas included.

Ulcers in the legs and feet may be the result of not being able to easily feel pain when exposed to injury (thorn pricks). Pain is not detected because the nerves that carry pain impulses to the brain (warning the foot of injury) have been damaged by the lack of blood supply, a consequence of blockages of tiny capillaries that supply nutrition and oxygen to these delicate nerves. If vision is also impaired, as is common in diabetes, this makes a stronger case for not allowing these patients to cut their own toenails because of the risk of infection and injury. A prick from the thorn of a rose tree can land the diabetic in hospital fighting for his or her survival.

Having diabetes should not be viewed as a death sentence. It is ironic that everything the diabetic is supposed to be doing to keep the condition under control and the person in good health are precisely what every person should be doing viz., maintaining normal weight, exercising, not smoking, keeping blood cholesterol down and avoiding sugar and other foods containing a high glycaemic index.

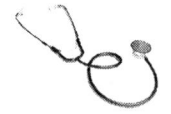

DIARRHOEA

Diarrhoea means watery stools and 'watery' means – not just loose or thin – but 'like water'. It is the number one killer of children in developing countries, responsible for just under 25 % of deaths of children under the age of 5 years.

The fluid that constitutes diarrhoea does not come from water or food that has been ingested, as is often believed. It is being channelled *from* the body i.e. precious water from the blood in the rich circulation around the intestines is being poured back into the gut. Picture a hosepipe with holes along its length and water being poured from the outside *into* the pipe. This is the risk in diarrhoea as dehydration will set in very quickly, especially in infants, young children and the elderly.

Under normal circumstances fluid taken orally is absorbed through the stomach and small intestines and taken to the kidneys by the circulation where the impurities are removed and passed into the urine and recycled water is returned back into the circulation. When diarrhoea is present the water that is put back into the circulation is finding its way into the intestines as a result of inflammation or infection of the intestinal lining.

The common causes of diarrhoea are:

- Infection: commonly due to viruses, Salmonellae (food poisoning) or other pathogens (organisms causing disease) like amoebae (amoebic dysentery) and giardiasis (infection caused by giardia – another bacteria that may invade the gut). Many food borne illnesses result from unhygienic handling of food and are, therefore, largely preventable. It is unreliable to depend on the *taste, sight or smell* of food to tell whether bacteria are present. Furthermore, these are the very senses that may be impaired in the elderly and not quite developed in children.

- <u>Drugs:</u> – may also cause diarrhoea. Some antibiotics may affect the gut by causing loose stools and, at the other extreme, profuse diarrhoea with blood and mucus, as the lining of the gut sloughs off. This is a serious condition and requires urgent hospitalisation and discontinuation of the offending drug/s.

- <u>Inflammation:</u> – In diseases such as Crohn's and Ulcerative Colitis which are generally termed 'Inflammatory Bowel Diseases' - the symptoms are those of cramp-like abdominal pain, intermittent diarrhoea and blood in the stools. Such bouts may occur 4 – 5 or more times a year .The frequency of these episodes gives the clue that these are not common bouts of gastroenteritis and warrants investigation – not another course of 'Imodium'! If the condition deteriorates there may be weight loss and fever accompanying the diarrhoea – sometimes requiring hospitalisation and, occasionally, surgery for resection (removal) of severely inflamed intestine. Blood noted in stool always needs further investigation and diagnosis.

Any drug that causes a loose stool that was not there before the drug was taken may be a result of the medication and warrants informing the doctor. The offending drug may need to be discontinued. Antibiotics kill off good bacteria in the gut and allow others to flourish and produce toxins that can cause serious symptoms and possibly death. This has become a major problem in hospitals with a bacterium called Clostridium difficle that appears to be vying with MRSA (Methicillin Resistant Staphylococcus Aureus) for notoriety.

Conditions that cause loose and but not watery stools do not often lead to problems with dehydration. At the first sign of diarrhoea avoid all solid foods and dairy products. Ignoring this may unnecessarily prolong the diarrhoea and worsen abdominal colic.

The treatment of diarrhoea in any age group is taking a 'rehydration mixture'. This is made up of eight teaspoons of sugar and half teaspoon of table salt mixed with one litre of water taken from the kettle – boiled and cooled. Taking a 'glucose' drink *without* the addition of salt is useless because the glucose helps the salt get absorbed. The watery stools lose a lot of salt and it is this missing ingredient that is responsible for the *weakness* and lightheadedness that accompanies diarrhoea. Losing excessive salt will upset the delicate balance in the body and cause serious side effects. For an adult the quantity of rehydration fluid should not be less than three litres per 24 hours - taken in *small amounts* (half a cup at a time every twenty to thirty minutes). This avoids overloading the stomach and reduces nausea and vomiting.

Children between one and two years of age should receive 1 teaspoon (5 ml) per minute of rehydration fluid. This is increased to 25 ml every 5 minutes once vomiting has stopped. If the diarrhoea is not profuse and the child is not dehydrated allow 50 - 100 ml per stool if less than 2 years old - and 100 - 200 ml per stool if older than 2 years.

Once the diarrhoea has settled allow the following fluids - depending on the known weight of the child:-

5 kg	=	20 ml / hr
10 kg	=	40 ml / hr
15 kg	=	50 ml / hr
20 kg	=	· 60 ml / hr
25 kg	=	70 ml / hr
30 kg	=	75 ml / hr

Breast fed infants have fewer diarrhoeal illnesses than formula fed and should continue with breast milk if they develop diarrhoea. Formula-fed infants should have their feeds made up to half-strength for twenty-four to forty-eight hours after the first watery stools; the diarrhoea usually settles down within this period. Watery stools lasting longer than this require medical attention.

Medication in the form of a suppository may be necessary to control fever, nausea or vomiting. Vomiting that occurs once should not be a major cause for concern and if another follows this soon after it is usually 'part of the same vomiting spell' and should not be seen as separate bouts of vomiting. The stomach will not 'rest' until all its contents are brought up. This is undigested food the body is wise to be rid of as the gut is inflamed and, therefore, unable to process it.

An animal that is unwell instinctively refuses to eat to allow the inflamed gut to rest. Man is guided by the fear of hunger and starvation and forces himself to eat or the child is unwittingly coerced into doing so only for it to be vomited shortly afterwards. If there is doubt about the health of the gut it is safer to err on the side of caution and rest the organ by using only the rehydration mixture. Twenty-four hours without food will cause no harm provided this mixture is taken. If the stool *should* become diarrhoeal the treatment ('no solids') would already be well under way. The sooner the fluid and salts being lost in the stools are replaced the quicker the patient will recover. However, if vomiting recurs after a period of sixty minutes or longer and, especially if clear fluids given after the first episode of vomiting are also brought up, it is likely that it may persist. Further time should not be wasted and a doctor's advice sought.

Vomiting in the presence of diarrhoea is a double insult to the body and will quickly lead to dehydration. A suppository is an efficient and painless method of administering an antiemetic (emesis = vomiting). If a loose stool flushes out the suppository before it could be absorbed through the lining of the rectum it may have to be replaced with another. A period of at least thirty minutes is required to allow the suppository to be absorbed from the rectum. Its insertion should be timed for soon after a motion is passed. If vomiting persists hospitalisation and intravenous fluids will become necessary. The fluid in the 'drip' is simply a combination of sugar, salt and water.

Many subjects are afraid of the idea of having a foreign object inserted into the rectum – what with the increased awareness and incidence of 'sexual abuse'. However, the pain from an injection may linger for up to twenty-four hours whereas the suppository is entirely *painless*. A soft plastic packet or 'Glad Wrap' used as a glove, if the latter is not available, will avoid contamination of the fingers from the anal area. The introducing finger should gently follow the suppository into the rectum or the medication may not get past the anal sphincter (valve) and the bullet shaped drug may fly out and will have to be replaced. A small amount of Vaseline smeared within the anus will facilitate entry of the suppository. Avoid applying the Vaseline to the suppository itself or it will make it too slippery and difficult to manoeuvre. The ideal position for a child is to lay the recipient on the left side – so that the patient is not witnessing the procedure too closely. Furthermore, it is easier to steady the upper-most leg in this position than have both of them free to kick out at the 'operator' if the patient is lying supine (on the back). To self medicate – sitting over a small mirror with good illumination will help guide the suppository. The operator's hands must be thoroughly washed after the procedure.

The sugar in the rehydration mixture provides the calories and also helps to stop the diarrhoea. The salt replaces that which is being lost in the stools. Loss of this salt (sodium) may lower the blood pressure and cause dizziness. This is more prone to occur when the person tries to get out of bed too suddenly (to visit the toilet). To avoid this - first sit up, put out the legs, stand and then after one feels steady enough begin walking (these trips will understandably be frequent!). Salt is not normally good for high blood pressure but in the setting of diarrhoea it plays an important role. Plain water or any fluid that does not contain salt is not addressing the basic problem, which is the loss of salt and water. Diarrhoea and any situation where excessive amounts of salt are being lost, as in strenuous exercise, should be the main reasons for drinking so-called 'sportsmen's drinks'. The salt content of these mixtures is high – making it not recommended for all and sundry. Many misguidedly use this as a 'soft drink', which it is decidedly not – especially for young children.

If a person is taking a diuretic (used to get rid of water and salt), especially the elderly, this should be discontinued until the diarrhoea settles or it will aggravate the dehydration.

A person with a temperature above 37 degrees Celsius, regardless of the cause of the fever, should be discouraged from taking any solid food to avoid possible nausea and vomiting. A single violent bout of retching may tear the lower end of the oesophagus and cause bleeding into the stomach and the vomiting of blood (haematemesis). This development will change a simple gastroenteritis into a complication of vomiting that will require hospitalisation and probably a (unnecessary) gastroscope.

In the presence of excessive vomiting (more than three or four times) it is advisable to add a pinch of bicarbonate of soda (or a pinch of 'Enos Fruit Salt') to the rehydration fluid, as bicarbonate is also lost during excessive vomiting.

As a precaution, if nausea persists and saliva wells up in the mouth in waves as a prelude to vomiting, it is advisable to drink a half litre or more (the more the better) of plain lukewarm water fairly quickly to give the stomach sufficient 'body' to help rid itself of its contents. This extra water will give it a 'tidal wave' effect to avoid a 'dry' vomit, which will be more difficult, causing more distress and adding a greater risk of bleeding. Emergency units use this manoeuvre to wash out the stomachs of attempted suicides to remove drugs that have been taken as an overdose.

If fever is present, especially in a child, it may be advisable to bring this down before offering fluids as the raised temperature may itself induce vomiting and further distress. Children do not take kindly to the 'trauma' of vomiting.

The presence of blood and / mucus in the stools implies a dysentery that often requires antibiotics. Diarrhoea that persists beyond the usual three to five days may be due to:

- Not observing a stricter 'fluids only' policy – avoid dairy products
- Introducing solids before the watery stools have become more formed
- Bacteria or other organisms (germs) causing the diarrhoea

Other measures may need to be taken such as: stools sent to the laboratory for culture, antibiotics and, if it persists for weeks, a possible colonoscopy, which involves a long tube with a light (and camera) being introduced through the rectum for direct visualisation of the large gut.

The use of 'Imodium' and equivalent drugs to control diarrhoea may seem convenient but these work by 'paralysing' the gut and while these may stop the diarrhoea, the virus or bacteria that was responsible for it in the first place now remains happily bottled up within the gut. More importantly, these drugs may cause the motionless gut to become distended to such a degree as to further compromise function of the gut. The occasional patient has had to have surgery and loss of parts of the gut (resection) all for the convenience of avoiding going to the toilet often. Diarrhoea may be the overriding concern of the patient but replacing the fluids and salts should be the primary objective.

One of the common side effects of codeine phosphate is constipation and this is useful in diarrhoea as it slows down the motility (movement) of the gut without paralysing it. Codeine can also bring down a fever.

An accompaniment of diarrhoea that sometimes causes much discomfort is abdominal colic. This often settles down once the gut has been restricted from solids. However, if it becomes overbearing an antispasmodic like 'Buscopan' may be used, bearing in mind the use or the need for this is not the norm and often leads to unnecessary (self) medication.

In severe constipation, as is common in the chronically bedridden or demented patient, there may be loose or watery stools, albeit in small quantities. This does not necessarily mean that the person has diarrhoea or that the constipation has been relieved. The rectum may become so gummed up with dry (inspissated) stool that fluid stools from above the congealed rectal 'mass' are finding their way *around* the obstruction to emerge as a 'watery' stool. A rectal examination will confirm the diagnosis of impacted stool and 'spurious' (false) diarrhoea.

Any change from the normal in the consistency of the stools, (diarrhoeal or constipated) occurring in a person of advancing years (after +/- 45 years) that persists for longer than two or three weeks needs a doctor's opinion. Such a change in bowel habit may be due to cancer of the gut.

This requires a colonoscopy (tube introduced into the rectum and advanced carefully up the large intestine and the interior of the gut visualised for any abnormalities). This examination is not normally painful and no anaesthetic is necessary. Once the tube enters the rectum the anus relaxes as would ordinarily happen with a normal bowel movement. The gut should be properly prepared using laxatives to empty out the contents of the gut to permit adequate visualisation. Some discomfort maybe experienced if it becomes necessary to introduce air into the colon to 'blow' away bowel contents if they obstruct visibility. This will end up (down) as loud farts after the procedure. Diarrhoea may also accompany HIV/ AIDS due to involvement of the intestines.

Once the stools have become more formed (i.e. not watery) it would signify the return of the gut to normal, but meals should be simple and taken in small amounts at frequent intervals. A soft boiled or poached egg, oats or bananas may be gentler on the gut when returning to oral feeds. This would also be the time to supplement with *Formula IV Plus* (one sachet daily) and *Nutrishake* (two scoops twice daily) to improve the nutrition that has taken a battering, given that the 'rehydration mixture' contains no vitamins and minerals - only salt and sugar.

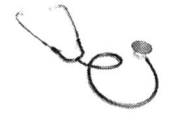

DIFFICULTY SWALLOWING (DYSPHAGIA)

A sore throat from tonsillitis or pharyngitis is not to be confused with the difficulty experienced in swallowing food. An infection in the throat and adjacent areas will cause difficulty in swallowing but this occurs over a period of a few days to a week and is often associated with pain and sometimes with fever.

Dysphagia that occurs over weeks to months and progressively becomes worse has a sinister implication. Initially the difficulty is with swallowing dry foods and solids (bread, meat) and later, as the condition deteriorates, soups and other liquids. This may or may not be associated with loss *of appetite* (anorexia) and *weight loss*. Until proven otherwise with further investigations this swallowing difficulty is most likely due to a malignancy i.e. cancer of the oesophagus (food pipe).

The disease needs a high index of suspicion. In an infection the difficulty is with solids *and* liquids, the person is unwell and the illness occurs over hours or days. Many a chance for effective treatment of cancer is lost because the patient often *takes long to get to the doctor* because of the *insidious* nature of the symptoms. Repeated courses of antibiotics are not the solution and should raise the concern that further investigations are required.

Acid reflux (backflow of acid from the stomach into the oesophagus) over years can result in a stricture (narrowing) of the lower end of the oesophagus. Though the cause is benign (innocent) the complaint is that food tends to get stuck in the area behind the lower end of the sternum (breastbone). It may present as dysphagia *without* cancer being present. The investigation performed is a gastroscopy. Biopsies (samples of tissue for examination in the laboratory) can be taken at the same time.

Food that tends to get 'stuck' anywhere in the chest after it is swallowed implies an obstruction along its path from the mouth to the stomach. This symptom also demands early attention. Apart from malignancy the obstruction could be due to a condition in which the lower end of the oesophagus, before it opens into the stomach, becomes narrowed due a 'thickening' of the muscular layer of the oesophagus (achalasia = failure to relax). The main complaint is early satiety: a few mouthfuls and the person feels full. This mimics a *stricture* of the oesophagus. The treatment is the same for both conditions i.e. stretching the narrowed part with 'balloons' inserted via the gastroscope. This may be done over several visits.

The gastroscope is a thin long tube (the thickness of a ring finger) with a 'camera' at its end. Just before the tip of the tube is a deflated balloon that, once it is positioned at the site of the narrowing in the oesophagus, is distended with air - forcefully stretching the stricture. An analogy that comes to mind is a bicycle pump with a balloon tied to the lower end of the pump.

Fear of cancer should never be the reason to delay seeking advice because sooner or later, as the 'blockage' becomes narrower and narrower *no food or water* may pass through the narrowing – forcing one to seek medical attention. If the diagnosis *is* cancer the delay may cost the chance of successful treatment.

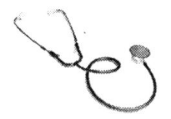

DRINKING WATER

Water is defined as: *'a clear liquid, without colour or taste, which falls from the sky as rain and is necessary for animal and plant life'*.

In many parts of the world this is rapidly disappearing. There are countries that have already been rationing water for decades. Those blessed with adequate supplies should be conserving them now instead of waiting for shortages to appear before introducing water restrictions. The cost of water will not easily be a deterrent to curb its use or abuse. The poor will suffer and the rich will simply pay the extra and maintain their water sprinklers, swimming pools, and Jacuzzis.

Thirst is a very fine tuned sensation necessary to maintain the delicate balances between the fluids outside the cells of the body and that within. Cells cannot perform their functions without water. An infant needs about 150ml/kg daily while a 10kg baby will require about one and a half litres per day. However, any condition that leads to increased water loss like diarrhoea, vomiting, fever or hot weather will require additional water. Infants and the elderly can become dehydrated very quickly. Illness and certain medications can also alter the fluid requirements of the body. Diuretics, commonly used in the elderly for high blood pressure, increase the excretion of water through the kidneys.

The elderly have other special problems. Ingested fluids like tea, coffee, soft drinks, fruit juices make up about one litre of the required fluid intake and another litre is obtained from food. The elderly are prone to dehydration because of: –

- Reduced food intake (affordability or availability)
- Lack of appetite due to chronic illnesses to which they are more susceptible
- Medication which they are more likely to be prescribed
- Physical or mental disabilities that makes them dependent upon caregivers for their fluid intake – a patient with Alzheimer's disease, especially in the later stages of dementia, may need frequent reminders to eat or take fluids
- Deliberate 'restriction' of fluid intake to reduce the production of urine and avoid more frequent visits to the toilet, changes of underwear, incontinence pads or bedding
- An impaired sensation of thirst due to age, illness and drugs.

Looking at or tasting it cannot tell the quality of the water. Chlorine, added to our drinking water by local municipalities, effectively kills bacteria but does nothing for the chemicals that already lurk in it. These chemicals find their way into the water by being washed off the farms where ever-increasing quantities of fertilisers and insecticides are being used. An increasing population creates an increasing demand for greater supplies of food. The addition of chlorine and the boiling of water cannot remove these chemicals and the latter are being increasingly blamed for some of the diseases of the last century. The only effective method of removing these impurities is through proper filtration; most cheap filters are ineffective but they lull the user into a false sense of security.

Drinking bottled water should be viewed as a business more than a deep concern over mankind's welfare and, as such, is open to the vagaries of manufacturers. Create the need and trust entrepreneurial skills to do the rest - 'Alpine mountain air' has been canned for sale! Nonetheless, it has correctly identified that something needs to be done to remove the chemicals present in our drinking water. Chlorine is known to cause cancer. It has also been linked to miscarriages, stillbirths, birth defects, strokes and heart diseases.

The air passages (nostrils and sinuses included) normally produce up 2 to 3 litres of mucus daily in order to perform their functions. Our fluid intake should at least replace this by taking in small quantities through the day. Physical exertion and the weather will dictate further increments. Taking any medication, and particularly non-steroidal anti-inflammatories (for arthritis) and antibiotics, should make it mandatory to increase the fluid intake. During the night the kidneys slow down the production of urine. Medication taken in the evening will linger longer in the kidneys and place them at possible risk from the presence of the drug. Taking extra water before retiring will help to flush out the drug. This may mean having to empty the bladder during the night. Similarly, in gout the levels of uric acid are high and taking extra water can reduce the damage it can cause the kidneys. It is not often appreciated that the quantity of urine that the body produces is determined mainly by excess protein and salt and by limiting their intake, the output of urine may be reduced.

The total protein requirement of the body is about 90 gm for the entire day (about 30 gm in each meal). The body has no way of storing protein and, therefore, it has to be taken at each meal. Eating a 500gm steak is simply forcing the kidneys to excrete the extra 470 gm of prime beef through the urine. Fats and carbohydrates are excreted in the stool but proteins are passed exclusively through the urine. Accordingly an important part of the management of kidney failure is restricting the intake of protein and salt. Should one wait for the kidneys to fail first before lessening their workload?

Any form of physical exertion like walking, washing clothes, mowing the grass, or having sex, increases the metabolism of cells in the body to produce the extra energy. This in turn produces heat which is lost mainly through sweating and the lungs. The sweating loses heat by evaporation. All this will use water making it necessary to help the body replace it by drinking extra water (not fruit juice and soft drinks – these often contain added salt that will make one thirsty all over again). Only water can effectively satisfy a thirst.

Alcohol is a diuretic, making the kidneys excrete more urine. Hot weather causes greater loss of fluids through sweating. Drinking alcohol before exercising in warm conditions will compound the dehydration. Coffee also has a diuretic effect. The drinking of water should be anticipated *before* the sensation of thirst is felt because by the time the message comes through that one is thirsty the body is already dehydrating. No person who is exercising in any form should be without a water bottle. How many joggers carry water bottles?

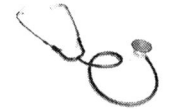

ECZEMA

Eczema, asthma and hay fever often coexist. The cause is not well understood. Eczema may be the dry, scaly type or the wet variety. Common sites that are affected are the elbows, knees, behind the earlobes and around the eyes. Sometimes the entire body may be affected. It can also be aggravated in pregnancy, particularly, in the later months. They can resemble a fungal infection and often an antifungal ointment is erroneously used. If treatment has not shown an improvement within seven to ten days the diagnosis should be reviewed. Be wary of using a trial and error approach in treating a fungal infection by mistaking it for eczema. The steroid ointment used in the treatment of the latter will spread the fungus and mask its appearance. Steroids in ointment or cream form (dry eczema use cream, wet eczema - ointment) is the mainstay of treatment but should be used sparingly and for as short a period as possible as they can further damage skin.

It may be more efficient and cost effective to cover the affected area with 'Cling wrap' to keep the medication from being absorbed into the clothing. This is especially useful at night. The caution is "Use very sparingly" and avoid the face and eyes.

The psychological effects of having eczema on exposed parts of the body must not be underestimated and should be actively addressed as the skin is the largest and most visible organ. The problems that arise when it involves food handlers also deserve special attention. The use of disposable gloves (not latex) for affected hands have additional benefits.

For more extensive skin involvement a short course of oral steroids (prednisolone) may be more effective than topical preparations. 'Aloe Vera Gel' is a useful alternative that avoids the unpleasant side effects of conventional medicine, given that eczema is a chronic condition that may wax and wane. This product may be an added bonus in pregnancy when, or in an infant in whom, one should be wary of using drugs.

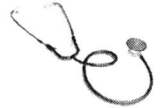

EGGS

Keep in refrigerator to maintain freshness. Never buy if they are cracked. If they should break before they can be used seal the crack immediately with cellophane tape. To make an omelette break the eggs individually before collecting in a common container - this will avoid losing all of them should one egg be rotten. Boiled eggs may have a healthier advantage over fried ones because they are not exposed to the altered carbon structure of the oil that occurs with the intense heat of frying. Frying will increase the calorie content of the egg by virtue of the oil or butter. Never eat raw eggs. While this may be a popular source of protein for bodybuilders and boxers there are easier and healthier ways to achieve this (using a protein supplement). Raw eggs and those with cracked shells are at significant risk of being contaminated with Salmonella bacteria responsible for food poisoning. The use of raw eggs (in 'egg-flips') poses a similar threat.

Next to brain, eggs have the second highest source of cholesterol. There are many *alternative* sources of protein and the inclusion of eggs in one's diet should not have to exceed more than one per week. Avoid creating the problem in children so that cholesterol-lowering drugs do not become necessary later. Avoid buying the large ('jumbo') eggs – they have bigger yolks and therefore more cholesterol. Duck's eggs, different from hens, should also be avoided as they are favourite carriers of salmonella bacteria. To test if eggs are fresh float them in water and discard if they sink. Also, if they are held up against a light source they should be transparent – indicating healthy eggs.

Organic eggs may not be the healthier alternatives they are promoted to be as their shells are thinner and more porous. Because of this they are not easily cleaned, as detergents used to wash non-organic eggs may be absorbed through the more delicate organic shells. Bacteria from the hen's droppings may cling to the shell of the unwashed 'organic' egg.

Avoid recipes that call for a lot of eggs. Chefs who think nothing of adding up to six eggs/more to a dish are cooking up problems.

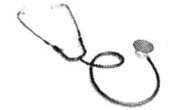

EXERCISE

Exercise should be made compulsory at school level. Teach children young. Teachers and physical education instructors should teach exercises their pupils can take with them into their adult lives. The simplest and most user-friendly form of exercise is walking: no fancy or expensive equipment is required and any age group can participate.

Enrolling at a gymnasium has a role to play but there are limitations. It can be expensive and enrolling does not automatically guarantee attendance. The gymnasium addresses one aspect of exercise i.e. the physical side and pays little attention to the brain which in turn does little to relieve the stresses that turn on the adrenaline and steroids, which caused the stress in the first place. The busy executive who hurries to the gym during the lunch break and 'works out' and then rushes back to work is paying attention to the tyres of the car but ignoring the engine i.e. the brain. At a gym there is little time to socialise. Each person is there for a specific reason i.e. exercise and, having paid for the facility, will expect to get maximum benefit for the money, effort and time spent. If a person is overweight and unhappy with his or her perception of the body image that he or she will be displaying to all and sundry at a public gym there is even less likelihood such a person will attend easily. Will this also prevent them from walking in the open?

Partners should encourage participation. Husbands who do not have a weight problem (and can 'eat whatever they like') sometimes defend themselves with "My wife walks too slowly" or "She is not really an exercise person". Could it be that some husbands feel uncomfortable to be seen in public places (even on dance floors – "She hates dancing") with their overweight wives and, conveniently, do not look beyond the lame excuses offered by their embarrassed partners? If one wishes to get rid of the partner then not exercising or discouraging it is one way of ensuring an earlier death for them from cardiovascular disease. But be warned – death is not guaranteed. One could be taking care of a stroke victim.

Studies have shown that the risk of heart attacks and strokes can be reduced by almost 40% with regular exercise and it matters little at what age it is started. Clearly, habits learned early will carry more easily into later life before the couch potato grows too big to move.

Walking in the open field or road or beach brings one closer to God and nature and people. The pace is less frenzied. The chance to reach another human is a lot easier than when one is busy tearing up the kilometres on a static exercise bicycle going nowhere and staring at nothing or one's reflection in a mirror with one eye on the clock –"Have I done ten minutes yet?" Greeting a fellow walker outdoors will have one's own happy smile returned with a carefree "Wonderful morning isn't it?" Can one compare a gymnasium with an early morning walk on a beach with the fresh smell of salt in the air, the sound of seagulls and the waves lapping on the sand? While one is walking and enjoying God's earth one can find a discarded plastic bag – there is always one to be found – and help to pick up litter that stares one in the face crying "Please sir! Can you take me home with you?" However, walking outdoors and enjoying Mother Nature should not make one fall victim to a mugger or worse, which is a reason to walk with a partner. Invest in a shock-stick for self-defence and avoid deserted pathways.

Dog owners who allow their pets to run loose in public places should be heavily penalised. Their pets are known to themselves only. Who can tell what is going through an animal's mind when it passes an innocent bystander? After it has attacked somebody and the calf muscle or one's behind lies butchered the pathetic comment the (guilty as charged) dog-owner may muster is "Gee! Little Butch" or

"Poopsie-Whoopsie has never done this before!" Dog owners should also be penalized and their privileges revoked for allowing their pets to create 'obstacle courses' by defecating on public walkways. There are more than fifty types of worms transmitted by doggie–poo that could find their way onto carpets and thence into the mouths of toddlers. Is this the equivalent of feeding toddlers dog excrement? That one cannot *see* the mess on the pavement does not exclude the presence of the parasites on the shoes.

The walk should cover a distance of:

- at least SIX kilometres - THREE times a week done within ONE HOUR each time (ten minutes per kilometre) or
- THREE kilometres every day done within THIRTY MINUTES each time.

The principle is to keep the heart beating at a constant rate for that length of time. A river that has never known a flood will not develop its smaller tributaries. The smaller branches of the main coronary arteries will not be encouraged to develop without the constant flooding effect that regular exercise can offer. These small branches can help to 'by-pass' blood past a blockage (coronary thrombosis / heart attack) provided one has been exercising (cardiovascular-type). Weight lifting will not achieve this cardiovascular benefit and is not recommended for patients with narrowed arteries (angina). The tension generated from the lifted weight is transmitted along the arteries of the muscles that are being trained all the way back to the heart. This could precipitate a heart attack or make angina worse.

Any pain or discomfort experienced in *any* part of the body, be it in the chest, calf muscle or any joint, is not a signal to continue exercising even harder. Slow down or stop. This pain is the only way the body has of warning there is a problem. Ignore it at one's peril: one could be setting the stage for a heart attack or torn hamstring or an overuse injury to a joint or ligament. It is not worth the trauma and could cost one's life. Undue shortness of breath experienced during exercise could also signify a heart attack. Any person contemplating an exercise programme should first consult a doctor. MOTs (road-worthiness) should not be compulsory for cars alone.

If coronary artery disease is not an issue a fitness programme should include some form of non-aerobic exercise using light weight lifting (dumbbells) or resistance-training equipment. This helps build muscle strength (the framework of one's car) whereas aerobic exercise, like swimming or walking, improves the cardiovascular status (the engine). The overall strength of the muscle may help prevent the fall that can result in a fractured hip. A joint is helpless without the muscle to work and support it. A simple inexpensive one kilogramme dumbbell carried while walking will marry the two forms of exercise and may also provide a deterrent against muggers.

Energy can be utilized with exercise and any form of the latter helps - parking one's car furthest from the entrance to the shopping mall, using the stairs instead of the lift, helping to wash the dishes after a meal, pulling in the tummy muscle whenever one can remember to do it, standing instead of accepting a kindly chair - all help to burn calories.

Exercise releases endorphins in the body. These substances are responsible for the great feeling one gets after exercise and resemble morphine used in the treatment of pain. The 'high' that regular joggers experience can also become 'addictive'! These endorphins can help lift depression, relieve stress and help one sleep better. They may also help to lighten the burden of chronic pain.

Exercise helps to improve circulation in every part of one's body whether it is the back (to alleviate back pain) or the penis (to help sexual dysfunction). Panting and puffing and having to suspend activity in the middle of sexual intercourse are hardly the picture of a romantic evening. Lack of exercise may contribute to sexual dysfunction and for this the treatment is not 'Viagra'!

One may choose to exercise in company. This could encourage exchanges of ideas, stimulate debate, share recipes, discuss problems, and eat up the kilometers. Exercising outdoors could also earn one a whole hour by oneself. The time could also be used to renew ties with God or nature or plan the day ahead or view problems in a different light. This is best done in the mornings when only one's sleeping time is 'compromised' and the air has not yet been polluted with deadly carbon monoxide fumes from car exhausts. To this end a good wind helps - along with choosing a route away from heavy traffic. There would be time afterwards for a shower before going to work.

Walking on roads does have hazards that can cost life or limb. Beware the pavement. The computer-like brain determines the pace and pressure with which each step is taken. Suddenly one crosses a road and to get back onto the pavement the brain is lulled by the previous subconscious calculations and does not lift the foot high enough to clear the height of the pavement and the unwary walker goes flying forward. If age has made one less agile the hands will miss saving the face, and if one does succeed in protecting one's self by outstretching the arms a fractured wrist is near guaranteed. Of course, if one should break a hip in a stumble, one may never walk easily again.

Avoid crossing a busy main road as one can misjudge the speed of vehicles – use a pedestrian crossing or regulated intersection. Cross briskly without running as the latter carries a risk of tripping. Beware the cyclist who is often not considered as traffic. Looking around as one walks will help exercise one's neck but watch out for potholes on the pavement and loose stones that can lose traction and send one sliding to the emergency unit.

Marvel at the sunrise. Admire the gardens and trees. Keep the back straight and examine one's shadow as one walks to observe the posture of the spine. Osteoporosis will curve the upper spine and incorrect posture will add to the deformity. Tighten the belly muscle (pubococcygeus) as one walks. To identify this muscle imagine halting in midstream the passage of urine. This muscle helps strengthen and flatten the tummy and the same muscle controls the bladder, vagina, back passage and muscles of the spine thereby alleviating incontinence, improving one's sex life, helping backache and assisting in childbirth. Do this simple exercise continuously and nobody will be any the wiser. Posing models understand its importance in producing flatter, svelte tummies.

Breathing plays a vital role in exercise. If one is still puffing unduly after some months of regular exercise a doctor's advice should be sought. The lower one thirds of the lungs are hardly used and could be likened to running on one leg. For every third or fourth building one passes on the walk one should take in as big a breath as possible through the nose. Mouth breathing may seem easier but this does not allow the air to be warmed or filtered of dust particles. Then let the air out very slowly through pursed lips until all the air is exhaled that is physically possible. This ensures that the whole lung and the bases of the lungs in particular are utilised for providing the oxygen necessary during exercise.

Asthmatics should use their inhalers at least fifteen to twenty minutes before exercising.

Dress warmly because it is easier to peel off if necessary. Sudden changes in body temperature are best avoided. As one builds up heat from the exercise loosen clothing (unzip or open the front) but taking them off may change the temperature too precipitously. Avoid walking in the rain as the risks of injury and starting a cold or worse are higher.

If one suffers from angina or has had a heart attack in the past, always keep the chest protected from the wind and cold. Jumping macho-style into cold water is similarly to be avoided. Many of the deaths from shipping disasters in icy waters are as a result of heart attacks precipitated by the sudden exposure to cold water. Strenuous exercise soon after eating should also be frowned upon as should taking alcohol prior to exercise (swimming). Avoid unnecessary exposure to sunlight and wear long sleeves, a hat and sunglasses (to prevent cataracts) or, better still, exercise *before* sunrise. Walking in the evening exposes one to the day's collection of toxic (carbon monoxide) exhaust fumes. These same fumes gather on fruit and vegetable sold by roadside vendors. Examining the tailpipes of vehicles will provide more graphic evidence of what engines spew out.

For the kind of exercise advocated above, have a banana or bowl of oats thirty to forty-five minutes before. Taking fruit juice or water before a walk should not make it necessary to find a toilet along the way because more of this fluid would be lost through perspiration.

Regular exercise also stimulates the bowels to move better and prevents constipation. When walking take small steps and avoid grinding the heels into the hard road surface. This avoids putting unnecessary strain on the spine, hips, knees, ankles, small bones of the feet and the ligaments that support their long arches. Experiencing pain anywhere requires an explanation and possibly rest and, failing this, a professional opinion. Avoid exercise if pain is present.

Ever observed elephants doing push-ups? Man is the only mammal that deliberately exercises. Animals incorporate their life styles to provide the physical workout they require. Animals in captivity must mimic man in more ways than visitors to the zoo and the keepers of their charges imagine! In trying to achieve a healthy balance between domestication and an earlier death or risk of disease exercise should not be the cause of injury. If a fast bowler delivers at speeds of over a hundred kilometres an hour the momentum needed to generate this must end at the crease line. Consider the strain on the braking ankle and foot, never mind the arm that is trying to tear itself out of its socket in the delivery.

Jogging has the same penalty at a lower premium. The constant pounding of one's entire weight (anywhere from 70 up to 120 kg) being transferred from one foot to the other should make advocates of this form of exercise/ passion/ addiction/ employment/ exploitation/ madness sit up and take notice. And be around their protégés when the latter eventually develop abuse or overuse-type of arthritis and watch them swallowing anti-inflammatory drugs and preparing for steroid injections and joint replacements. Joints were not designed for the sudden twists and turns in activities like squash, badminton and tennis. No artificial prosthesis can replace one's own natural joint. Parents who encourage (force) their children to engage in ballet and gymnastics may well be sacrificing them to a lifetime of arthritis. One sees them in the rheumatology clinics and orthopaedic surgeons' rooms.

Muscle should be warmed (circulation improved) and stretched before being subjected to rigorous exercise. Walking initially at a slower pace will achieve the first requirement. Then gently stretching and holding the stretch for a few seconds at a time will help prime the muscle and prevent injury. Watching a cat or dog arise from sleep, and the body stretching that follows, should teach their less learned earthly inhabitants that jumping out of bed, as is sometimes advertised on television by manufacturers of beds and mattresses, is not what nature recommended. Five to ten minutes in bed (before arising and assuming the erect position) should be spent stretching – like a cat.

After the exercise stay warm and keep moving. A tracksuit helps retain body heat. Avoid peeling off too soon and refrain from eating for at least 45 minutes to an hour afterwards. Fluids on the other hand should be taken even before one starts the exercise. If one waits for thirst to first appear one has missed the boat. Small sips should be taken throughout. No person should exercise without a water bottle in hand. Bottled drinks aimed at 'sportsmen' should be used by those engaged in heavy or vigorous workouts. They contain a lot of salt and should not to be used as soft or cool drinks and for this reason to be avoided in children.

Exercise should generate a sense of well being and happiness. The contorted faces of dehydrated joggers hardly lend themselves to this frame of mind.

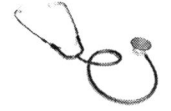

GOING FOR AN OPERATION

The thought of any operation may bring on feelings of fear and pain and misgivings that something 'might go wrong'. Any person expecting to have any surgery (or any invasive procedure or test) should be informed whether there is an alternative.

The following points should be clarified: –

- The precise nature of the operation
- What is the prognosis
- Who will be operating – trainee registrar or consultant
- The expected duration of hospitalisation, how long the recovery period is expected to be
- The surgeon's and anaesthetist's fees, hospital and theatre fees where applicable – can the same operation be done elsewhere at lesser cost
- The cost of medication – chemotherapy
- Whether a general or local anaesthetic is envisaged and if an epidural is an option (the anaesthetic is introduced through a lumber puncture and the patient is awake through out the operation – bearing in mind that the patient will then be privy to everything that is being said and done during the procedure!
- The possible complications that could occur (not all of which are predictable) even if it means that the patient may see the operation in a negative light, and, if complications did

arise, what measures would be taken and what long term implications could there be

- Analgesia after the operation
- Need for physiotherapy or appliances – wheelchairs, crutches
- The convalescence afterwards – at home or nursing home
- Activities that may be restricted after the procedure – sexual intercourse, lifting heavy weights, driving, climbing stairs, walking, bending, sporting activities and hobbies
- Return to work and any special limitations/precautions
- Is the will up to date
- Is there a need for a 'living will'

The following information should be given to the anaesthetist or surgeon: –

- If any medication is being used currently or been discontinued in the past.
- Past history of illnesses both recent and old
- Allergies to drugs, anaesthetic agents, iodine, other disinfectants used to swab the skin before the operation and certain dressings/plasters
- Previous anaesthetic difficulties or complications (problems with the neck, presence of dentures and crowns, last visit to the dentist, ability to open the mouth

The anaesthetist assesses whether the person is medically fit to undergo the procedure. A consent form must be signed by the patient before the procedure can be performed. This will specify the name of the operation - bearing in mind that, depending upon the circumstances at the time, changes may be made in the best interests of the patient at the discretion of the surgeon and anaesthetist.

An hour or so before leaving for the theatre 'pre-medication' in the form of a tablet is usually given to allay anxiety. In theatre expect to have a drip put up through which fluids and medication will be administered. A needle is inserted into a vein usually in the back of the left (to keep the dominant arm free and remember to inform the staff if one is left handed) hand or wrist or, failing that, in front of the elbow. Expect to feel a muted prick when a vein is punctured. The more anxious the patient feels (especially when finding a suitable vein is difficult) the more nervous the doctor may become and this state of affairs may cause the veins to become even more elusive. And still on this point: it does not help to be viewing the procedure. Rather think of the nurse or the last time you went fishing or were appraised by the receiver of revenue! For children and the very squeamish a local anaesthetic cream can be applied an hour or so before the needle is inserted.

Preoperative measures (depending on the circumstances): –

- Daily walks up to three km per day for thirty minutes or about six km three times a week covered within an hour. Check with one's doctor about a planned physical activity. Exercise helps to boost the immune system and the circulation.
- Smoking should most emphatically be stopped as early as possible. Failing this the number should at least be cut down. This can influence the outcome of the operation in terms of the anaesthetic and the risk of clots in the veins of the legs (deep vein thromboses) and lung complications that are more common in smokers. Stopping smoking, even one week before an operation, has been shown to improve the outcome of the anaesthetic. One yoga exercise requires a deep breath to be taken and held for as long as is physically possible and then let out slowly, over as long a time as possible, by pursing the lips together. This helps to move air from the bottom one to two thirds of the lungs which are normally hardly ever utilised – unless one is exercising vigorously.
- Zinc – 30 mg daily – to prevent infection
- Vitamin C daily – slow-release form because this vitamin is excreted very quickly from the body and, therefore, should be provided throughout the day (helps in wound healing).
- Omega 3 – at least 3 capsules daily

- Vitamin E 200 IU. – 1 capsule daily
- Formula 4 Plus – 1 sachet daily,
- Calmag (calcium/magnesium supplement) – 3 tablets daily

The above should be taken for at least four weeks before the expected operation and the Omega 3 and Vitamin E discontinued for at least a week before the actual procedure. These would be restarted three days after the surgery or once the risk of bleeding has settled. These two supplements help to 'thin' the blood and prevent thromboses. Omega 3 is a powerful anti-inflammatory and also helps reduce the recovery time of tissue injuries - regardless of the cause.

The trauma of the surgery will increase levels of free radicals in the body. These are the by-products released from cells when they are damaged. These free radicals cause further damage to normal cells. Vitamin C and E are powerful antioxidants that mop up the harmful free radicals reducing the trauma of surgery. Overall, the post-operative recovery may be significantly improved.

A 'general anaesthetic' entails the use of an injection to make the patient unconscious. This is given via the cannula (needle) introduced into the vein in the hand or forearm. This cannula also provides a portal for intravenous fluids as the patient would have been starved for at least twelve hours before the anaesthetic. 'Nil per mouth' is intended to keep the stomach empty to prevent the risk of its contents being vomited during the anaesthesia and the operation. The consequences of inhaling acid-containing vomitus into the lungs has serious and, often, life threatening complications.

Once the patient has been 'put to sleep' breathing is 'assisted' with a machine (ventilator). This is connected to the patient through a tube (endotrachael) inserted through the mouth and past the vocal cords into the bronchial tube. Post-operatively it may cause a sore throat and hoarseness. A simple throat gargle made up with warm water and salt may be adequate and can be used as often as necessary. Proprietary lozenges and gargles contain a local anaesthetic, the effect of which usually wears off within 20 – 30 minutes.

After the operation, and with the surgeon's permission, every attempt should be made to get out of bed early to improve the circulation, prevent the formation of clots in the large veins at the backs of the legs (deep vein thromboses) and assist in deep breathing to get air into the bases of the lungs as described earlier. Chest physiotherapy will help prevent lung infections especially in the frail and elderly.

The hospital stay should be as short as possible because of the inherent risk of contracting a 'hospital infection'. Hospitals have their own colonies of bacteria, many of which are drug resistant and difficult to treat (MRSA, Clostridium difficile – 'C diff')

Keep visitor numbers to a minimum as one cannot identify who might be harbouring an infection. Those who are unwell should be discouraged from visiting patients in hospital. Infants and young children should also be kept away. Visitors should sterilise their hands before and after entering the ward. Shaking hands and kissing the patient should be discouraged and sitting on or touching the patient's bed avoided. Try not to overstay one's visit and spare a thought for the person in the next bed. Tokens of appreciation for nursing staff should preferably be with fruit rather than biscuits and chocolates - Florence Nightingale needs to be fit to do the job.

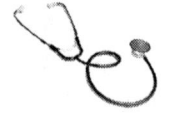

GOUT

An inflammation in a joint is called 'Arthritis'. Gout is one type of arthritis. It may occur in any joint but commonly in the joint where the big toe meets the foot (metatarsophalangeal or 'mtp' joint). It often begins suddenly - usually at night. The pain can be very severe, often requiring an injection of an anti-inflammatory drug: a sleeping tablet would be a blessing.

The following precipitating factors should be identified and avoided

- Minor injury (stubbing the toe)
- Foods like fish with dark flesh (mackerel, sardines)
- Offal (tripe, kidneys, liver)
- Alcohol
- Drugs like thiazides ('water tablets') used in hypertension (high blood pressure) and aspirin

A joint that swells could be due to gout. The blood test that measures the level of uric acid in the blood may help establish the diagnosis but does not exclude it if it is normal. If the swelling recurs at another time, not necessarily in the same joint, this makes the diagnosis more likely to be gout. Asthma and gout share a common characteristic: they are recurrent.

One method of confirming the diagnosis is by aspirating fluid from within the affected joint and identifying microscopically the uric acid crystals that cause gout. Aspiration involves inserting a needle into a joint – usually the knee. The idea of a needle being stuck into a joint may sound horrendous but the procedure should only be as painful as having an intramuscular injection.

The importance of the aspiration: –

- To exclude an infection in the joint
- The fluid can be examined for uric acid crystals - the presence of which is the only certain way of confirming the diagnosis of gout
- It avoids the need for unnecessary dietary restrictions if the cause is not gout
- Ensures correct treatment is prescribed
- If the problem recurs the diagnosis will have been already established

Gout has implications mainly for joints, tendons, cartilage, and bursae. The latter are pads present over bony prominences e.g. over the point of the elbow – designed to protect the bone against injury; 'housemaid's knee' is another example of a pad protecting a joint when kneeling on floors. However, when gout occurs in the presence of hypertension (high blood pressure) there is a greater risk to the kidneys - and both conditions merit more stringent control. It is often, mistakenly, advised that all 'acids' should be avoided in the prevention of gout: the acid in tomatoes and oranges is ascorbic acid not uric acid and ascorbic acid is Vitamin C and the latter does not cause gout.

There are a few, uncommon, medical conditions where cells are being rapidly destroyed. In leukemia white blood cells are broken down in large numbers and purines are released from these cells. These are converted by the body into uric acid. If a white blood cell swallows uric acid and releases it within a joint the acid acts like a foreign body and irritates the joint. The end result is inflammation i.e. gout. A swollen joint requires expert medical opinion – not the neighbour's anti-inflammatory tablets that were left over from his last attack of gout.

Gout that has been present for many years (chronic) may lead to the development of small bead-like swellings commonly situated over the edge of the upper ear lobe. They contain a thick, cheesy substance that harbour the uric acid crystals. These may also occur over the upper part of the back of the forearm (close to the elbow) and maybe pea sized or bigger. These do not usually require any intervention but, unfortunately, do not disappear with treatment of gout. They can be unsightly.

As with any joint that is inflamed the influence of bed rest should not be underestimated. The affected joint should be elevated to help reduce the swelling. Anti-inflammatory drugs, preferably by injection initially, and thereafter orally, are the mainstay of treatment - response to ordinary pain tablets is not as effective. Medication should be continued for at least a week after the pain has subsided.

If gout occurs several times in a year it is advisable to use a drug called 'Allopurinol' on a daily, long-term basis to prevent gout. It should not be started during an acute attack (it could make the joint *more* painful!) but may be continued if one should have the misfortune to still have one. Episodes of gout may occur even if preventative medication has been diligently taken. If discontinued it should not be resumed until a week or more have passed after the pain has subsided. Soda Bicarbonate ('Citro Soda') makes the urine alkaline (opposite of acid) and this helps to make the uric acid more soluble (dissolves better) and therefore easier to flush out of the kidneys into the urine. Taking extra fluid as a matter of permanent habit also helps reduce the damage of gout crystals to the kidneys.

Taking omega 3 (3 capsules daily) may help prevent or reduce the inflammation that occurs in gout. These may be increased to 3 capsules twice daily during the acute phase and then reduced once it is over. Omega 3 is not a drug and does not have the side effects of conventional anti-inflammatory agents (drowsiness, stomach inflammation, ulcers [occasionally complicated by bleeding] and damage to the kidneys).

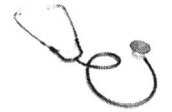

HEAD INJURIES

Two crucial points about head injuries may be used as a guide to the level of concern that such an injury should generate:

1. The nature of the injury
2. Change in the mental state of the victim after the accident.

A bleed within the skull (Subdural Haematoma – within the skull but *outside* the actual brain) may remain without symptoms for up to six to twelve months. A clue might be a change in the personality of the person – the accident being long forgotten or passed off as trivial! The thyroid gland, if it is underfunctioning, may also produce similar personality changes and gradual loss of memory. A simple blood test would exclude this diagnosis.

The nature of the injury and the circumstances surrounding it are also important. The skull bones are quite thick, almost a centimetre or more. Striking the head against an open cupboard door as one sits up from a squatting position may cut the scalp but such a force may not easily crack the bone. But an injury to the head involving movement e.g. being thrown out of a moving vehicle or falling from a height, may generate sufficient force to fracture the skull. Being struck on the head with an object – iron bar, brick, bat or baton may also break the skull.

Any change in mental status soon after an injury e.g. drowsiness, confusion, unconsciousness of any severity needs urgent medical attention. A skull X-ray is only useful if a fracture is suspected - its absence does not exclude its possibility. As they become more readily available CAT Scans and MRIs are much more sensitive for detecting fractures (not seen on plain X-rays) and evidence of brain injury or bleeding.

Bleeding from a scalp wound can be profuse because, unlike other parts of the body, the bleeding vessels in the scalp are unable to retract (seal) because scalp tissue is dense and inelastic. A firm pressure dressing over the wound will help stop the bleeding. In an emergency a clean handkerchief folded into a wad may be effective. Most scalp wounds require stitching and, as with all wounds, the earlier this is done the less likelihood of infection setting in. Meningitis (infection of the lining of the brain) is a serious condition and should not become a complication of a simple head or scalp wound.

Bleeding from within the ear/s after a head injury has serious implications and will require examination with an auriscope or otoscope (instrument for looking into the ear). If it is not due to a wound of the external ear canal the cause could be a ruptured eardrum or, more importantly, a fracture of the base of the skull (upon which the brain rests).

Although bleeding from a wound may have stopped, if there has been any exposure to road/garden dirt or manure – this will have to be meticulously debrided (cleaned) and anti-tetanus vaccination administered.

Head injuries that occur in the setting of an alcoholic binge or medication-induced drowsiness pose a special a problem: such victims should be seen in hospital. A head injury (and there may not be external signs of one!) can masquerade as the effects of debauchery. Drunks ending up in a police cell overnight have been found the following morning dead from an unsuspected head injury (bleeding within the skull).

A fit (Epileptic seizure) occurring after a head injury, and if a previous history of epilepsy is not available at the time, must be assumed to be a first-time seizure and requires hospitalisation. Victims of head injuries, depending on the nature of the damage to the brain, may have a lifetime risk of developing epilepsy; the more extensive the damage the higher the risk.

Symptoms and signs ('symptoms' are what the patient complains of and 'signs' are what the doctor finds during the examination) that should alert one that something is amiss after a head injury are:

- Inappropriate drowsiness
- In a child – irritability (e.g. restlessness and persistent crying)
- Nausea, vomiting or worsening headache (aggravated by coughing or sneezing)
- Inappropriate behaviour
- Confusion or difficulties with memory
- Loss of consciousness for any length of time
  - Watery discharge from the nostril. In contrast, a runny nose will produce a rather thick mucous. Crying may allow tears to escape into the nostrils via the tear duct. But this will cease once the crying stops! Fluid from the brain (cerebrospinal fluid – this is the same fluid that is obtained in a lumbar puncture) can leak out through the nostril if the base of the skull has been fractured.
- Blood from one or both ears (from within the ear canals)

If these should occur the patient should be seen in hospital as soon as possible. Bradycardia (slow heart rate) – pulse rate taken at the wrist (behind the base of the thumb) of 50 beats or less per minute would also be an important (late) finding.

Headache after a head injury (unless it has the features described above) is often a worrying symptom for the victim but is quite common in this situation and rarely requires more than simple analgesics like paracetamol. Avoid taking more potent drugs that may cause drowsiness (e.g. codeine and non-steroidal anti-inflammatory drugs like ibuprofen) as these may mask the picture of raised intracranial pressure (high pressure within the skull).

A compulsory part of a Driving Test should include at least seven days attendance in an Acute Brain Injury Rehabilitation Unit. During this period the aspiring road user is obliged to help one victim of a road traffic accident to

- Shave
- Brush the teeth and clean the mouth
- Wash the face, upper half of the body and then the lower half
- Ensure that the morning enema has been administered and the bowels appropriately emptied and the disposable sanitary pad correctly positioned
- Brush the hair or what is left of it after the accident / operation on the brain
- Dress the patient
- Hoist or slide the patient onto a wheelchair
- Make certain the body straps are in place
- Secure the bladder catheter to the side of the leg
- Measure, empty and dispose of urine that collected overnight
- Wheel the patient to the breakfast area
- Feed breakfast - spoon by spoon

This is the routine each morning for most victims of road traffic accidents who have been brain injured. This is the reality drivers need to see before the head is injured. This is the side car manufacturers need to see when they advertise their products on television - for they will not be present when breakfast is served! Car manufacturers should have their products banned from television (remember the 'Camel' cigarette advertisement?). They glamourise cars as though these were toys – appealing to immature macho egos - rather than acknowledge that their products have the potential to become instant killing-machines.

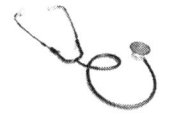

HEADACHE

Headache is the commonest symptom experienced by all people at some time in their lives (backache could command second place!). Self-medication with painkillers is sometimes used for years before a cause is sought; the sufferer often believing a headache to be a trivial symptom.

There are two categories of people who suffer from headache:

- those who are having it for the first time (acute) and
- others who have had it for years (chronic).

Headache occurring for the first time that stays for longer than one or two days in any age group and *without any other symptom* needs an explanation – and that means seeing a doctor. If it is part of an illness that has headache as one of the symptoms e.g. sinusitis there will be other clues that the headache is not isolated. In the initial stages there may not be other symptoms.

A headache + a temperature (any level above 37 degrees Centigrade) may be treated symptomatically on condition the patient can bend the neck forward without causing pain in back of the neck. If forward bending (flexion) of the neck produces pain this could mean meningitis. This is serious and demands urgent medical attention – let the doctor decide whether the painful neck is due to a throat infection and not meningitis.

Headache of recent onset i.e. weeks or months in a person not prone to them requires a medical opinion - the age of the person does not matter. This symptom in a school-going child may be neglected or overlooked. Hypertension knows no age barriers and tumours in the brain can occur in children. There may also be a more benign explanation like poor eyesight.

Chronic headache needs a diagnosis if this has not already been established in the past. Taking analgesics (pain killers) daily and over weeks and months can themselves cause headache and foster a cycle of pain-tablet-pain. Only by discontinuing them can the cycle be broken and the path cleared to resolving the headache. Headache, as is commonly believed, is *not* a common symptom of high blood pressure and it is not surprising that hypertension has been labelled the 'silent killer'!

Migraine is common and children are not immune. There is often a family history of migraine (more common in women) and stress has been known to precipitate an attack even though the cause has been identified as a spasm of the arteries in the brain.

There is no test or investigation for migraine and the diagnosis is based on

- Chronicity (recurring over long periods),
- Association of nausea, vomiting and sometimes
- Abdominal pain
- The need to lie down in a darkened, quiet room
- Visual changes – objects appear blurred.
- A family history of migraine – especially in mothers
- Warning symptoms before an attack that the sufferer learns to recognize - peculiar smells, flashing lights

The pain can be very severe and simple analgesics are often not effective. Nausea and vomiting may be controlled by suppositories or by injection (vomiting will preclude the use of oral medication). Of the two alternative routes a suppository is not painful. *Omega 3* (three capsules a day) and *Calmag* (three tablets daily) may help reduce the number and severity of the migraine attacks.

Headache often raises the possibility and concern of a 'tumour' in the brain. This is not always an easy diagnosis – and a CAT Scan or MRI may exclude the presence of in intracranial tumour.

The following features relating to headache should prompt medical advice:

- A recent onset in a person not prone to them
- Disturbed sleep
- Present in the morning on waking
- Associated with nausea, vomiting and aggravated by coughing/sneezing
- Associated with drowsiness or blurred or double vision
- Associated with changes in personality
- Accompanied by convulsions (seizures / fits)

A headache occurring in a young person, often a man, and situated at the back of the head, and of recent onset may be due to a cerebral aneurysm. In this condition there is a weakness in the wall of an artery in the brain (congenital weakness) causing it to bulge out and produce a swelling (aneurysm). More commonly there are no warning symptoms of its presence and often comes to attention after it has ruptured. The result is often a massive bleed within the brain making survival the exception. The headache is sometimes precipitated by physical exertion, or the onset of hypertension may exert pressure upon the weak spot in the arterial wall and produces signs and symptoms. If it is detected before this catastrophe occurs the aneurysm can be sealed off with a metal clip with good results. While it may not be practical or even necessary to investigate every headache with a CAT Scan or MRI a careful history and high index of suspicion can avert potential disasters. The medical profession has been known to brush off trivial (crucial) symptoms for up to ten years before a frustrated patient or next of kin insists on further tests or referral to a specialist.

Headaches situated at back of the head and neck could also be due to problems arising from the cervical spine. Some of the nerves arising from this part of the spine also supply the head. The scalp is a thick muscle that is attached at the back to the muscles of the cervical spine. Any tension on the neck and shoulder will be transmitted to the top of the head resulting in a 'tension headache,' a symptom commonly associated with stress and anxiety. Headache after a motor vehicle accident in which the head suffers a concussion is not uncommon provided it is not accompanied by drowsiness, nausea and vomiting or confusion. These symptoms require urgent medical attention. They could represent a rising pressure within the head secondary to haemorrhage within the skull or brain.

It is worth reiterating that headache is a *symptom* not a diagnosis. The cause needs to be established before easily reaching for a painkiller.

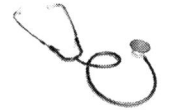

HEART ATTACK

Pain experienced anywhere in the body is nature's way of warning that there is a problem. A toothache is not an indication to take analgesics except as a temporary measure. This pain is being produced by infection/inflammation. Pain from a heart attack is caused by blockage of blood flow in one or more of the arteries of the heart (coronary arteries). For an organ that must work non-stop, from before birth to death, it boasts one of the most inadequate systems of blood supply. If the narrowing in the coronary artery is complete and no further blood can flow through it this will result in a full blown 'heart attack'/ myocardial infarction.

The causes of the narrowing may be due to:

- 'Plaque' that has been building up over time on the inner walls of the artery thereby gradually reducing the lumen (inner diameter of the artery) and
- Spasm of part of an artery.

If the spasm can be relieved either spontaneously or with medication the damage to the heart may not be as severe as if the blockage was complete. If the narrowing is incomplete (partially blocked) and there is a demand for blood (and oxygen) that cannot be met the result will be pain and this is called 'angina'.

If any part of the heart does not receive blood for longer than a few minutes that part may 'die' and, if the victim survives, the part that was compromised of its blood supply will result in a scar. The heart muscle does not tolerate scar tissue as this will compromise its function as a pump; the smaller the size of the scar less the damage to heart muscle.

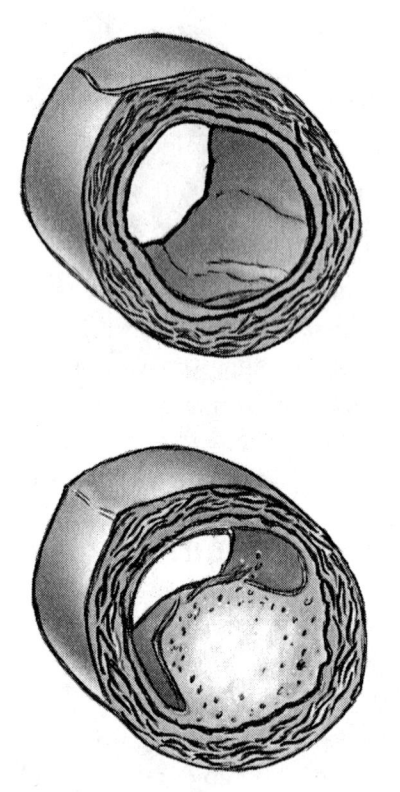

ATHEROSCLEROSIS: NORMAL ARTERY & CLOGGED ARTERY

Pain relief is of paramount importance. Pain stimulates the release of adrenaline that in turn makes the heart beat faster. This increases the demand for more blood and oxygen than the narrowed artery may be able to supply. An outburst of anger may make a similar demand of a compromised coronary artery and result in a heart attack.

Measures that may reduce the extent of the damage or scar are:

- immediately stopping whatever activity the victim was engaged in at the time of the attack (the initiating event)
- stopping smoking immediately instead of lighting up when the circulation is already compromised!
- lying down, remaining calm and breathing in deeply and exhaling slowly through pursed lips - anything that makes the heart beat faster will demand more oxygen and this the heart cannot supply at that moment
- loosening tight clothing and staying warm – shivering will stimulate muscles to contract and cold will precipitate spasm in vessels
- calling for assistance instead of being a 'macho man' and pretending it is just a 'wind' and everything will be 'all right'
- not going out for a jog to work off the pain!
- if one has been participating in a group activity (marathon) - to stop in the middle of it
- placing a T.N.T. tablet under the tongue or spraying two squirts of the liquid version of T.N.T (GTN) under the tongue - if this has already been prescribed or is available. One should be lying down or be seated before using this medication as it tends to drop the blood pressure and cause dizziness and lightheadedness. This will aggravate the situation further.
- calling a doctor or getting to the nearest hospital if the TNT tablet or spray is not effective within ten minutes of having used them twice or thrice in succession
- immediately taking a tablet of aspirin if it is available
- breathing oxygen if this is available

Clues that may help identify the pain of a heart attack

- It is situated in the centre of the chest/breast bone – the further from the centre of the chest that it occurs, e.g. over the left nipple, the less likely it is to be angina

- It is burning in character – never sharp or needle-like or stabbing. It may also feel like a tightness or constriction in the chest and can sometimes mimic 'heartburn'
- the pain may radiate to the left shoulder or arm, sometimes down to the hand or upwards into the neck or lower jaw and, rarely, the back of the chest
- it lasts for longer than a few seconds or minutes – up to 15 to 30 minutes or more
- is not made worse by breathing
- classically occurs during or soon after physical activity – chopping a tree, jogging or other physical exercise, during sexual intercourse especially in the setting of a clandestine affair!
- it maybe associated with sweating, shortness of breath, palpitations (fast heart beat) and lightheadedness/dizziness.

In women and diabetics none of the above may apply. There may be only an unaccustomed tiredness or shortness of breath and no hint of aught serious.

Pain that fits the above description or if there is doubt about the nature of it requires medical attention. While this is being arranged give the patient an aspirin tablet as an emergency measure to help 'thin' the blood and prevent more clots from forming within the arteries.

If this is not the first attack and the patient has been prescribed sublingual nitrates use it immediately (TNT – trinitrate tablet or GTN spray – glyceryl trinitrate - placed under the tongue or sprayed under it). Take the precaution to lie down before administering GTN spray or bystanders will *really* believe the patient has taken a turn for the worse and cause the 'victim' even more anxiety – at a time when reassurance is paramount. A common side effect of GTN is headache for which paracetamol can be taken. However, the headache does not last long and becomes less troublesome with continued use of the drug. After using the sublingual (under the tongue) spray keep the mouth closed and breathe through the nostrils for at least a few minutes - until the medication has been absorbed. It may cause a burning sensation in the mouth - ignore this.

On arrival at the hospital expect the following to happen fairly smartly:

- A doctor will take a brief history about your symptoms and an ECG (Electrocardiogram) will be requested. Any current medication and pertinent details about your medical background (family history, risk factors like – smoking, high cholesterol, hypertension, diabetes and previous cardiac problems) should be disclosed. Bring all current medicines or a recent prescription.
- An ECG entails leads being attached to the arms and legs and also to the front of your chest. A hairy chest can expect to be shaved so that the leads can be attached to the skin. There is no risk of being electrocuted by the procedure. The strip of paper recording will be analysed and, if it is appropriate, a diagnosis of a heart attack may be made. A decision will then be taken whether a clot-busting drug (thrombolytic) is to be used.
- A needle (plastic cannula) will be inserted into a vein in the arm and while this is being done blood will be taken for tests, one of which may help to confirm a myocardial infarct (heart attack). The plastic cannula will be left in the vein and secured with special adhesive tape. This portal allows medication and fluids to be easily administered and, in an emergency, can be life-saving.
- The ECG leads will be connected to a monitor that has the 'ECG' recordings shown continuously on a (TV-like) screen. A thimble-like instrument (oximeter) will be fitted to the tip of a finger – this reads the oxygen levels of the body continuously. A blood pressure cuff will also be placed around the upper arm
- Morphine for pain will be given through the drip and oxygen will be administered through a face mask. The morphine will make one relaxed (on cloud nine) and

drowsy/sleepy. It can sometimes cause vomiting but this is anticipated and a further injection given to alleviate this.

- Once the patient has been stabilised he or she will then be transferred to an ICU (intensive care unit) or coronary care unit where a new set of nursing staff will take over. Further management will depend on whether the pain settles down or not and whether any complications occur. Other procedures may include – an angiogram, by-pass operation, balloon angioplasty, cardioversion, and insertion of a pacemaker.

Angiogram: used to ascertain any narrowing of the coronary arteries. A needle is inserted into a large artery in the groin (femoral) and through it a thin catheter is threaded upwards towards the heart and into the coronary arteries. The progress of the catheter is followed on a monitor screen. Once the correct position is reached (coronary artery) a dye is injected through it and X-ray pictures taken as the dye flows though the arteries of the heart. If there is a narrowing and the cardiologist feels that the narrowing can be widened a balloon (built into the tip of the same catheter) is inflated. This is called balloon angioplasty and may avoid the need to have a bypass operation.

By-pass Operation: this literally means the blockage in the coronary artery is 'by-passed' by using a length of vein from the leg (the ends of the leg vein are tied off - this can be done to veins only and not arteries because the blood in the veins would flow through other branches and circulation is not compromised) and joining it to the affected coronary artery (one end above the blockage and the other below it) effectively *by-passing* the obstruction. The narrowed or diseased segment of the artery is not removed. There is no guarantee that the transplanted vein will survive i.e. remain patent but there is a good enough success rate to warrant this procedure if the indications are carefully weighed up.

Cardioversion: If the heart rate is very fast and irregular (atrial fibrillation / ventricular fibrillation) the heart will not tolerate this for long. The problem becomes magnified if the heart has suffered a previous insult (failure, enlargement, previous heart attack). This may be reflected by symptoms of generalised weakness, shortness of breath, dizziness or chest pain (if the coronary arteries are diseased).

In atrial fibrillation there is a risk that blood within the heart chambers is being churned like a 'milkshake mixer' and may produce clots in the blood that could travel out of the heart and lodge in peripheral arteries - in the brain such a clot may result in a stroke. To avoid this complication the rhythm can be jolted back to normal by 'shocking' the heart with an electric current. This procedure is usually done in theatre and the patient is given a short-acting drug by injection to sedate the patient so that he or she will not feel the pain of the shock and will not remember much afterwards. This procedure could save a lifetime of medication and the need for monthly blood tests.

Pacemaker: If the heart rate is too slow insufficient blood will be pumped out to the body. This happens when the impulses or messages that regulate the speed at which the heart beats are not being sent out fast enough. The speed is then determined automatically by impulses sent from an electronic device (pacemaker) smaller than a small cigarette packet that is implanted into the soft tissue of the chest wall and connected by thin electrodes to a chamber or chambers of the heart. If for some reason one needs a faster heart rate than is set on the pacemaker (running for the train) the pacemaker will allow this to happen and once the rate settles down the device will capture the pre-set rate. This is called a 'demand pacemaker'. A pacemaker requires regular check ups. A 'medic alert' bracelet stating that the person has a pacemaker should be carried at all times. Once a pacemaker has been fitted a CT or MRI Scan cannot ever be performed because of the risk of causing an explosion. In the event of death the pacemaker must be recovered before burial or cremation.

In another condition called ventricular fibrillation the lower two chambers of the heart (ventricles) beat very fast and no blood is effectively pumped out of the heart. Accordingly, there will be no detectable pulse and if this irregularity cannot be corrected within minutes ('shocked' back to normal) death will occur. CPR (cardiopulmonary-resuscitation) may keep the circulation going until a defibrillator is available. This is the emergency that most commonly kills in a heart attack – when CPR and shocking the heart could save lives.

Precautions to be taken after the heart attack (rehabilitation)

- Definitely no smoking. Even one cigarette is tempting Lady Luck for another heart attack. Smokers who survive and have another heart attack should have blood tested for cotine/nicotine (for the presence of tobacco) and if found positive should be discharged from hospital and refused further treatment – let alone another by-pass operation!
- Avoid strenuous exercises especially lifting (spare wheel in a puncture) or pushing (stalled on the motorway without petrol). Climbing two flights of stairs is almost the equivalent of normal sexual intercourse in terms of stress and strain. This part of the 'return' to normal need not be denied because of unfounded fears. Often the partner is more afraid than the patient to initiate intercourse for fear of precipitating another heart attack. It is well recognised that such activities engaged with partners outside the marriage carry a greater risk of a coronary event.
- Avoid big meals – redirects precious blood from the coronary arteries to the stomach.
- Avoid exposing the chest to sudden changes of temperature, jumping into or swimming in cold water is not recommended. Deaths in shipping disasters (Titanic) are commonly caused by shock precipitated by icy water.
- Exercise regularly, starting out gradually – 1/2 to 3/4 of a kilometre at least three times per week and increasing to cover five kilometres within an hour after one or two months. Reassurance will come from the 'stress test' (treadmill test) done as part of the post-heart attack follow-up. The patient is exercised on a tread mill and while this is in progress a monitor will continuously record any changes that may occur as the heart is 'stressed' by the exertion. Be prepared to exercise quite hard otherwise vital information that can determine prognosis and the

benefit from any exercise programme will be wanting. Take along appropriate shoes for jogging. If any chest pain is experienced during the 'stress test' the doctor or attending staff must be notified at once. Weight lifting as part of an exercise programme is not recommended. The weight transmits the tension all the way back into the coronary arteries.

- Medication for angina and high blood pressure must be taken regularly. Do not court disaster by proclaiming that the chest pain one is experiencing is a 'wind' or 'indigestion' especially when a diagnosis of one or more diseased arteries has already been established. Men find it more difficult to acknowledge that they have a 'heart problem' and in trying to maintain a macho image shoot themselves in the foot. It is more prudent to place a TNT tablet or GTN spray into the mouth when pain occurs than to be stoical. Furthermore, taking GTN 'in error' will not do any harm provided it is taken lying or sitting down and one can tolerate the headache that often accompanies the medication. This is not a serious side effect.

- Eat more fish and less red meat and dairy products. Lose weight gradually but with determination. Body fat, like any other tissue in the body, must be supplied with blood and oxygen even though it serves no useful function. Compare with a maid that does no work but is paid regularly with hard-earned cash. Get rid of the fat (and the maid).

- Taking Omega 3 – 3 capsules twice daily, Vitamin E 200 IU. – 1 capsule daily, Vitamin C – slow release form – 1 tablet daily and 'Lipotropic Adjunct' – 2 tablets daily can help reduce and may prevent further heart disease. Every person, starting as early as high school, should be taking Omega 3 and Vitamin E (200 I.U.) daily to prevent heart disease and strokes and a host of other illnesses. Prevention will always be better as there is very little that medicine can cure.

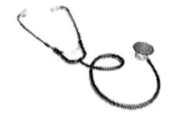

HEARTBURN

This is a common symptom - often treated in a cavalier manner with antacids. The underlying cause is the presence of stomach acid or food containing acid making contact with the lining of the oesophagus (gullet / foodpipe).The latter is not designed for acids, unlike the stomach. The result is a burning sensation in the middle of the chest that may mimic a heart attack. This differentiation can sometimes be difficult and warrants further investigation. To complicate matters further heartburn and cardiac disease may co-exist, and long term acid reflux (backward flow from the stomach into the oesophagus) may lead to cancer in the oesophagus.

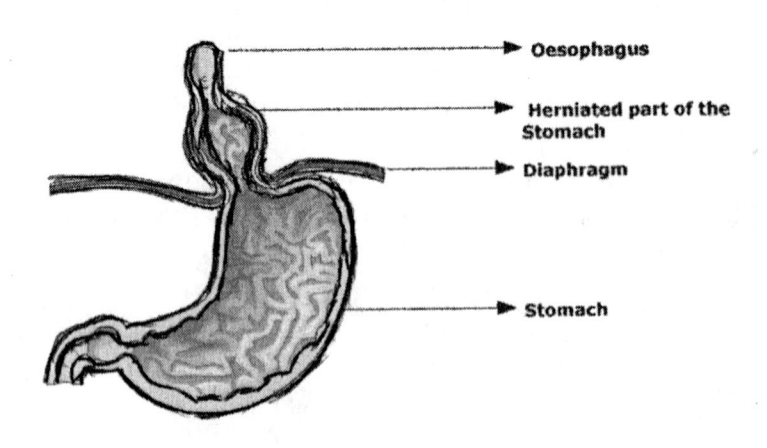

HIATAL HERNIA

Contact between the stomach acid and oesophageal lining may occur in several ways. Hydrochloric acid is very similar to the acid used in swimming pools – except the one in the stomach is much less concentrated. The oesophagus passes through an opening in the diaphragm (muscular wall that separates the chest from the abdomen) before it joins the stomach. This opening acts as a valve to close off the upper end of the stomach after food has passed through. If the opening in the diaphragm is too wide (called a hiatus hernia – hiatus means 'opening') then the diaphragm cannot perform its function as a valve, and food and acid escape back into the oesophagus. This may occur more easily when the person lies down flat after a substantial meal.

The evening meal is usually the biggest and may be eaten late. Sleep is disturbed by a burning, excruciating pain. Though the condition is called 'hiatus hernia' surgery is not an easily recommended option and the success rate depends on careful patient selection.

The following alternative measures may help: –

- Meals should be kept small and at more frequent intervals
- Eating fairly early so that the stomach is not loaded at the time of retiring and the food has been digested and passed out of the stomach with less likelihood of regurgitation (reflux) of food back into the oesophagus
- Avoiding fatty meals because they take longer to be digested
- Sleeping on higher pillows to avoid lying supine. The latter makes it easier for the hernia to slide upwards and drag the upper part of the stomach and its junction with the oesophagus through the widened opening, allowing the acidic stomach contents into the oesophagus
- Losing weight – a tight roll of fat around the abdomen will push the stomach and its contents more easily into the oesophagus
- Bending down to tie a shoelace will also 'squash' the stomach contents into the oesophagus and should be avoided

- Taking an antacid before a meal once the diagnosis has been confirmed (with a gastroscopy). This neutralises the stomach acid and coats the lining of the oesophagus protecting it from the acid
- Avoiding neat (undiluted) alcohol – 'tequila sunrise' can be a hernia's nightmare!
- Avoiding foods that have been shown (from personal experience) to precipitate or aggravate heartburn.

Swallowing air through the mouth while eating (and talking) may cause the stomach to become bloated. The gas will eventually find its way up in the form of gastric flatulence and this belching may force gastric contents into the junction of the upper part of the stomach with the lower part of the oesophagus producing heartburn. Gastric flatulence is mainly due to eating too fast and swallowing air with the rapid mouthfuls of food. Gas that is belched out is due to air that has been swallowed. That which goes out the back passage is produced by bacteria responsible for fermentation (within the large gut) of certain types of carbohydrates e.g. raffinose present in beans. Heartburn occurring for the first time in a middle-aged person should be investigated with gastroscopy. A person suffering from persistent heartburn, having been investigated and found to have a hiatus hernia when the symptoms first appeared, should have a repeat gastroscopy because changes can occur in the oesophagus that may not have been present before. Any change from the usual symptoms should also prompt earlier re-investigation and not the endless repeats of antacids. What was initially an inflammation of the oesophagus (oesophagitis) over time could transform into a malignancy.

Taking neat alcohol (spirits) on a regular basis (tequila/whiskey) may set the stage, by its irritant effect, to cause changes in the lining (epithelium) of the throat, oesophagus and stomach leading to ulcers that may require follow up. In the lower part of the oesophagus cancer can spread from the stomach. An early symptom that should not be ignored is a burning sensation on swallowing hot liquids felt in the area at the lower end of the breastbone (sternum). The incidence of cancer is higher in cigarette smokers. See chapter on Hiatus Hernia.

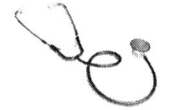

HERNIA

A hernia is the protrusion of a part of the gut through an abnormal opening or weakness present anywhere in the belly (abdominal wall). The common sites where such abnormal openings exist are

- In the groin on either side (inguinal hernia)
- Anywhere along the middle of the front of the belly (e.g. umbilical hernia)
- Less commonly over the upper parts of the thighs close to the groin (femoral hernia)

In the male foetus before birth the testes (testicles) lie within the abdomen and close to the kidneys. From this position they travel down on either side to the lower part of the abdomen and pass through an opening in the groin close to a ligament called the inguinal ligament. The latter forms the boundary between the lower abdomen and the thigh. Once each testis has passed through its respective openings the body closes the gap. However, these apertures are always weak spots in the abdominal wall and if pressure within the abdomen is raised (through obesity, pregnancy, constipation or chronic cough) this may gradually force part of the gut (pictured as a string of sausages) to protrude through the weak spot and, in time, produce a 'hernia' - sausage pushing its tip through the point of least resistance.

Initially, this is visible in the standing position only (internal pressure within the abdomen is higher when upright) and disappears on lying down, or it may protrude when the pressure is momentarily increased e.g. during coughing. As the opening becomes enlarged over time the continual thrusting of the 'sausage' (gut) becomes visible externally as a swelling. If the gut should become trapped within this narrow opening the blood supply to the part of the intestine trapped within this 'ring' may become compromised and lead to gangrene of the ensnared gut. This becomes a surgical emergency and a race to save as much gut as possible.

To avoid this - a hernia should be assessed by a surgeon before this situation arises and a decision taken early about further management.

The presence of *pain* over the swelling, no matter how trivial, warrants urgent medical attention - this may herald the first sign of strangulation of the gut/hernia..

A previous operation with the incision made along the midline of the front of the abdomen may also result in a weakness in the wall through which a part of the gut may try a 'jail break' (picture the sausages imprisoned within the belly and continually searching for a weak spot through which to escape!) and result in a hernia. Similar weaknesses may occur from obesity and multiple pregnancies. Another common site for a hernia is around the navel (umbilicus) usually seen in young children as part of an incomplete closure of the opening through which the umbilical cord passed. This will also require surgical closure. The wearing of 'trusses' to contain a hernia was born out of desperation at a time when surgery was not an easily available option. The underlying principle of the operation is based on closure of the opening.

An unusual strain (lifting a heavy object) may cause sudden herniation ('protrusion') of part of the gut through a narrow opening compromising the circulation to the trapped intestine. This will result in sudden pain and lead to gangrene of that part of the gut unless the blood supply can be restored quickly.

A swelling in the upper part of the front of the thigh may also be due to a hernia – femoral hernia. In this situation the intestine finds its way ('herniates') through a weak spot in the thigh through which the femoral artery, vein and nerve normally leave the abdomen to reach the thigh. This is a more serious hernia as the gut can strangulate more readily than with an inguinal hernia. In comparison with men femoral hernias are more common in females but the commonest in the fairer sex are inguinal hernias.

A hiatus hernia is the protrusion of the upper part of the stomach (still part of the gut) as it pushes its way upwards though a wider than normal opening in the diaphragm. Unlike the other hernias the oesophagus normally enters the abdomen through this aperture. This is very rarely treated surgically. Heartburn is the presenting symptom suggesting its presence and it usually occurs after lying down following a large meal.

The underlying problem in a hiatus hernia is that acid from the stomach is finding its way into the oesophagus (gullet/foodpipe). The lining of the latter is not designed to tolerate this acid.

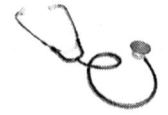

HYPERTENSION

High blood pressure is a common condition and no age group is exempt. It has very few, if any, symptoms and is often called 'The silent killer'. Unless the blood pressure is taken with the appropriate equipment (sphygmomanometer) there is no way of knowing that the pressure could be high enough to cause a stroke. Headache is not a common feature of hypertension as is the popular belief and, if present, should be a reminder that something is amiss. Self medication with analgesics should not be the order of the day without the cause being ascertained.

Blood pressure is recorded as two figures (like a 'fraction') – one above and the other below. The top figure is called the 'systolic' pressure and the lower the 'diastolic' pressure. Each time the heart beats once the contraction pumps out blood into the arteries with a certain force to get it out to all parts of the body: this is the systolic pressure. Once the contraction is over the pressure that remains in the arteries after the blood has been pumped is the diastolic pressure.

If the analogy of a double storey house is used (in a very simplistic attempt at explaining how hypertension works) - in order to get water up to the top floor a certain amount of force or pressure is required. If the diameter of the pipes carrying the water is narrowed (constriction or narrowing of the arteries) more force or pressure will be necessary to get the water to the second floor (rest of the body).

Drugs that relax the arteries can reduce high blood pressure. Factors that narrow the arteries and increase blood pressure include smoking and high cholesterol levels.

Other contributing to hypertension are

- excessive salt intake
- stress
- diabetes
- obesity
- lack of exercise.

high blood pressure damages blood vessels throughout the body, and every part is dependent upon blood supply for its normal function – whether it is the penis, the brain, kidneys or the toes. The initial injury is to the tiny capillaries – vessels so small they are thinner than a spider's web and can only be seen under a microscope, and where the cells in the blood have to move single file! Damage to these small vessels supplying vital organs do not produce symptoms and no test is available that will detect it in the initial stages. Left untreated for long periods the increased pressure will eventually damage the organ. Therefore early intervention is important. Treatment is for life unless advised otherwise by a physician. Changed circumstances and an improved risk profile may bring the pressure back to normal and obviate the need for treatment but the proof of the pudding will lie in the cuff around the arm.

What can one do to improve the blood pressure in addition to taking medication (not in place of it)?

- More effective stress-coping mechanisms
- Reducing the intake of salt
- Cutting down on animal fats (saturated fats) and dairy products (the latter are also animal fats)
- Quitting smoking and, failing this, reducing the number of cigarettes / using 'Nicotine' patches
- exercising regularly
- reducing cholesterol and LDL fats (bad low density lipoproteins)
- reducing the intake of alcohol – one glass of red wine or one tot measure of spirits has been shown to be beneficial to

the heart – this has potential for abuse or putting on weight from the empty calories supplied by the alcohol.

Young patients (under 30 to 35 years) who develop hypertension require further investigation for possible causes for the high blood pressure, as these may be amenable to treatment e.g. a narrowed artery in the kidney. Elevated systolic blood pressure in the elderly was, until a few years ago, considered benign. This policy has changed – those who were left untreated later suffered more strokes than those who received medication.

Normal blood pressure is about 120/80 mm Hg. (measured against a column of mercury) and this should be the target figure for most ages and both sexes. In an elderly person the systolic (top figure) pressure should not exceed about 140 mm Hg. If there is any doubt about the pressure or the person cannot relax easily when the pressure is taken (called 'white coat hypertension') or the person is known to be anxious - a 24 hour ambulatory blood pressure recording may be more informative.

The blood pressure cuff is applied to the arm and is connected to a digital recorder worn around the waist on a belt. The pressures are measured electronically over a 24 hour period during which recordings are automatically taken every half hour. If they are abnormal the times during the day or night when they occurred can be identified and appropriate steps taken to avoid precipitating or aggravating factors. The investigation is worthwhile as unnecessary treatment with expensive drugs (that can have significant side effects to boot) can be avoided.

Once the diagnosis has been established treatment must be taken every day and at the same time each day. Any side effects of the medication, regardless of how trivial they may appear, warrant at least a telephonic discussion with the prescribing doctor. Sexual dysfunction is quite common with certain drugs and should be mentioned candidly. Other common side effects may be headache, dizziness, tiredness, cough and throat irritations, worsening of asthma, passing urine more frequently and dry mouth. With most antihypertensive drugs there is a risk of dropping the blood pressure if one suddenly assumes the erect position. This can cause dizziness and possibly a fall complicated by a fractured hip or skull.

This is the typical scene: in the middle of the night husband (on treatment for hypertension) jumps out of bed to use the toilet. He takes five to ten steps to the toilet, passes about 500 ml of urine (which will drop the blood pressure further), feels faint and then has a black-out, gashing his head on the toilet pan as he falls. Then it's a frantic call to the GP or visit to the Emergency Unit.

To avoid this – first sit up in bed, put out the feet, then stand and once it feels okay (no lightheadedness) proceed. Jumping up to answer the phone has a similar hazard. Blood pressure normally takes a few seconds to adjust to the erect position after the body has been lying horizontal through the night. This can take longer to adjust if the person does not exercise regularly as blood from the legs need good muscle tone to get it back up to the heart again. This adjustment also takes longer with age (the arteries become harder) or if medication is being taken for hypertension.

The organs that suffer most in hypertension are the heart, brain and kidneys – heart attacks, strokes and kidney failure respectively. The most devastating complication must surely be a paralysing stroke occurring in one's latter years, when children have left, and the spouse, often afflicted with one or more chronic illnesses, is left the challenging task of playing nurse to a partner. The spouse has no experience in the management of a disability that may well tax a professional carer.

One of the difficulties in the treatment of hypertension is convincing a seemingly fit person who has no symptoms to take medication (often with undesirable side effects) for the rest of his or her life. And therein lies the potential for life threatening complications.

Any person at any time of his life who has been told that his or her blood pressure is 'slightly high' has the seed sown for possible future hypertension and should have regular check-ups and seriously address the factors that could prevent it. Examining the urine and the eye (using a special instrument called an ophthalmoscope) at intervals is as important as taking the blood pressure. The eye (looking through the pupil with the ophthalmoscope) is the only site in the entire body where blood vessels can be studied to give clues if they are being damaged by hypertension (diabetes or other diseases).

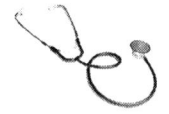

IN–LAWS

In–laws are the parents of the husband *or* the wife. They are not the parents of the wife *and* the husband and no attempt should ever be made to force this issue upon the newly wed wife or husband.

Convention has it that the wife ('forcibly') *inherits* the parents of the husband and his parents 'adopt' the new wife as their 'new' daughter. This concept is more often than not fraught with difficulties. That there are relationships between the wife and the husband's parents that work wonderfully well is beyond question and may function better than with her parents, but these are often the exceptions.

Problems are sown early when the prospective bride does not meet the expectations or approval of the future in–laws. If any of this should be disclosed to the future daughter-in-law it could make relationships difficult, if not impossible and may set the tone for the rest of the life of the marriage. The spoken word will forever be remembered! To change this later will require a mountain of 'reconciliation' and effort if the future is to be made workable and trouble free.

In-laws-to-be often forget that their son may well marry this person they do not approve. The parents of the husband may rely on their son's sense of 'duty and obligation' to his parents to place themselves first – before the interests of his wife. This is unfair to the wife and is tantamount to blackmail. If the son is a spineless adult, whom the domineering parents reared to marriageable age, he most likely would side with his parents and make life difficult and often hellish for the rest of the marriage. The prospective bride should be aware that this husband is married to his parents and will not easily be married to her.

The bride-to-be should also understand that she is never going to become the equivalent of the husband's sister and, as such, there may be constant jockeying for poll position. Do not easily expect to become the in-laws' daughter. If the relationship allows this to happen count it as a bonus. At the very first introduction to the new 'family members' keep an open mind. Do not make hasty judgments about them and *never* voice these opinions or views to the husband: "If you have nothing good to say – say nothing".

On the other hand, the husband may make any comment about his own family. Do not adopt the same views or give any clue that one shares them regardless how strongly he feels about his family and friends or how often he repeats the sentiments. This is a trap for the unsuspecting wife and will forever colour whatever discussion or argument that may follow in the future. The approach of the wife should always be supportive and positive about his family no matter what he may say to the contrary. Encourage him to change his views and be positive. As far as is physically possible try not to live with in-laws no matter how tempting the prospect may seem and regardless of how much money could be saved by living with them, even if it is a temporary arrangement. The latter may stretch longer than expected and leaving may turn out more awkward than anticipated.

The addition of a grandchild should bring joy to grandparents and the respective parents. If undertones of simmering animosities exist before the arrival new power struggles may develop after the baby is born. There may be conflicting views on matters as diverse as the best gynaecologist in town, the softest napkin and what works best for cradle cap. It is difficult overnight to adopt or be adopted by new in-laws and, in the time it may take to get to know them and for them to know one's self, relationships can flounder and much dirty underwear be laundered.

The expectations of all parties concerned may be unrealistic. The wife is outnumbered and she may find herself trying to cope with up to ten or more members of the husband's family (each with his or her own personality and personal problems) let alone trying to adjust to being married and have a husband with his own needs and expectations. It might be better to struggle and live in rented accommodation than be tempted by the husband and his promises of "It will only be for a short while and look at all the money that could be saved".

These decisions should be taken well in advance of the wedding. Better to be forewarned than to go through unpleasantries and sometimes divorce because of in-laws who do not approve of the wife, or the husband who makes his parents the main priority in his life and still expects to have a happy union with his wife. The husband should understand that, while he is not expected to 'divorce' his parents on his wedding day, in the true scheme of things his wife is the next step in the evolutionary ladder, the bearer of his children.

Having sex in the room next to the in-laws may not be in the best interests of all parties concerned. If brothers-in-law are sharing the same house this may have its own drawbacks. The young bride will always be fair game and the potential for discord ever present, both real and imagined.

Relationships between daughter-in-law and the members of the parents family should be allowed to develop over time and hasty opinions and judgements avoided.

The husband's clan will outnumber the wife and the personalities, whims and fancies of each member may only surface over time. In this period of adjustment delicate bonds should not be disturbed and damage from discord should be minimized.

The ability to listen with sincerity and have a genuine interest in the other person is paramount and is universally applicable – beginning with the husband. This is not a skill that is acquired overnight or without practice, and even though it may have been missed in the formative years when adults did not listen as a child it can be learned. One should be open to change and be teachable.

Avoid complaining to the in-laws about their son regardless of what he may be doing that is 'wrong'. This will not endear the wife to his parents. He is of their flesh and blood – "How dare she speak of him that way"! She may not receive any support or sympathy from this quarter and run the risk of creating a permanent rift between her and the in-laws. Injustices within the marriage must be addressed but not at the cost of alienating herself from her husband and his parents. He will not take kindly to being ridiculed or belittled in the eyes of his own family because he cannot rid himself of them - even if he so wished.

In such situations if an objective discussion with the husband cannot resolve the issue the assistance of an arbiter or marriage counsellor should be enlisted. Constant nagging is useless and resorting to this implies that the partner is no longer listening. If he is not listening there is little point in pursuing such an approach Find a new strategy or seek professional help.

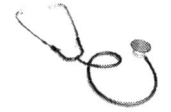

INFERTILITY

The marriage vows do not say aught about fertility and yet nature intended a coupling between the sexes to ensure that the species line is continued. The rest of the trappings of 'marriage' are of our own creation.

How often do marriages flounder because of infertility? How many parents and in-laws of newlyweds have put pressure one way or another when no news of pregnancy was in the offing? Friends and next of kin are also not averse to jibes - "When are we to hear the patter of tiny feet?" - giving little thought to the anguish the couple may already be experiencing without the added stings and slings of the seemingly concerned.

If the main reason for marrying is procreation then couples are advised that, in addition to a certificate of clearance for the HI virus, a valid sperm count report and normally functioning reproductive system should become the order of the day! If this is not to be then couples should understand that the ability to successfully produce (healthy) progeny is not guaranteed by either partner. Guilt and blame for a pregnancy that does not materialise should not rear their ugly heads. Love should be the overriding factor on which marriage should be based – not the results of a positive pregnancy test.

Most infertility clinics rely on some intervention to overcome the problem. Why are more and more couples facing infertility? Alas, for most pregnancy continues to remain a 'hit and miss' affair. There is little planning given to the conception and then, if they are unfortunate, the ensuing pregnancy. Men are defensive when the issue of whether the cause of the infertility lies with their sperm and often see this as a direct attack on their manhoods. A sample of sperm produced at the laboratory is a simple, inexpensive and non-invasive test and it may establish early on the integrity of the testicle. If the sperm are normal the next priority would be to establish whether the ovaries are producing eggs during ovulation and for this the services of a gynaecologist are required. Blood tests may also be necessary to exclude other causes of infertility e.g. a malfunctioning thyroid gland.

There are several reasons for the shrinking size of the modern family. Where the law of nature once dictated that the fittest should survive, and accordingly parents had up to a dozen children, today's smaller numbers of one or two make it imperative that these few are the *best* the couple can produce.

The role of *nutrition* in both the production of and maintenance of the sperm and egg is almost completely ignored. The casual advice to "Eat healthily" is laughable when one considers that to get one dose of Vitamin E, which plays an important role in reproduction, one would have to consume 250 slices of white bread or 4 ½ cups of peanuts or 375 gm of peanut butter per day! It is physically impossible to meet the daily requirements with food alone.

Respected members of the medical profession and people in learned capacities pooh-pooh the idea of supplementation and joke about producing 'expensive urine'! Should it make a difference to one's nutritional status if both partners ate hamburgers every day three times a day for three months? Would this affect their nutrition in general and that of their reproductive organs in particular?

Sperm and eggs do not materialise out of thin air! Nutrients, vitamins, trace elements, enzymes, proteins, fats and carbohydrates are all required, in the first instance, to produce the cells (each sperm and egg are single cells) and, thereafter, maintain them in storage until they are required. These cells are not made instantly the moment intercourse takes place. Sperm cells have a distance to travel from their site of origin and nutrition is necessary for their safe and effective journey from the storage sac (under the prostate gland) via the penis to reach the vagina and thence the uterus. There it must timeously meet the egg that has been carried from the ovary, down the fallopian tube and into the uterus. At their final destination nutrition or fuel is also required for the union of sperm with egg.

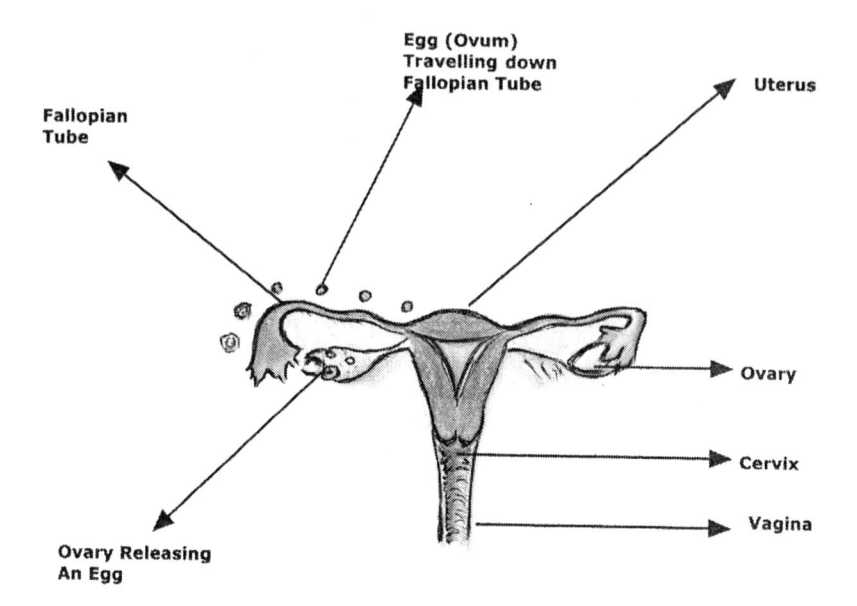

FEMALE INTERNAL GENITAL ORGANS

Although oysters have long been prized as aphrodisiacs – the truth is they contain high concentrations of *zinc* and the testicles and ovaries use zinc in the production of sperm and eggs respectively. Furthermore, they should be eaten two to three days *before* intercourse takes place because sperm are made in advance in the testicles and stored in specialized 'ejaculatory sacs' situated below the prostate gland.

Zinc also helps in the overall growth of the infant through to adulthood and in the development of its reproductive organs. Fruit and vegetables of the 21st century are mass produced with the addition of fertilizer to enrich a soil continually raped of its trace elements e.g. zinc, selenium and molybdenum. The potato looks the same but its nutritional value has decreased over the past 50 to 100 years because the soil can only supply what the farmers add to it. Zinc and its role in reproduction is the furthest thing from the farmer's mind.

Factors that influence sperm dysfunction: –

- The testicles lie outside the body hanging in a sac (scrotum) of loose skin between the legs and nestling in a mound of coarse pubic hair well away from contact with heat generated by the body. The latter adversely affects sperm and this makes it imperative that heat in any form should be avoided
- A hot bathtub could be 'cooking' the sperm – making a shower a healthier alternative
- Wearing tight Jockey-style underwear generates and traps heat
- Similarly, sleeping in such underwear is not recommended
- Children being encouraged from an early age, when the organs are still developing, to wear heat generating underwear
- Wearing skin-hugging 'Lycra' shorts and generating extra heat during exercise

Riding a bicycle, with the testicles straddling the seat and being bounced off it with every stroke of the paddles.

- Shaving pubic hair and losing an effective cooling system and directly exposing the organs to heat from the body – will contribute to sperm damage, deformity or their dwindling numbers.

The use of a lap top computer generates heat that could be the equivalent of barbecuing the testicles under a grill!

The erect posture that man has adopted has another price to be paid apart from that related to the spine. The testicles are more vulnerable to injury whereas quadrupeds have them well out of harms way. Furthermore, natural cooling (cf. the water-cooled radiator in the automobile that relies on motion and air movement to effectively cool the engine) is less efficient when long hours are spent sitting at a desk at work and then hours spent sitting in front of the television. This can hardly make for ventilation the way Mother Nature intended! Exercises (minus the heat-generating-type shorts) like walking and swimming are healthier options.

The missionary position (male on top) during intercourse is ana-tomically ideal for sperm to be deposited closest to the cervix (open-ing of the womb). This can be improved upon by placing a pillow under the buttocks of the female – this tilts the cervix upwards and creates a 'well' for the sperm to collect at the back of the vagina. Once ejaculation has occurred the thrusting movements of the male should be stopped with the penis held as deeply as possible within the vagina; this may also prevent damage to the sperm. In addition, the penis should not be extricated from the vagina immediately after ejaculation so that all of the ejaculate may be discharged. The female should not change position for at least thirty minutes to prevent the precious ejaculate from leaking out of the vagina. Under these cir-cumstances the usual advice to empty the bladder soon after inter-course may be ignored!

Other factors contributing to the decline in fertility are: –

- Cigarette smoke
- Preservatives added to all processed meats
- Refined foods like white bread, white sugar and maize-meal
- Exposure to irradiation (from often unnecessary X-rays)
- Lack of exercise and couples choosing to have babies later

More sperm are being deformed and reduced in both numbers and motility than ever before – the numbers of couples that attend 'infertility clinics' and the increased number of miscarriages bear tes-timony. The sperm and egg, like other cells of the body, have walls or cell membranes that surround them. The integrity of these walls will determine the function and well being of the cells. Vitamin E, Omega 3 fatty acids, the plant sterols and lipids contained in Formula IV Plus and Zinc supplements all play a role in maintaining the health of the cell wall/membrane. The same wall can prevent a virus or cancer causing agent from entering the cell.

These supplements should be mandatory for any couple that is planning a pregnancy and should be taken by *both* partners for 2 to 3 months *before* conception takes place and, thereafter, by the mother for the full *duration* of the pregnancy. This supplementation becomes even more important for the infertile couple. These are not drugs and, as such, will *not* interfere with any fertility programme - fertility clinics would have their clients believe otherwise.

The fees charged for investigating infertility and the measures used to ensure a successful conception are exorbitant. Will the medical profession try to improve the basic nutritional status of the unfortunate couple before embarking on these more expensive alternatives? The August 2002 issue of the Journal of the American Medical Association made the bold comment that the cure for cancer is a long way off because the current amount spent in the United States each year 'researching and treating' this dreaded disease is a staggering $100 billion! What will happen to this money if a cure is found?

The most fertile period each month in a female's reproductive years is the middle two thirds of her menstrual cycle. This is the window in the cycle of four weeks when sexual intercourse should be planned. The intervals between sexual intercourse are important in the male even though the testicles are capable of producing one hundred million sperm a day. Every third day should be adequate – allowing sufficient time for the numbers of sperm to improve.

The best time for intercourse is early morning because

- Chores and stresses of the day are still to be
- The bodies have been rested
- The number of free radicals from tobacco (this sperm-damaging toxin should have been discarded already!) and environmental pollution is lowest – free radicals damage sperm
- Testosterone levels are highest
- Erection is the firmest.
- Children are still asleep

This may require an alarm clock and retiring earlier.

While all these measures play a role in improving or trying to overcome the problem of infertility there is a human element that should not be ignored – that falling pregnant should not become the reason for living and being together. Couples need to be supportive of each other especially in the face of pressure from next of kin and friends, all the other hundreds of unwanted pregnancies and all the other mothers who seem to fall pregnant at the drop of a sperm.

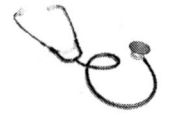

IRREGULAR PERIODS

While it is normal for periods to appear at fairly regular intervals (on average once every 28 days) each female will adjust to her pattern give or take a few days earlier or later than the expected day. It is important to know if menarche (the first period) has occurred and the age at which it did – the average being about the start of the teen years. There has been a tendency for menarche to occur at an earlier age, in keeping with the earlier sexual maturity of girls. This adds to the pressure facing young girls having to deal with bursting curves and the physical capability to bear children yet without the additional benefits of age and experience. This may also have a bearing on the age at which virginity is lost and an unwanted pregnancy risked. The persistent male in heat will find her easy game. Once menarche has been reached the periods may disappear after being present for a few months. There is no immediate cause for concern as they usually return to normal after a time that may vary from one female to another. However, if the periods have not reappeared after about the sixth month a gynaecologist's opinion should be sought.

Bleeding that occurs more than once in a 28 day cycle is acceptable if it occurs for only two to three cycles. If this pattern persists beyond that and, if there are no reasons for avoiding it, the oral contraceptive may be used for two to three months and then be discontinued. This may return the periods to a normal pattern. If the irregularity recurs a gynaecologist's opinion may be necessary, as other medical causes need to be excluded (anemia due to lack of iron, thyroid disorders). If one is taking an oral contraceptive and a day is missed or for some reason was not absorbed (as during a bout of diarrhoea) 'break through' bleeding may occur. More importantly, the contraceptive protection may be lost. In such situations an extra pill should be taken immediately. Using the 'injection' method of contraception ('Depo-Provera') may also result in scanty periods and, much to the inconvenience of the user, cause intermittent or daily bleeding or spotting. This is a common 'nuisance' side effect of the injection but usually settles down after a few months of continued use.

Strenuous and sustained physical activity (marathon training) may alter the periods, causing them to become irregular and even disappear. The solution: reduce the level of activity.

Irregular periods, excessive hair (on the face), problems with infertility and obesity may be part of a condition called Polycystic Ovarian Syndrome. A drug commonly prescribed for diabetics (metformin) has been shown to benefit this condition and improve infertility. It requires referral to an endocrine clinic (dealing with hormones) or a gynaecologist.

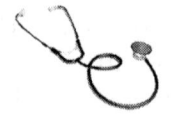

LOWER ABDOMINAL PAIN

There are not many causes of lower abdominal pain. The surgeon arbitrarily divides the abdomen into 9 equal quadrants – three above, three in the middle and three below.

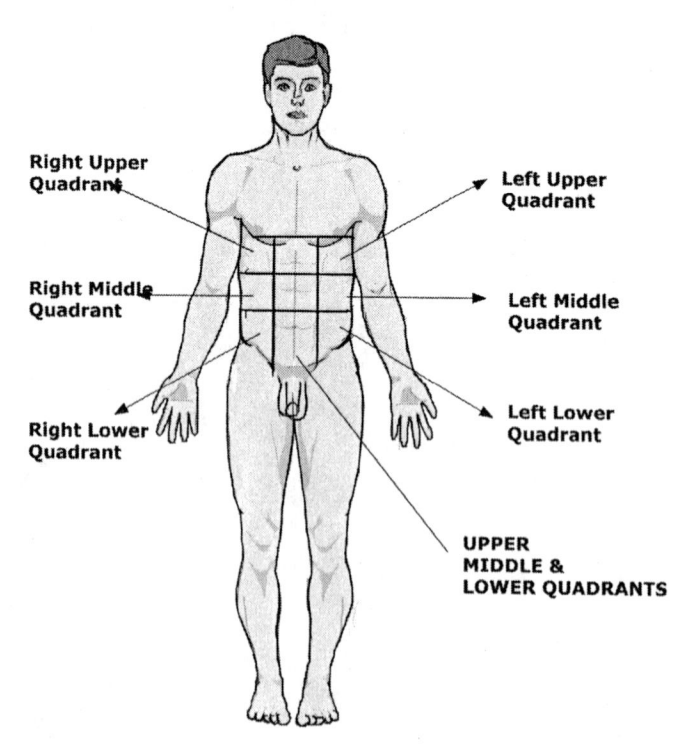

Right Upper Quadrant

Left Upper Quadrant

Right Middle Quadrant

Left Middle Quadrant

Right Lower Quadrant

Left Lower Quadrant

UPPER MIDDLE & LOWER QUADRANTS

THE NINE QUADRANTS (SQUARES) OF THE ABDOMEN

The lowest three form the lower abdomen – the right, left and middle quadrants.

The *right quadrant* contains the

- appendix
- caecum (beginning of the large intestine and where the small intestine ends) in both sexes
- right ovary and the tube that leads from the ovary to the womb (fallopian tube) in the female.

The *middle quadrant* contains

- the bladder (both sexes)
- prostate (males) and
- the uterus (in females).

The *left quadrant* contains the

- rectum (both sexes)
- the left ovary and fallopian tube (females).

These quadrants help in ascertaining the most likely problem relative to the organ present within that particular area or square – "Show me where the pain is?" Has this motive behind the question.

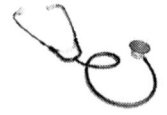

LOWER BACK PAIN

Through evolution Homo sapiens, better known as 'man', has adopted a more erect posture but this relatively new position on two limbs instead of four has not kept pace with adaptations to the spine.

When man bends down the muscles of the spine, instead of contracting to support the vertebral column, are relaxed. The brunt of the strain required to keep the person erect and prevent him from falling forwards onto the face as he bends down is now placed upon ligaments that run down the entire spine – one set in front (anterior ligament) and another behind (posterior ligament). These ligaments are not designed for 'weight lifting' let alone supporting the spine in the bent position. Ligaments have a poor blood supply compared to muscles and have inadequate healing capabilities. It is hardly surprising that lower back pain is such a common ailment. Any measure that can strengthen the back or brace the spine when bending should be almost mandatory to make up for Nature's shortfall when man assumed the erect position

The muscle that plays an important role in supporting the lower back is called the *Pubococcygeus* (pew-bow-cock-siege-yes). It extends from the pubic bone in front (situated just above the penis in the male and in the lowest part of the belly in the female) to the coccyx – the tail end of the lower spine. The muscle can be identified by inserting a finger into the vagina (or anus) and squeezing onto the finger as hard as possible or by attempting to stop the passage of urine in midstream. Tightening the pubococcygeus as hard as possible will help contract and reinforce the muscles of the front of the lower belly, the vagina, back passage (rectum) and the lower back.

Each person should be taught how to almost continuously contract this muscle from a very early age – as diligently as learning the 3 Rs.

Strengthening this muscle will

- Protect the lower spine, its cartilages ('discs'), ligaments and muscles
- Improve the tone of the sphincters (valves) of the bladder and urethra and help prevent incontinence of urine
- Improve the tone of the anal sphincter and prevent incontinence of faeces
- Improve one's sex life by alternatively contracting and relaxing the vagina and penis in the respective partners
- Control contractions during childbirth – helping to relax when the uterus is not contracting and reinforcing the contractions of the uterus when it does and
- Tone the muscles of the belly, which normally get hardly any exercise at all.

Each morning the back and lower limb muscles should be stretched before attempting to get out of bed. Muscles are blissfully unmindful whether the telephone is ringing or that there is someone at the door. Cats and dogs arise by first stretching the entire body – we could learn much from observing those from which we seek to be so different.

The last ten minutes before arising from bed, as one contemplates the day ahead, should be spent in stretching. The muscles of the spine and in particular the lower back and the cervical part (neck) are some of the largest in the body. Much of the injury to them is caused by jumping suddenly out of bed and expecting muscles that have been in a thoroughly relaxed state during almost eight hours of sound sleep, to contract instantly to accommodate a change in posture from supine to 'spring-chicken' erect! One of the commonest causes of muscle injury in sport and exercise is inadequate stretching of muscles. Stretching may be more important than the actual exercise.

The following situations should immediately ring alarm bells so that the body is proactively protected: –

- Lifting supermarket parcels out of the trolley and into the boot
- Bending down to pick up young (and sometimes not so young) children
- Bending down to lift sleeping children to be carried to the car or to bed
- Carrying the bride across the threshold (could bring the honeymoon to a painful end)
- Lifting the spare tyre out of the boot and then carrying the flat one back into the boot
- Pushing a stalled vehicle
- Lifting furniture
- Lifting up patients and invalids
- Digging a hole in the garden
- High jumping
- Carrying children on the neck/shoulders
- Standing at the sink washing dishes
- Bending down to use the bathroom sink
- Bending the lower back to wash clothes or children in the bathtub
- Lifting heavy objects held away from the body
- Bending down to tie shoelaces or remove or put on shoes and stockings and
- Slouching while sitting long periods at a desk or computer keyboard where the desk or chair are often too high or too low

During pregnancy the ligaments in the lower spine and the pelvis are being primed for childbirth by becoming maximally relaxed and stretched to allow for the impending miracle of nature. These ligaments are very susceptible to injury given that the uterus size has increased tremendously as the pregnancy advances and puts greater strain on the lower back. A non-pregnant uterus is about the size of a small adult fist. For a heavily pregnant mother to bend down from the waist and pick up her last born infant (or young child) or other heavy weight off the floor is begging for back injury and, possibly, even surgery in later life.

Another important cause of lower back pain is obesity. This is becoming a contender for the dubious title of the 'second biggest silent killer' – high blood pressure/ hypertension currently holds poll position. Obesity has no symptoms and its presence is only known when a complication arises and, even then its causative role may go unnoticed. Death Certificates do not commonly list 'Obesity' as the cause of death! This 'role' has yet to be properly recognized and dealt with. In one way or another, obesity is linked to diabetes, hypertension, heart attacks and strokes, cancer, fractures and other injuries to which the obese are more prone than their normal-weight peers. The extra weight is carried around the waist and invariably this tends to drag the body forwards and this has to be countered by the spine and its ligaments, which receive little help from the back muscles.

Sedentary jobs and poorly designed chairs that offer little support to the lower spine contribute to poor posture, which, in time, may alter the mechanics of the small bones that make up the spine. These abnormal stresses are passed onto:

- The ligaments
- The small joints (facet joints) that exist between one vertebra (bone of the spine) and the one above and below it
- Cartilages that lie between the vertebrae acting as cushions
- Muscles

These 'discs' as they are popularly known have been blamed for many of the ills that befall the spine but the small joints (facet joints), ligaments and muscles share the responsibility . The 'disc' or cartilage can be likened to a rectangular biscuit with a centre of jam. If there is an abnormal strain placed upon the biscuit (cartilage) e.g.

bending at the waist or lifting a heavy weight off the floor, the hard part of the biscuit may crack either in front (where the bending is producing maximum pressure) or on the side of the biscuit. The soft jam leaks out through the crack and eventually lies in front, on one or the other side or behind the hard part of the biscuit and in this position exerts pressure on the delicate spinal cord (front) or the nerves (sides) that come off the spine between each vertebra.

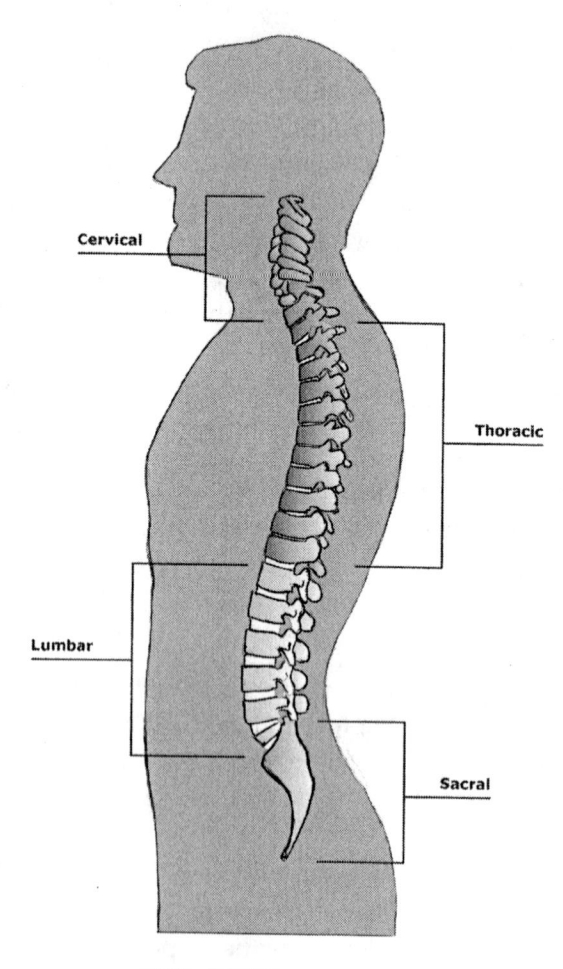

Cervical

Thoracic

Lumbar

Sacral

THE SPINE

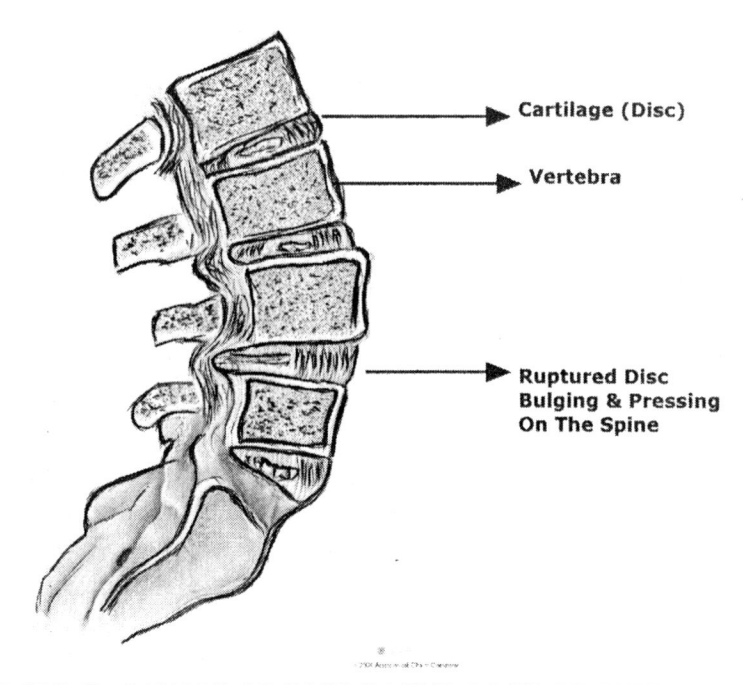

Cartilage (Disc)

Vertebra

Ruptured Disc
Bulging & Pressing
On The Spine

THE SPINE: CAUSES OF PAIN IN THE BACK OR EXTREMITIES

The spinal cord will not tolerate any pressure effect upon itself and will quickly produce pain and signs of weakness depending on the level at which the pressure is being exerted. This is serious and should be treated as an 'emergency'. If the pressure is on the spinal nerves there will be pain and pins and needles sensation on the part of the lower limb that was being supplied by that particular nerve.

From the lumbar spine (made up of five vertebrae) one nerve from the left and one from the right leave the spinal cord between each of the five vertebrae (i.e. five nerves on either side of the lumbar spine) and travel downwards to join the nerves from the sacrum (tail part of the spine) to eventually become part of the largest nerve in the body. This is the sciatic nerve that runs down the middle of each buttock carrying nerves in the lower limb down to the furthest toe.

Pins and needles sensation in the legs (paraesthesiae) and pain may not be indications for surgery as an immediate procedure but *any signs of weakness* of a muscle or group of muscles or disturbance of bladder or bowel (incontinence) is serious and requires urgent referral to hospital.

Pain that does not respond to 'conservative' measures (bed rest, analgesics and anti-inflammatory drugs, physiotherapy, sometimes traction, Omega 3 and Calmag) after a reasonable trial period (4 to 8 weeks) may need surgery for relief. The patient may 'demand' it out of sheer desperation if the pain becomes intolerable and intractable! While surgery may be effective its success cannot be guaranteed.

Current trends in the management of lower back pain do not recommend long periods of bed rest – two to four days as opposed to the seven to fourteen days of not so long ago. Backache that is accompanied by any difficulty in walking (ataxia) or incontinence of urine or stool is a relative emergency as the problem could be a lesion (tumour) of the last part of the spine ('cauda equina' – this means horse's tail because the last part of the spinal cord is unlike the part above it). Picture the spinal cord as a long thick asparagus with branches at different levels all the way from the top to the bottom and the last part as the root of the asparagus that is split up into a number of branches.

Backache may also occur in a person who has psoriasis, which is an inherited skin rash that commonly affects the fronts of the knees, backs of elbows, scalp and ear canal, and sometimes the entire body, producing a whitish or silvery scale that can be scraped or flaked off with a fingernail. Backache in a young man associated with a burning sensation in the penis during micturition (passing urine) and a gritty sensation in the eyes may have a condition called Behcet's syndrome.

Backache in a young person (school age) and for the first time in an older person (50 and above) needs a diagnosis and often X-rays of the spine and pelvis. Radiology is not recommended for every person with back pain because the information gained from this investigation does not always influence the immediate management unless worrying symptoms (that the patient feels) and signs (that which the doctor finds on examining the patient) exist to justify the investigation. It exposes the body to irradiation and should not be done as 'routine' simply because of backache as there is a risk of triggering cancer. Only radiographers and radiologists are qualified to take X-rays and to report on them, respectively; beware the charlatans who are making a business (killing!) out of taking beautiful pictures of zips on trousers and commenting on the state of the spine!

The sudden onset of back pain while lifting a heavy object may be due to a ruptured cartilage (disc) – the biscuit has cracked and the jam (soft centre of the cartilage) has leaked out and is pressing upon the asparagus (spinal cord). This requires fairly urgent medical attention.

An injection (anti-inflammatory) is painful but may help to transfer the pain from the back to the side of the thigh. This is where all intramuscular injections should be given and not on the buttock; the latter site is 'undignified' especially for a female patient and there is a small but real risk of damaging the large sciatic nerve that runs beneath the buttock whereas the side of the upper part of the thigh has no important structures that can be injured.

In addition to the anti-inflammatory agent a combination-type of analgesic (paracetamol+codeine) works better than if either was taken alone. However, codeine is the 'sister' of morphine and has a potential for addiction. Other side effects are drowsiness and constipation.

The following adjuncts in the treatment of backache may also help:

- Hot water bottle (without burning oneself)
- Massage – without applying pressure directly upon the spine
- Electric blanket on the mattress
- The mattress should not sag in the middle – placing a firm board under it helps if the mattress itself is not already compressed by the weight of the patient
- Lying on the floor with the buttocks against the bed and the legs on the bed – like a chair lying on its back – may help take the pressure off the spine
- Tightening the Pubococcygeus as often as possible and especially when any movement is anticipated – getting up, sitting down, about to sneeze or cough
- Regularly stretching the muscles of the spine (like a cat)

- Stimulating (passive) sex will get the blood flowing to the lower spine and pelvis, take the mind off the pain and, more importantly, stimulate the release of endorphins that are chemically related to morphine.

Omega 3 – 3 capsules twice a day and *Calmag* 3 tablets daily are supplements that will add another dimension (and these are not drugs) to the management of back pain. Omega 3 works as an anti-inflammatory and helps to repair damaged tissues thereby reducing the recovery time. *Vitamin C Slow Release* – 1 daily and *Vitamin E* (200 I.U.) – 1 capsule daily are both powerful antioxidants that can 'mop' up 'free radicals' that are produced when tissue injury occurs – as in the inflammation in the structures of the back.

Physiotherapy is not usually advised in the acute phase but may be useful once this is over. Traction does not have universal approval but is an excellent way to keep the patient (literally) tied to the bed to ensure 'strict bed rest'.

Prevention is, as always, better than cure (not that medicine has much it can cure anyway!). To remove the spare-tyre from the boot roll it out instead of lifting. To return the flat one into the boot stand the tyre against the bumper, kneel on the ground, tighten the pubo-coccygeus as hard as possible and lift the lower end of the tyre off the ground and flip it into the boot. This avoids having to lift it.

If the spine is envisaged as the legs or supports of a crane at the dockside and the arms as the 'arm' of the crane the latter has a heavy weight behind it to counterbalance itself or it will topple forward. Similarly, if a supermarket packet is lifted from the trolley with the arms outstretched the spine has to exert a counterbalancing action backwards to prevent the parcel from pulling one into the trolley face forward. If the parcel weighs five kilogrammes this must be coun-terbalanced by a weight greater than this and this places the spine, along with its ligaments and muscles, under strain. Holding the par-cel close to the body (i.e. close to the spine) reduces the distance from the centre of gravity,(which runs vertically through the centre of the spine), making the counterbalance less and therefore less stressful to the back. The message: objects to be lifted should be held as close as possible to the body.

Gardening enthusiasts can prevent unnecessary strain to the back:

- Stretch the muscles of the back, arms and legs before engaging in any physical activity
- Get up at intervals and stretch some more and walk about to get the circulation going
- Dig a hole in the garden by kneeling on a firm foam cushion, not by bending from waist level – as is the common practice. This brings the work surface (the hole) closer.
- Weeding should be done from a seated position on a low stool keeping the lower back erect (a cold draft will cause the back muscles to go into spasm resulting in a stiff, painful back).

Before alighting from bed stretch (as described above), roll over onto the side of the body facing the edge of the bed, drop the feet and legs over the side and, as these are lowered, the arm closer to the bed is used to prop oneself into the sitting position. Stay seated for at least 30 seconds to allow blood to adjust to flowing vertically from a previously horizontal one. This simple manoeuvre places less strain on the back. It also prevents sudden changes of blood pressure that can cause lightheadedness and a risk of falling, especially if one is taking medication for hypertension.

To pick up a child from the floor help the child (not lift) to climb onto a chair or equivalent height and then, while simultaneously tightening the pubococcygeus muscle, carry the child off the chair holding it close to the body. Furthermore, it is less of a strain to carry the child over one or other side of the hip rather than in front of the abdomen – the latter position puts more stress on the lower back. Carrying the child on the shoulders is ill advised because it subjects the entire spine to the extra weight.

In everyday situations that commonly abuse the back the following measures may help:

- Wash basins are positioned too low to spare the lower back. To bring the face closer without straining the lower spine spread the legs apart and, in this position, bend both knees, while simultaneously tightening the pubococcygeus muscle.
- Washing dishes at the kitchen sink would be less of a strain on the back if one foot is placed on a low stool and the feet are alternated. If no stool is available stand with the feet planted firmly apart.
- Washing clothes in the bathtub can be done by kneeling on a firm foam cushion at the side of the tub and leaning into it.
- To tie a shoelace place the foot on a chair while simultaneously tightening the pubococcygeus muscle
- Instead of bending the spine use the 1st and 2nd toes as 'pincers' to pick up appropriate objects from the floor.
- Do not put anything down that will have to be picked up again later
- To pick up a box or other object from ground level kneel down and assess its weight by gently tilting the object to ascertain an easy lift. Then placing one knee on the ground, lift the object with both hands and bring it close to the body (remembering to tighten the pubococcygeus muscle) and then stand.

Gauging the weight of the object by tilting it (not lifting): –

- Alerts the brain to adjust the effort accordingly
- Calls for back up if it is too heavy to be lifted without injury – trying to impress the new bride and carrying her across the threshold is not healthy for the spine and this practice should be discouraged – or the honeymoon may end on the doctor's couch!
- Looks more professional and avoids the sudden realisation that the attempt should not have been made, which would be too late to back out without losing face

As for pushing the stalled car and lifting heavy furniture – *don't*! A useful tool in support of saving one's back from injury lies in a simple statement - "I'm sorry I'm not allowed to do that!" and no further explanation is necessary.

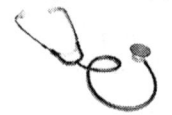

MARRIAGE

Time has changed the significance of this 'formal agreement' between a man and a woman to live together according to the customs of their religion or society.

The twenty-first century no longer acknowledges that marriage has to be 'formal'. There is not the emphasis on a ceremony or the document that seals the priest's blessings 'before God or the law'. The 'agreement' has been replaced by a tacit approval that two people who so desire may live together.

Also relegated into the history book is the understanding that the so-called 'union' should be between a 'man and a woman'. Gay and lesbian 'marriages' have become more acceptable, recognising that companionship and sexual union between same sexes can also be successful. Customs have had to bow to pressure from people more concerned with being in a happy relationship than their 'religious and societal' differences (that may have kept them apart in the past). The emphasis has moved from marriages where happiness had been sacrificed for other priorities like 'staying-married', children, financial security, the sake of the family and friends etc.

To this sea of change should be added the terms 'husband' and 'wife' and, given that relationships have been allowed to cross sexual barriers, this would seem appropriate. These terms should be scrapped and more neutral descriptions adopted that would bury the stereotyping these two words have created for centuries. 'Wife' was intended to mean the female 'partner' in a marriage: little can be further from the truth because 'partner' implies equality and there is little that is equal in many marriages. From early childhood the seeds are sown of future inequalities in marriage. The adults/teenagers that 'marry' are products of a mould that has been cast long before the two people meet. How does the developed product change roles at this late stage when they are married? These roles have been indoctrinated from a time when little John mowed the lawn and practiced driving the family car in and out the driveway whereas sister Jane helped with the dishes and mastered the skills of sewing and cooking. How do these roles, skills and interests developed in childhood change simply because two people find each other in adulthood and decide to live together? How easy it is for John after he has 'wed' to watch television while his wife darns his socks and does the dishes or dinner. And Jane may well wonder how her role is little different from John's wife's and yet she married a man of her own choice.

John does not introduce his work business partner to people with the rejoinder "Who is subservient to me and is available to do my bidding at a moments notice because that is how the business agreement was designed". The term 'wife' in the introduction "This is my wife" immediately conjures up a picture of a person who can cook, clean, procreate, care for the home and in-laws, cater for parties, play nurse when John is down with the 'flu or the children have diarrhoea and have vomited all over the carpet, bring in the washing from the line when rain threatens the clothes she has washed, tidy the lounge quickly when visitors drop in unexpectedly on Sunday morning , engage in scintillating sex and move on to getting breakfast ready while John recovers from his spent testosterone, remembers when the library books are overdue and picks up the children from school. And none of this even begins to address the role of the 'working wife' who goes out to supplement John's income.

John's introduction to people as "Husband" immediately defines his masculine sex, the boss, the decision maker, the driver of the car when the family goes out, the protector of the family – whether it is an intruder in the middle of the night, the receiver of revenue or the irate neighbour next door, the provider of income, of love, of sperm and a strong arm when aunt Martha dies, 'The do it your self know all things mechanical expert', the one who gets to make decisions like which programme is best on television, where the family goes on holiday, knows when the overdraft limit has been reached, why the exchange rate is falling, why there is no petrol in the car and is the one who tells junior about the facts of life. Until mothers and fathers re-examine the roles they assign to their offspring, either from their own upbringing or personal experiences, the status quo of future Johns and Janes and their stereotyping as 'husbands' and 'wives' will mar future relationships between prospective men and women. Husbands will continue to live out their programmed roles and wives will follow suit. Nevertheless, the rules are changing – women do not wish to be seen as the 'wife' of the past.

Husbands may be less anxious to see the changes rung in, not only because they may have been 'indoctrinated' from childhood but their changed role in a relationship may mean the loss of 'privileges' they would much rather hold on to. The new 'partner' in today's relationship will be working harder. But a beginning has to be made because women are changing beyond anything their parents ever expected. One sees this in the number of 'marriages' that fail and the reasons for their failure. When divorce threatens or becomes a reality do the parents of the separated partners re-examine the formative years of their children and challenge the stereotyping they created for the now divorced couple?

Changes in the childhood of young people need to be introduced as a matter of urgency because these are the future adults who will in a short time (ten to fifteen years) come to meet others with whom they may decide to enter into a 'partnership'. The end product on the conveyer belt is running into trouble faster than changes are being made earlier on the production line that will help them cope with the changes that 21st century living are forcing onto them as adults.

If relationships are to survive longer for the sake of future men and women and children (who suffer incredibly when partnerships break up) and if the ranks of divorced men and women are not made to swell even more – then John must understand that the soccer that he played with a passion before he decided to enter into a partnership with his new found mate must not be used to cover for all the missed suppers and birthdays at home and the late nights and alcoholic binges at the club after the game. The idea "Why should I relinquish my activities just because we are 'married?'" perpetuates a stereotyping of the typical male cultivated and nurtured in childhood – something that he cannot afford to continue into a 'marriage' or more appropriately a 'partnership'.

John will have little knowledge about his wife except that which he will see and know for himself from the moment he sets eyes on her. For anything further than that he will have to rely on the hearsay of his wife and anybody who is familiar with her formative years before he met her – her parents, brothers, sisters, relatives, friends and, perhaps, photographs.

There may be things about his 'wife' that she may find difficult to divulge. How does she describe that the reason she cannot handle her boss is because her own father beat her whenever she did anything wrong or that her uncle raped her in the garden shed when nobody was looking and therefore she cannot have sex with the light on or feel comfortable with his body? Only love and understanding and the assistance of a therapist, sought early rather than late, may resolve such and other problems.

How many partnerships recognise that, just as the electrician is best qualified to fix the wiring in the house, a marriage counsellor is the one best qualified to help with difficulties that may arise in a relationship between two people? How often does the husband cling to the image of the 'macho male' who believes that he can "Handle it himself" and that "It's no big deal" and "I don't need to spill my guts to a total stranger" and "Since *you* think there is a problem then *you* go to the therapist" and "I don't need no hot shot counsellor telling me how to run my life" and "I went once – how many times do you want me to go?" How often does he see this as a betrayal more than an attempt at getting the person best qualified to do the job of fixing the 'wiring' in a relationship?

Physical violence in a partnership has no place whatsoever – that is the long and short of it. Human beings do not eat grass, fly or put salt in tea – it is not the done thing. Hitting one's wife is not the done thing. More often than not it is the 'husband' who is responsible for the perpetration. If it ever should happen that a man did inflict such abuse (whether he used his hand, head, fist, foot, penis or voice it matters little) by the wildest stretch of the imagination this could be 'allowed' to happen once and only once.

If it should happen a *second* time that is the signal to move out of the relationship no matter what he says or does. Break this rule and one must be prepared for future violence because the *third time is simply a matter of time* before it happens again – and again and again.

A man may be forgiven the first time but it can never happen a second time. Furthermore, the atonement for the violation must be overwhelming and sustained and every effort made to reconcile, preferably with the help of a psychologist or marriage counsellor. Any reluctance to seek professional help should be seen as an attempt *to cover up* and even *deny* that there may be a problem. Agreeing to see one should allow for open discussion. Attending a single therapy session is tantamount to not attending at all! But this may be used repeatedly in future altercations – "I went as you told me to and it did nothing! I don't need to go again".

No amount of bribery of any kind, repentance or promises to be better and that "It will never happen, again I swear it" should be accepted. The *only* next step after the second assault must be the appointment to the psychologist and a strict adherence to the therapist's plan of treatment and follow up. Any departure from this must be seen as a serious breach and the likelihood that an amicable future is unlikely.

The reasons for the violence are of no consequence. It could also be that the other partner 'aided and abetted' and made the 'violence' the culmination of a number of aggravating factors; but the overriding point is the abuse has taken place.

It has been said husbands or men, in general, do not know how to communicate the way women do. This sentiment ignores that, as boys, the luxury of crying out their troubles was not seen as acceptable behavior – not quite as their sisters could. A crying boy was not viewed too kindly by the male parent let alone by the boy's peers. To the father a crying son symbolised the 'sissy', viewed with embarrassment and a sense of failure. This same boy becomes the adult husband. When does the adult learn how to verbalise or communicate? - Certainly not in the middle of an argument with his partner.

It is often ill understood that there are important physiological differences between men and women where sex is concerned. The reasons for the 'misunderstanding' may have their roots buried in childhood, in school and in the teenager's own attempts to find answers to questions that arose out of their burgeoning gonads. It may well be that women have much to learn about these differences and ignorance about them makes relationships more difficult.

How does the young teenage girl educate herself with knowledge about sex that will help her cope in the setting of a sexual relationship in or out of a marriage? If the education was adequate (and it is not) why are there so many unwanted pregnancies and so many divorces?

It is still easier for the medical profession to enquire about a patient's diabetes or high blood pressure than their sexual history. It is not often that the primary reason for the consultation is sexual discord – though this is gradually changing. Victorian inhibitions, religious and parental influences and other factors all play a role in making candid discussions about sexual problems difficult. The medical profession needs to overcome these hurdles so that the consultation encourages frank discussions.

Sex is the one aspect of a relationship that no person outside of it may be privy to. If a problem did exist with whom would it be discussed? And who will divulge "Excuse me my wife refuses to give me sex!" What male ego will be able to take the battering of such an admission?

Neighbours, friends and relatives may have knowledge of the state of the finances of a couple and who is having an affair with whom and how much alcohol people are guzzling, but who will get to know that Jane is refusing her husband sex because he: –

- Comes home late
- Is usually drunk
- Gives her no money

- Pays more attention than is becoming to the young thing in the miniskirt
- Refuses to allow her to go out to parties or to work or to visit her mother
- Refused to take out the garbage
- Did not lend a hand with the dishes and watched television until the late movie ended and then wanted passionate intercourse while she was exhausted and trying to sleep.

The husband does not have a mistress and he is not about to pick up the classifieds and call an escort agency. And he may not care to masturbate – why should he resort to that when Jane is right there next to him in bed with her back turned towards him and snoring to boot; totally oblivious to the yearning in his loins that refuses to settle down no matter which way he tosses and turns?

How will his conscience allow him to wake her up either deliberately or by 'accident' as he introduces his icy feet close to hers in the certain knowledge that this is known to lighten her slumberous state? How does he impose his own selfish needs upon this dear wife who worked all day, tended to the kids and their dozens of needs, cooked supper and washed up afterwards and who now is deservedly claiming her well earned rest and sleep? Should she be expected to throw in good five-course-sex into the bargain?

At the time all this mental anguish is taking place Jane's husband has only one overriding concern – to relieve the mounting tension that has been building up in his private parts. Beginning with the blonde bombshell he met at the office and fueled by the fact that he has been 'dry' for four days and that late movie with the naked couplings, all of which have added more determination than ever and now he is faced by this familiar derrière that has all the hidden potential to come to life and put him out of his misery. But Jane is sound asleep and blissfully unaware of the erection quivering in the background. Should he wake her and will he be the 'son of a bitch' if he did? And if he does not she will remain fast asleep and he will stay awake and she may never know that he desperately needed sex.

The morning after he finally dropped off to sleep and the testosterone remained 'unspent', Jane does not understand why he could not pick up the kids from after care like he always does, did not put out the bin and he knows it is the day the garbage truck comes by, say she looked beautiful in her new blue suit and did not kiss her before leaving for work. Jane is certain in her own mind that the reason for his behavior cannot be that he did not have sex last night because they did it only four nights ago! How often does he need sex anyway? Why had he not helped with the children or the washing up after supper then she might not have been so tired afterwards? Why didn't he wake her up nor do something himself? Why must she always be the one to initiate sex?

On the other hand, she may also "Thank God he crossed his legs and slept it off" because she certainly was in no mood for sex last night! And even if she did let him 'come from behind' she hates the wetness that forces her to get up and go to the toilet and didn't the doctor say she was not to go to bed after sex without emptying her bladder first? All of this will disturb her sleep.

What stands out amidst this sea of dilemma is that there is no "We" or "Us" – it is all "I", "He" or "She". As long as this status quo remains the individuals see each other as separate and not belonging to a partnership where there is a 'team effort' instead of a pair of race horses each pulling in different directions. Business partners will be more productive if they worked in harmony with each other. They can maintain their identities but the common goal should be the success of the venture (marriage) where the benefits of the partnership are shared.

New ways must be constantly found to make the partnership or marriage work – just as in a business. This takes some effort. Every now and again 'board meetings' are necessary to reassess progress, iron out problems, and reward the achievers and give recognition for jobs well done. How many marriage partners remember to say anything good about each other or show appreciation for the effort each puts into the partnership? The true merits of each partner will only become noticeable when one or the other becomes disabled, diseased, divorced or dies. While all the yesterdays are important for determining the quality of today the yesterdays have no other value save the memory of them. It is the now and the immediate future that counts.

What is often missing is advance planning so that sex does not become a hit-and-miss affair, where there is an excellent chance of missing out if each partner is expecting the other to understand the unspoken. The husband expects that the wife will know that having had sex four times last week has little bearing on the moment at hand. It could just as well be that the four times never happened – today's need for sex has no bearing on what happened yesterday. Yesterday has been long forgotten but the wife is expecting that it should hold good for x number of nights to come. This is physiologically erroneous and probably responsible for much of the ignorance of the sexual needs of each partner.

Sex for the male happens at two levels: one takes place in the brain and the other at the level of the penis - seeing the blonde with the miniskirt will only make an immediate impression at the cerebral level. John will not get an erection because he laid eyes upon her. As long as it is happening at this level he is safe in fantasising and technically, he is not having an affair because nobody except he is aware that the blonde has created any impression at all. If the blond in question and he were to sneak into a closet together the deed is as good as done and no amount of explaining to the contrary will matter after that as the arousal becomes penile.

No matter how strong John may be in terms of his fidelity, if the circumstances are made convenient then anything is possible and the safety factor should be that the circumstances must, as far as is physically possible, never be made 'convenient' for an illicit relationship to happen. The level of arousal can be changed from the cerebral to the penile very quickly. It can happen within minutes of entering the closet. The secret John should have learned is *never* to enter that closet or his goose is well and truly cooked. His brain will have no difficulty in changing gear from fantasy to the reality of an intercourse, more so because the mental imagery has already been introduced by prior visual stimulation. All that remains is to change mental to physical.

Each partner should understand the mechanics and the power of their sexual urges to never allow themselves into a situation that can lead to sex. Do not bring the chocolate into the house and then expect not to want to eat it! The power of the will is not that strong and it is safer not to put it to the test. The instinct to have sex is more powerful than any willpower, social mores, conditioning and partnerships can put up in defence – even presidents are not immune!

Jane, on the other hand, is generally protected by the fact that sexual arousal is a slower process and requires much more genital arousal than is available at any given moment. It will take a lot more foreplay than stepping into a closet will afford to prepare her vagina for intercourse Sexual arousal for her will not happen urgently unless she has been *primed* before she enters said closet. What is depicted in movies, where both partners have a passionate quickie, is more to titillate the voyeur than happens in reality. This is not denying that it does not or cannot happen but this is not the norm – women generally need much more to get them sufficiently aroused before they can have passionate sex. What holds in these situations of illicit sex that makes it so exciting is the age-old thrill of the 'chase'. The moment ejaculation has occurred the whole 'affair' will seem so pointless in terms of the price that may have to be paid. It is the chase that is exhilarating more than the actual ejaculation because that orgasm that moments before seemed the most important event of the decade, will pale into nothing the moment the last thrust dies out.

When sex is expected to be a five course meal on each occasion time, tiredness and lack of motivation or interest may militate against intercourse taking place at all. Where John's basic sexual need is considered there does not have to be a five course meal – a quick sandwich may suffice but this requires an understanding of the differences in physiology between men and women. It also has to do with love and understanding and not allowing thoughts of "Why must I?" "Why should I?" creep into a relationship.

If "Why should I?" does rear its head whenever compromise is necessary it no longer becomes a relationship based on an understanding that there are physiological differences between men and women. The easier choice of ignoring these differences exist is the basis of much of the discontent that mars many relationships - resulting in so called 'sexual incompatibilities'.

One basic tenet that is often missing in most marriages and relationships is the ability to listen with the intention to act upon or take cognisance of what is being said. This is different from listening and doing nothing. People who live together for a period, even if it is for a weekend may find that Friday night when the relationship is "new" may not be quite like Sunday morning after having been thrown together for 48 hours. The newness and novelty of the meeting becomes familiar and everyday boring. The darling of one's passion becomes a mother and along with this all the responsibilities that accompany parenthood – couples stop listening to each other. Married partners cannot pack up and go their separate ways once the weekend is over. Re-introducing that mystery of Friday night becomes part of the work required to keep the relationship alive and interesting; the scintillating dialogue of the honeymoon should not be allowed to grind down to the Sunday bore.

To an extent communication between two people, who have been living together for a length of time, does not all have to be verbal. The ability to pick up messages from body language and little hints and signals requires that both partners must be in tune with each other. It does not work well if one partner, for whatever reason, chooses to ignore a signal and then defends the omission with the reply that nothing was verbalised. Couples who can use this marital telepathy and combine it with adequate verbal signals can cut out the many molehills in the valley of a thousand hills that are strewn across the paths of many marriages. It requires thinking and planning ahead: John's wife is late from work – John then gets on with preparing supper and organizes the kids. This is a far cry from "Where the hell were you?" and "Couldn't you phone and say you were going to be late?" and "The kids haven't been washed or fed yet!" This is the same John who will later wonder why it is his wife's rear end he is staring at - when he should have been having mind-boggling sex!

The influence of hunger and alcohol in a partnership also deserve special attention. If supper is served at 6 pm and an argument erupts at midnight or thereabouts it is possible for blood glucose levels to fall below normal levels. Obviously this will depend on the amount and type of food that was eaten. A fattier meal would take longer to digest and a meal based mainly on carbohydrates will have 'disappeared' sooner. This effect is compounded if no supper is received or eaten or if alcohol was taken earlier (before the quarrel). Alcohol itself can lower the blood sugar and, if the liver does not supply the extra glucose to make up the shortfall for not having eaten supper or the increased demand for glucose that occurs during a heated argument, the blood sugar may fall even lower. The more adrenaline one produces the more glucose is released from the liver.

A low blood sugar will make the person irritable, restless; have difficulty in concentrating (in diabetics glucose levels may fall due to medication) become agitated and outright aggressive. This is hardly the setting for a 'discussion' let alone an argument. The message is simple make certain that one is not dealing with a low blood sugar when having a 'discussion'! To add to the confusion these discussions may go on for hours into the night and the blood sugar levels, which were normal at the outset, may fall four hours later when the argument has become heated or shows no signs of settling. Smother the argument with a welcome snack. It has been said before that "The way to a man's heart is through his stomach!".

Every long-term relationship or partnership should have a basic plan for sex. Both partners should have used this 'basic plan' over the years – finding out likes and dislikes, what works and what does not. This staple diet should be recognised and respected for what it is and the 'routineness' of sex should not then be an issue.

To prevent the basic 'sex plan' from becoming boring every now and again it should be revised or added to for the sake of variety and keeping interest alive and fidelity in check. Couples who ignore the need for change may well find the spark gone out of their marriage and a risk of straying – to get elsewhere what they could not get at home. And yet the wife has been known to say, with righteous indignation, "But I gave him all the sex he wanted". The basic plan may have vegetated into the garden variety of humdrum sex.

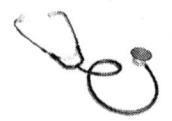

MIDDLE ABDOMINAL PAIN

Pain across the middle of the abdomen is commonly related to the large intestine. If it is *colicky* (coming in spasms or waves), is associated with diarrhoea or a loose stool (not watery) its link to the large gut and 'gastro-enteritis' is very likely.

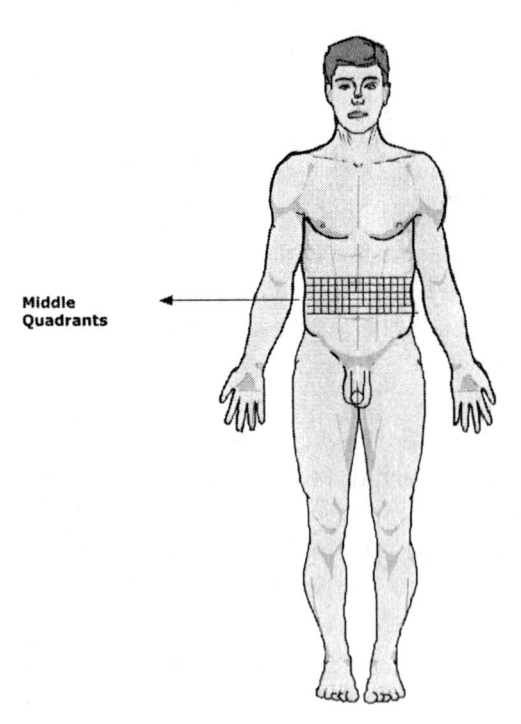

Middle
Quadrants

THE MIDDLE QUADRANTS OF THE ABDOMEN

A dull persistent pain in the centre of the belly (middle quadrant) or just above it especially in a person who *also* suffers from hypertension (high blood pressure) should make one suspect the large artery - abdominal aorta. An aneurysm (dilatation of an artery) of this vital vessel may produce such pain and have catastrophic, often fatal, consequences if it ruptures. Most of these aneurysms, (called 'triple As' - AAA - abdominal aortic aneurysm)are completely 'silent' (have no symptoms) until they rupture (bleed).Ultrasound examinations (used in pregnancies) can diagnosis such an aneurysm and an elective (planned) operation as opposed to an emergency can prevent a life threatening outcome.

An umbilical hernia is due to a weakness of the umbilicus or navel through which a segment of gut gradually pushes through and produces a swelling. This may not be visible at all times and could be 'pressure dependent', initially appearing only when the pressure within the abdomen is increased e.g. in the standing position or during straining when constipated. The hernia may cause pain in the region of the navel and this may be aggravated by attempts to sit up (increased intra-abdominal pressure). Umbilical hernias in adults do not resolve without surgery. If left untreated they enlarge with time and run the risk of becoming strangulated (portion of gut is trapped within the narrow opening of the hernia and its blood supply cut off). This is a surgical emergency – the trapped gut can become gangrenous.

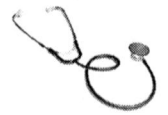

MUSCLE CRAMPS

This is a common condition in which a muscle or group of muscles go into spasm i.e. a state of *painful contraction*. While it is usually short lived (minutes) it can be quite crippling at the time. They may occur at rest and particularly at night after a day of unusually strenuous exercise. The precise reasons for the cramp are unknown.

It may occur during exercise and is the nightmare of the long distance runner. Muscles that have not been 'primed' for use, i.e. not been allowed to be gently stretched before and after the exercise, will be more prone to spasm – this stretching is as important as the actual exercise. Cramps may also plague pregnancy and those on medication with diuretics ('water tablets')

It has been observed that if the lower limbs are exposed to cold a sudden random movement may trigger a cramp resulting in a hard contraction of the affected foot or leg muscle. The contraction cannot be relaxed voluntarily and only by massaging or vigorously stretching the muscle will it relinquish its vice like grip!

Observing a cat or dog arise from sleep, stretching itself from head to tail, should teach that animals instinctively observe the protective value of priming muscles before putting them to use. The media often carry advertising for mattresses that suggest that jumping out of bed like a spring chicken is the macho way to start the day. How often has one jumped out of bed slavishly to answer the shrill demands of the telephone or doorbell giving little thought to muscles that have been asleep for hours? It is little surprise that backache supports the livelihoods of so many branches of the medical fraternity.

After a night's sleep, and before one gets out of bed, five to ten minutes should be spent stretching oneself – emulating a cat. With a bit of practice this can become a pleasurable way of arising and should be done lying on the back, left and right sides and finally on the belly.

These stretching exercises should also be done before any physical activity – pushing the car, digging a hole in the garden, having intercourse or preparatory to lifting an object. Athletes and weightlifters better understand the importance of the 'warm up.

Five minutes spent first gently warming up the muscles (running slowly on the spot), and giving the circulation a gentle kick-start and another five spent slowly stretching the muscles and holding it in the stretched position for thirty seconds at a time, and the same routine followed after the exercising is completed, will help to protect the muscle from injury and cramps.

Maintaining adequate fluid (water) intake is also often neglected and, if the exercise is strenuous and salt is lost from heavy sweating, sodium (table salt) will need to be replaced along with water to prevent cramps. It is not often appreciated that muscle cramp (pain) is the body's warning device to 'force' one to stop the insult to the muscle to prevent more significant injury from taking place.

Of all the nutrients calcium is most often deficient in the diet and the swing away from the fat and salt laden cow's milk will make calcium deficiency even more real.

Nature did not intend man to meddle with the milk of the cow. While skimmed milk has a lowered fat content and the calcium content is normal the fat is necessary for adequate absorption of this mineral from the gut. Furthermore, any calcium supplement or dietary calcium requires the correct concentration of magnesium and Vitamin C for optimal absorption. The company that manufacturers the product determines its quality and efficacy. Athletes who exercise regularly will lose calcium from their bodies and this is another reason for additional supplementation.

Though laboratory testing of magnesium levels in the blood may reflect 'normal' levels muscle cramps may remain enigmatic, often responding to calcium *and* magnesium supplementation.

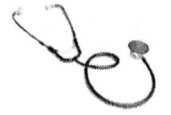

NECK PAIN

Pain in the back of the neck may arise from muscles in the area or the cervical spine. Muscle pain usually has a precipitating cause – e.g. sleeping awkwardly may put the neck muscles into spasm and the head is tilted towards the inflamed side. Movement of the neck on the affected side will be painful.

A cold draft (driving long-distance with the window down) or working with the neck in an abnormal/awkward position (painting the ceiling) may also produce this 'wry neck'. However, there should be no fever accompanying this pain. Fever and pain and the inability to bend the neck forward or put the chin on the chest makes the diagnosis meningitis until proven otherwise. It is safer to have a doctor decide whether there is an underlying reason like tonsillitis to explain the fever and pain on forward flexion of the neck. Missing a diagnosis of meningitis will be disastrous.

A whiplash injury to the neck may occur in a road traffic accident when the vehicle is struck from behind. This may cause pain in the neck (without a fever) and this symptom could occur 24 to 48 hours after the accident. A medical examination is mandatory after a suspected neck injury to exclude trauma to the cervical spinal cord and its nerves. It may be prudent to have the neck X-rayed if such an injury is suspected. Any weakness of the arms, hands or fingers or sensation of numbness (inability to feel normally with the fingers) or pins and needles warrants medical attention as soon as possible. Any person involved in an accident (the nature of which may not always be apparent at the time) must be assumed to have a spinal injury until medical personnel have made an assessment and before any attempt is made to move the victim. A potentially treatable injury can be rendered disastrous.

Cervical spondylosis is a fairly common condition of advancing years. The cartilages ('discs') between the bones of the vertebrae become narrowed with time bringing the vertebrae closer together and thereby 'pinching' the nerves that leave the spinal cord on either side between each pair of vertebrae. Pain will occur in whatever parts of the neck, shoulder, arms or fingers that are supplied by the relevant nerve. All the nerves that supply these parts must come from the spine. For example, if the nerve that comes out of the spinal cord between the 4th and 5th vertebrae (there are 8 nerves in this part of the spine – called the cervical spine) is compressed or inflamed the pain will be experienced along the neck on the affected side down to the shoulder. This gives the clue at what level the nerve is being affected and which disc is probably causing the problem.

Though the pain may be severe, unless there is evidence of muscle weakness, the general rule in its treatment is to observe a conservative approach i.e. no operation until at least 4 to 8 weeks of rest, a collar around the neck, anti-inflammatory drugs, Omega 3 (salmon oil), physiotherapy and, possibly, traction have failed to relieve the pain. However, if there is any evidence of pressure or damage to the spinal cord (proven these days with an MRI or CAT Scan) then the decision to have surgery may be made earlier. If there is no improvement in the pain after a fair trial of a conservative approach surgery may be a welcome alternative. It should be understood from the outset that a successful outcome cannot be guaranteed. A 'wait and see policy' is often rewarded with a resolution of the pain, and unnecessary surgery avoided

Tension headaches have their origin in the neck muscles. The entire scalp sits upon the skull like a baseball cap worn back-to-front – the sun visor part being the neck muscles. If these are tense from stress or anxiety the spasm is transmitted into the scalp muscle producing the typical headache. It's no small wonder that massaging the neck muscles helps relieve the headache. Chewing gum and bruxism (habit of grinding the teeth when under stress or during sleep) may cause pain around the temples.

Neck pain requires a diagnosis to establish the cause. If it does not settle within a reasonable time (for the diagnosis that has been proffered) complacency should not become the order of the day. While neck pain may be common and tumours of the cervical spine are not this possibility should be considered when common does not behave as common should.

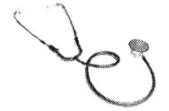

OSTEOPOROSIS

This term means 'bones with holes'. Bone has a unique feature not shared by any other organ. While the outline of bone grows to attain adult size the bone cells within it are continually making and breaking themselves down and this goes on throughout life. A fractured bone is beginning to heal itself the moment it breaks!

During the 'making' phase *osteoblasts*, the bone cells responsible for making new bone, need calcium and other ingredients like (magnesium, Vitamin C, Vitamin D, oestrogen) to assist in the process of repair. Women who are postmenopausal and those with inadequate calcium in their diet have empty 'holes' in the bones where calcium should have been deposited. The bones resemble 'Aero' or 'Crunchie' chocolates – the holes representing the areas where new bone was not formed. This is the basis of osteoporosis and it is not surprising that such bones break so easily, especially at sites that face maximum stress from weight bearing e.g. the neck of the femur (thigh bone) in the hip joint and in the lumbar (lower back) vertebrae.

Every year in the USA there are over 200.000 women who suffer fractures of the hip alone and of these 30.000 die. Death can happen at the time of the fracture as a direct result of it or later as a complication of the fracture. The elderly woman who breaks her hip and then lies immobile in bed is susceptible to chest and bladder infections, pressure sores, clots in the leg veins, constipation, and further loss of bone from the inactivity. One of every four women who sustain a fracture of the hip will die from it! And the main reason for this, and other fractures, is deficiency of calcium. Women ignore this mineral and may learn of its deficiency only when an X-ray for a fracture shows the bones to be osteoporotic. They pay dearly for this deficiency – sometimes with their lives.

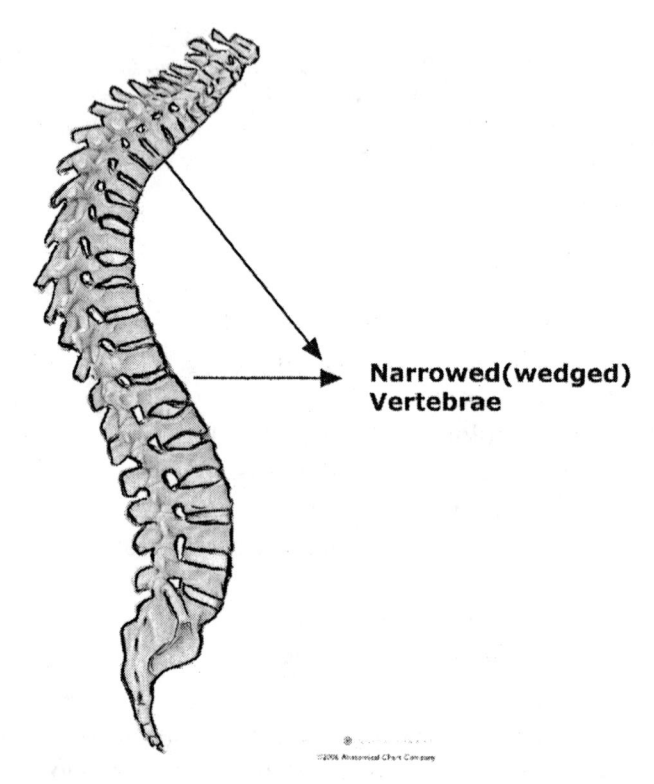

Narrowed(wedged) Vertebrae

VERTEBRAE SHOWING THE EFFECTS OF OSTEOPOROSIS

Females are at special risk for the development of osteoporosis because: –
- Calcium is missing (in adequate amounts) in infancy and through the formative years when the skeleton needs it most
- Menstrual periods lose further calcium (and iron)
- Pregnancies will lose calcium and iron to the 'parasitic' foetuses along with
- Breastfeeding,

- Menopause, with the cessation of oestrogen production by the ovaries, is the final insult depleting the bones of calcium.

It is often erroneously believed that the victim of a hip fracture always falls first and that the fracture is a consequence of the fall. This is not always the case. A slight stumble as one gets out of a sofa or in the bathroom or shower may be all that it takes to break the 'neck' of the thigh bone (femur) – where it turns upwards and inwards into the hip joint. This is a common and dangerous site for fractures.

The spine or vertebral column is the next major site of osteoporosis. Tiny fractures occur in the vertebrae and, given time and the stresses the back is subjected to, will contribute to increasing the curvature of the spine. Poor posture compounded by the weight of large breasts and obesity also causes significant loss of height, the thoracic spine (that part within the chest) tending to curve forwards. As this part of the spine gradually collapses it may lead to emphysema (a condition of the lungs more commonly associated with cigarette smoking) and difficulty breathing. The bent spine deforms the rib cage and prevents the lungs from expanding to their full capacity. If smoking is added to this the damage and disability are compounded.

The tiny fractures of the vertebrae mentioned above occur in the front parts of the bones and, with time, assume the shape of wedges. Picture a column of triangles of 'Nestle' cheeses place one on top of the other along their narrow edges with the narrow ends in front – and, as more and more vertebrae take on these shapes, the thoracic spine curves forward.

These fractures often present with back pain but may also occur without any symptoms – their presence suspected as the person gradually loses height. The only recourse at this stage is medication that may slow down or inhibit the normal breaking down process of the bone cells (osteoclasts) along with calcium supplements and exercise. For calcium to be made available to bone it must first be absorbed from the intestines.

Synthetic calcium preparations like calcium gluconate, calcium carbonate and calcium citrate have poor absorption rates. It has been estimated that of these preparations only about 8% gets absorbed while the rest ends up in the toilet.

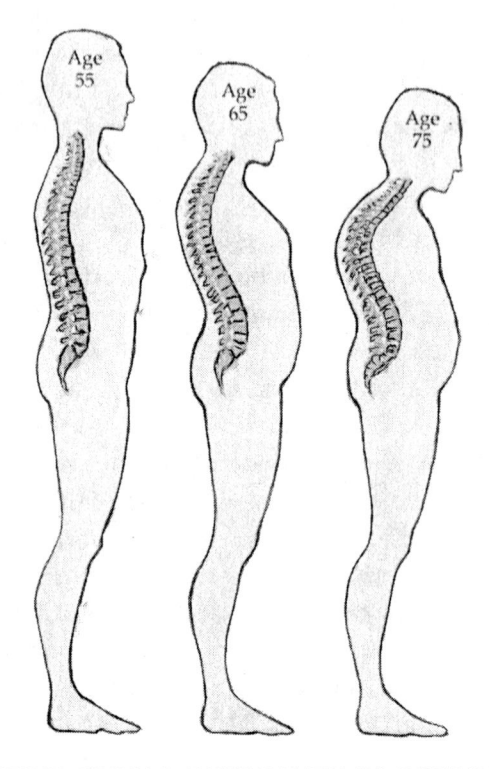

PROGRESSIVE SPINAL DEFORMITY IN OSTEOPOROSIS

Dolomite, which is a natural source of calcium, is mined underground from fossilised bone and has an absorption rate of 13 %. If it is a known fact that these calcium preparations are so poorly absorbed from the gut why are they prescribed? Calcium harvested from sea coral is also a natural source of calcium but contains all the pollutants of the ocean incorporated into the coral and these are not removed at the time of manufacture.

'Chelated Calmag' tablets (made from egg shells which are a natural source of calcium and contain no impurities) have an absorption rate of 76%! The darker downside remains unsatisfactorily answered:

could preventative medicine spell the death knell for medical practices, radiology, orthopaedic surgery, the drug industry and pharmacies, physiotherapy, acupuncture, the manufacturers of the prostheses and the hospitals? Prevention should be the goal because there is very little that medicine can cure.

Small-framed people and women, in particular, are more prone to develop osteoporosis. The typical patient is a small, elderly, fair skinned; woman who sits in a chair spending much of her time indoors knitting and drinking cups of tea. The lack of sunlight prevents the skin from manufacturing Vitamin D that is necessary for the absorption of calcium from the gut and tannin from tea further inhibits its absorption. Dark skinned women in warmer climates are less prone to this condition, being more exposed to sunlight and probably their tendency to be more active.

Anti-gravity exercises (walking – as opposed to swimming) plays an important role in the prevention of osteoporosis. The pressure effect of bone against the ground stimulates the bone cells to proliferate; this explains why swimming is not as effective as walking. Jogging, on the other hand, will increase the risk of osteoarthritis by exposing the cartilages of joints of the lower limbs to damage from the trauma of pounding them into the tarmac. If oestrogen, whether produced naturally by the ovaries or as hormone replacement therapy, lacks the presence of the bone building material i.e. calcium, osteoporosis cannot be effectively prevented. Oestrogen also helps to improve the absorption of the mineral from the gut and its utilisation by the osteoblast cell in laying down the bone. Vitamin C Sustained release, Vitamin D and magnesium supplements are also necessary for optimal absorption of calcium from the gut.

Leafy vegetables are rich in calcium but the mineral is present in a form that is tightly bound and therefore does not release the calcium in the gut to make it available for absorption. The bones found in canned fish are an excellent source of calcium (not all companies include the fish bones) and chewing the soft ends of chicken bones is also beneficial.

Osteoporosis is a preventable disease. Unfortunately, calcium supplementation from as early an age as one year is sadly neglected;

recourse to milk is relied upon even though to receive one adult dose of calcium requires the daily intake of 1½ litres of full cream milk. As mentioned above taking skimmed milk will not supply calcium because the latter needs the presence of the fat in the milk for its absorption. Nature did not intend for man or wily entrepreneurs to meddle with its blueprint. Furthermore, drinking 1½ litres of full cream milk daily may kill the person from coronary artery disease from the fat in the milk long before the bone will! Cow's milk was intended for consumption by the calf – not humans!

A pregnant mother will lose calcium to the foetus and, if the intake of the mineral is inadequate, the foetus will leech the calcium from the mother's bones, as it will not compromise itself. The number of pregnancies may match the degree of osteoporosis. Every pregnant mother should take at least 3 to 4 'Calmag' tablets daily and these should be continued until breastfeeding is complete.

Some very popular supplements prescribed to pregnant women would not meet the calcium requirements of a pregnant cat – some containing as little as 20 mg whereas the daily requirement in pregnancy is about 1500 mg! - This borders on sheer negligence. Just because a product is popular, is well-advertised and manufactured by a 'well known' company does not guarantee that the product works.

The time to begin taking supplements of calcium is as soon as the child can swallow safely; while the bones are developing and not when the hip breaks at 65!

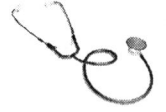

PALPITATIONS

This is a symptom experienced by people at some time or other from the fast heartbeat of a first love, to the pounding of the heart in an Acute Panic Attack or the rapid pulse rate accompanying an overactive thyroid gland. The rapid heartbeat may become noticeable as a thumping in the chest and sometimes the rate could be so fast that the heart may fail.

Heartbeats may become more noticeable when the subject is lying down on the left side as this position brings the heart closer to the left chest wall. Lying on one side or the other brings the artery in the temple area of the forehead in contact with the pillow, its pulsations reverberating against the pillow and made more audible to the ear.

If palpitations occur two questions need to be answered:

a) How many heartbeats occur in one minute?

Greater or less than 90 per minute:	If they are less than 90 the problem may be ignored.
	If the rate is greater than 90 the next question is –

b) Are the beats regular or irregular?
Can one tap out a regular rhythm - one, two, three, four? or
Do they go - one, two, three, four, five, six—seven – – – –
eight – – – – nine – – – – – – – – – ten – – – eleven, twelve,

thirteen, fourteen, fifteen, sixteen and so on i.e. there is no steady rhythm – one moment it is slow and the next it races away.

If the beats are irregular (atrial fibrillation) a doctor should be seen early as the palpitations may disappear and the diagnosis missed or delayed. This rhythm may cause symptoms of dizziness, shortness of breath, lightheadedness and sometimes chest pain. It may also create a feeling of panic. In this type of palpitation the heart is not beating very effectively i.e. it cannot efficiently pump out and receive blood. If allowed to continue in this chaotic manner it would eventually cause the heart to fail in its function as a pump.

The left side of the heart receives oxygenated (purified) blood from the lungs and pumps it to all parts of the body. The right side of the heart receives the 'used' blood back from the body and sends it to the lungs for more oxygen. This is supposed to be a smooth continuous action from birth to death. If the heartbeat is irregular and very fast the beats are ineffective and may lead to heart failure. This problem becomes magnified if the heart already has an existing problem e.g. angina, a previous heart attack or hypertension.

If the heartbeat is fast i.e. greater than 90 and sometimes reaching rates of up to 120 or more but are regular (not always easy to count when it is this fast) this is not as serious as the irregular pattern (atrial fibrillation) but may cause symptoms and warrants medical advice.

The structure of the heart may be likened to a house with two rooms upstairs and two downstairs. The rooms upstairs – right and left atria – (pleural of atrium) do not participate in any major pumping action. The rooms downstairs called ventricles – the right and left – do the major pumping (of blood). The rooms on the right and left sides are separated by a common wall.

- The right atrium (right upstairs room) simply receives blood from the rest of the body after the oxygen and nutrients contained in the blood have been used. It then passes it to the room downstairs – the right ventricle through an opening in the floor (tricuspid valve).

- The right ventricle (right downstairs room) pumps the same blood to the lungs
- The lungs saturate the blood with oxygen and this purified blood is then sent to the left atrium (left upstairs room)
- The left atrium then sends the same blood downstairs through an opening in the floor (mitral valve) to the left ventricle (left downstairs room) which plays the major pump as it sends oxygenated blood to every part of the body.

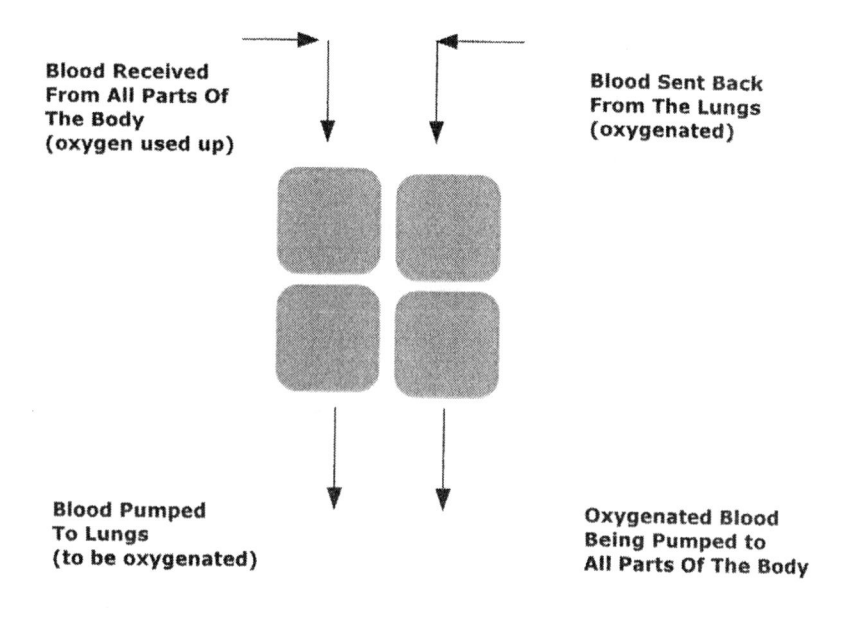

Blood Received From All Parts Of The Body (oxygen used up)

Blood Sent Back From The Lungs (oxygenated)

Blood Pumped To Lungs (to be oxygenated)

Oxygenated Blood Being Pumped to All Parts Of The Body

THE CIRCULATION

Palpitations with a heart rate of 120 or less but are regular do not usually imply heart disease. Often the underlying cause is anxiety as in an acute panic attack or other emotional setback. Another important cause of a 'resting' heart rate greater than 90 is an overactive thyroid gland. This condition is usually accompanied by warm, sweaty palms, shaky hands, excessive body sweating, being hungry all the time (in spite of eating extra food) and losing weight simultaneously. A simple blood test to measure the levels of the hormones made by the thyroid gland will confirm the diagnosis. Left untreated the strain on the heart may cause it to fail.

The best time to measure the heart rate is at night before one nods of to sleep because one is expected to be most relaxed at this time – the so called 'resting' heart rate. This is done by placing three fingers (use the middle 3 – index, middle and ring fingers) with the tips held in a straight line (place them on a table top to get them aligned) and place them along the wrist just behind the thumb where this digit meets the wrist joint. Count the number of beats in one minute using a watch with a 'second hand'. An electrocardiogram (ECG) is invariably required for confirmation of the diagnosis but it helps to know when to seek professional help based on simple observations of the heart rate. Palpitations are an important feature of anxiety. The sudden hammering of the heart if one is called upon to make an impromptu speech or is caught napping in the lecture room are all too familiar situations that generate anxiety and palpitations. The increase in the rate, often doubling the resting rate (which is about 70) to about *140 per minute,* is due to the sudden outpouring of adrenaline acting upon the nerves that control the heart rate. This may also result in sweating, faster breathing, a dry mouth, contraction of the stomach muscles, a sudden urge to pass urine and, pushed to its extreme (terrified) can make one incontinent of urine and stool! These episodes of palpitations are usually short lived.

The quickest way to slow down the heart rate is to take as deep a breath as possible through the open mouth, hold for as long as possible and then let it out as slowly as possible for as long as possible. This is a useful manoeuvre when faced with a sudden panic attack or impromptu public speech.

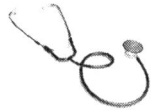

PERIODS

Every twenty eight days, throughout the reproductive years of a woman's life, the womb sheds the lining it was dutifully preparing (nest-like) to receive the fertilised egg. If fertilisation or pregnancy does not occur this lining (endometrium) shears off from the rest of the womb resulting in bleeding and the familiar 'period'.

The 'menstruation' consists mainly of blood, the lining of the womb and its secretions. This blood does *not normally clot* and if large clots are present implies that the bleeding is excessive and warrants a medical opinion. The average amount of blood lost per cycle is about 100 ml. In an average life span a female loses about 50 litres of blood from her menstruation. This is a significant amount of blood, iron and calcium lost into an average of 2000 sanitary pads. If conception has taken place and bleeding occurs this is a 'miscarriage' and, if nobody is any the wiser about the pregnancy, it goes undetected as though it was a 'normal period'.

Menstrual cycles are usually regular and minor variations in timing, number of days and quantity of bleeding are of little significance. However, any female of reproductive age who is sexually active and has missed a period, especially if they have been regular before, is considered pregnant until proven otherwise with appropriate tests using either urine or blood. In a pregnancy the urine test usually becomes positive about 10 days after conception. The blood test is more accurate for earlier confirmation of pregnancy. If the home pregnancy test (available from the chemist) is positive there is no need to have this test repeated by a doctor. However, if it is negative and if it is necessary to know as soon as possible, (which is almost always!), blood is sent for testing levels of bHCG (beta human chorionic gonadotrophin) – this is the hormone that is produced only by a viable placenta. For practical purposes, the placenta can only be present if the person is pregnant. The placenta attaches the foetus to the lining of the womb.

Menarche (the first period) is usually around the twelfth or thirteenth year and if menstruation has not occurred by then a medical opinion should be sought. An imperforate hymen closes off the vagina completely or may have a tiny opening preventing blood from passing out of the vagina. This is not a serious problem but requires minor surgery to widen the opening in the hymen. If this condition has been excluded and menstruation has not occurred by the late teens a medical opinion should be sought.

The quantity of menstrual flow is considered 'heavy' if there are large blood clots present – usually bigger than 2 cm in diameter. This amount of bleeding if allowed to persist for a length of time may lead to anemia due to loss of iron contained in the menstrual blood. The total bleeding time for a female from menarche to menopause could add up to a staggering total of almost seven years and fifty litres of precious blood!

Bone marrow is quite capable of adjusting to the increased demands that occur during menstruation unless the stores of iron in the marrow are borderline or low. In such situations the heavy periods can cause lightheadedness and tiredness from anaemia.

A 'D&C' (dilatation and curettage) is performed after a miscarriage to clear the uterus of products of conception. This procedure is mandatory to prevent infection from setting up within the womb and it is not unusual for the periods to disappear for a month or so after the procedure. If the periods are chronically irregular a D&C may be necessary to 'kick start' the uterus back to normal.

Theoretically, pregnancy cannot occur if menstruation has begun because the fertilised egg (ovum), if there is one around, would not have the appropriate lining of the uterus for implantation to take place but this is not impossible. If contraceptive precautions have been taken there is no medical reason for avoiding intercourse on the basis of the bleeding; this is matter of individual choice. A condom could eliminate the need to be celibate for the seven years of menstruation that an average woman would spend having her periods.

Menstruation is a normal physiological event and not the monthly 'curse' – the penance the fairer sex pays for being the child bearer. And, as with childbirth, the mother, relatives and friends may instill into the impressionable teenager, stories of discomfort and pain (dysmenorrhoea) with vivid descriptions of their own experiences. It is not surprising that dysmennorhoeic girls have dysmenorrhoeic mothers. A day off from school becomes a day away from work and time away from the unpleasant routine of household chores and other activities - including sex. A frank and sensible explanation of the changes that are about to happen to the young teenager as she accepts the challenges of her sexuality may prepare her for the time when she may awaken in the middle of the night in a pool of blood fearing a major haemorrhage that could cause her to bleed to death. The sight of blood (especially one's own) can be quite daunting.

Common symptoms of a period are a feeling of heaviness in the lower belly and back due to the contractions of the womb as it dispels the menstrual discharge. The earlier symptoms of passing urine more frequently and heaviness in the pelvis are due to the increased blood supply to the womb just before menstruation begins. During, or just before, a period constipation, heaviness, fullness and breast discomfort are quite common. Acne and migraine may be worsened.

Immediately before menstruation the body temperature falls a ½ degree or so due to withdrawal of progesterone and indicates that ovulation has not occurred. If the temperature, recorded each morning before arising from bed, shows an increase it may help establish that it has and prompt the introduction of sperm. The rising surge of oestrogen produced by the ovaries, in turn controlled by hormones from the pituitary gland in the brain, influences the changes that characterise adolescence.

Menstrual blood is usually very dark in colour and does not have an offensive odour. A forgotten tampon has been known to cause a smelly discharge from the vagina that can lead to infection within the womb. This could spread into the blood stream (septicemia) and cause a life threatening complication of using tampons. The treatment for this is *not* another 'antifungal cream' but urgent hospitalisation.

Women who use tampons to dam up the blood within the vagina for up to several hours (depending on personal preferences and levels of hygiene) also encourage bacteria to flourish in such an environment. In the laboratory, in order to promote bacterial growth for purposes of identifying a suspected organism, culture media can be enriched with 'nutrients' like sugar, egg-white or blood.

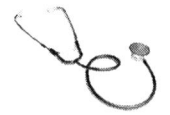

PILES (HAEMORRHOIDS)

Piles in the back passage are what varicose veins are to the legs. Veins are normally present in the wall of the rectum i.e. last part of the large intestines.

Conditions that increase pressure within the abdomen and predispose one to the development of piles are: –

- pregnancy
- obesity
- chronic constipation and
- chronic bronchitis and the cough that accompanies it

These pressures are transmitted to the rectum and the veins in the wall of the back passage causing them to become distended.

In the early stages they are engorged but remain within the rectum and are not visible outside the anus and are called internal piles. As the pressure is maintained the veins (there may be more than one and up to three) begin to protrude through the anus. Initially they can be pushed back manually into the rectum but later, as the condition invariably progresses, tend to remain 'outside'. This is called a 'prolapsed' pile and may suddenly become excruciatingly painful when the pile is tense with blood. The anal sphincter (valve) acts like a tight rubber band trapping blood in the veins outside the anus. Sitting becomes a nightmare, as will anything that increases the pressure within the pile – such as applying force in constipation (which is often the causative factor and a good illustration of how straining at defaecation (bowel evacuation) increases the pressure within the veins in the rectum.

With the 'western-style' toilet pan where the person is seated (and often leaning forward) the pants or underwear are often lowered to just below the knees preventing the legs from opening widely enough. This generates extra intra-abdominal pressure when trying to evacuate the bowel.

In contrast, with the 'eastern-style' toilet pan where the person squats over the pan which is situated at ground level, the rectum is aligned for easier evacuation, assisted by the added benefit of gravity and legs that, of necessity, are more widely spread out to make the squat more comfortable. Animals like cats and dogs adopt a similar 'squatting' position. The western toilet, regardless of gender, should be used with one leg removed from the pants or underwear. This would ensure a more comfortable evacuation with the legs wide open, maximum exposure and with the least amount of pressure - ensuring an easier bowel movement and, possibly, preventing the development of piles.

An acutely painful pile may 'push' the patient to have surgery with the promise of faster relief - resist this temptation. The pain will subside within a few days once the blood within the distended pile is resorbed by the body. However, if surgery is undertaken be pre-pared to have a 'gaping hole' in the anal area that will take weeks to heal, requiring sitting in pans of water (sitz baths) several times a day. Beware the surgeon overly keen to apply a knife to a painful pile. An alternative would be to have them injected with a chemical that occludes or clots up the vein as is done for varicose veins.

Once the swelling in an external pile has subsided the 'shell' of the pile may remain and is of no further medical significance. They do not become cancerous. If these 'skin tags' are very baggy, and there maybe several of them, adequate/effective toiletry can become diffi-cult. These can be removed surgically as a minor procedure without the inconvenience of weeks of sitz baths.

Piles can present as painless bleeding from the rectum and an important clue to the origin of the bleeding is that the blood streaks the sides of the (formed) stools and is not mixed with the stools.

The latter will imply that the bleeding has occurred higher up in the rectum or large intestine making it necessary to exclude another cause(?cancer of the gut). When it occurs for the first time a doctor's opinion should be sought – not simply to receive a prescription – but to try and identify a cause. A tumour present in the rectum (above the piles) may cause a pressure effect upon the underlying veins within the rectum and result in piles and bleeding. Blood on the paper during toiletry (as different from blood in the toilet pan) is usually due to a tear (fissure) in the folds of the anal sphincter and resembles the 'crack' seen in thrush affecting the corners of the mouth. The pain in this condition occurs during the passage of large constipated stools as the folds of the anus are then maximally stretched causing small tears in the delicate lining. Furthermore, the quality of the toilet paper and the vigour with which the toiletry is executed may also influence the development of fissures. Gentle dabbing as opposed to vigorous scrubbing is advised!

Cultures that advocate water and not paper as the medium of toiletry are gentler on the anal sphincter. 'Scheriproct' ointment is the treatment of choice for anal fissures. It contains a steroid that acts as an anti-inflammatory; other over-the-counter 'remedies' may not be as effective without it. This preparation is also available in the form of a suppository (to be inserted into the rectum) for bleeding or painful piles and fissures of the anus.

In an acute pile strong analgesics (painkillers) are required and a topical local anaesthetic cream applied to the pile should be used several times a day as the effect does not last very long. Standing, sitting, lying supine (on the back), sneezing, farting and straining to pass a 'constipated' stool will increase the pressure within the rectum and, therefore, within the pile and should be avoided.

An effective laxative ('Lactulose' syrup) will help to soften the stools. This preparation is relatively safe, as it is not absorbed from the gut into the circulation. The use of laxatives should be a short-term measure to help overcome the 'emergency' of the acutely painful pile. Exercise, adequate hydration, sufficient dietary fibre – soluble (oats) and insoluble (bran), - fruit and vegetables, the timeous heeding of the calls of nature - all help to prevent constipation.

Sleeping on the stomach or on the side without bending the thighs upon the belly (this may make the pile more tense) and a firm cushion or pillow between the thighs may lessen the pressure and, thereby, the pain in an acute pile. A sedative is recommended until the swelling subsides.

It may seem trite to point out that the stools in the toilet pan and the paper that is used in the toiletry must be *'seen'* to know that nothing is amiss. The colour of the stool and urine and the presence of blood in either give important clues to the state of one's health. Always look back! The western toilet pan does not encourage easy visualisation. While the passage of 'small' amounts of blood from bleeding piles is common and the presence of blood in a 'white' toilet pan can be quite harrowing to the viewer a blood transfusion is rarely required. However, chronic blood loss can lead to anemia (loss of iron) that can impair one's health. The situation will become more serious if the levels of iron in the blood are already lower than normal from other causes e.g. heavy menstrual bleeding or a dietary lack of iron (as in vegetarians).

A person who has been repeatedly troubled with piles can develop an *additional cause* for the rectal bleeding e.g. cancer of the rectum. The message is: not every haemorrhage may be due to the 'long standing' pile. And not every pain in the anal area may be due to piles - a rectal abscess can be missed.

A longstanding anal discharge should not be ignored simply because it is too embarrassing to have a doctor 'look down there'. And using a wad of toilet paper in the underwear – sometimes for months or years on end – is not the solution; the cause should be established.

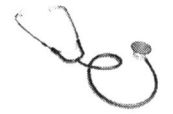

PNEUMONIA

This is an infection usually of one or more of the lobes of the lung.

The right lung has 3 lobes viz., upper, middle and lower and the left lung has 2 – upper and lower lobes. Picture the right lung as a two storey building plus basement and the left as a single storey with basement. The common types of pneumonia usually affect the basements (lower lobes) and more commonly the right basement and sometimes the first storey (middle lobe) of the right lung.

The effect of gravity and that the bronchial tube leading down to the *right* lower lobe is more vertical make this lobe (basement) more vulnerable to infection. It is easier for phlegm to track downwards into the lowest parts of the lungs. Picture a lift between the two buildings (described above) beginning at the top (mouth) - the next stops being the pharynx, larynx and trachea after which the lift separates into 2 – one going down into each building (lung).

A common starting point for phlegm on its journey to the basement is the sinuses (sinusitis) – the common attic of the two buildings. As it travels lower the infection becomes 'pharyngitis' – back of the throat - and if the vocal cords (voice box) becomes involved this is labelled 'laryngitis'.

The bronchus divides into two: the right and left bronchial tubes and infections here are called 'bronchitis'. Further down and the lung becomes the site of infection (pneumonia).

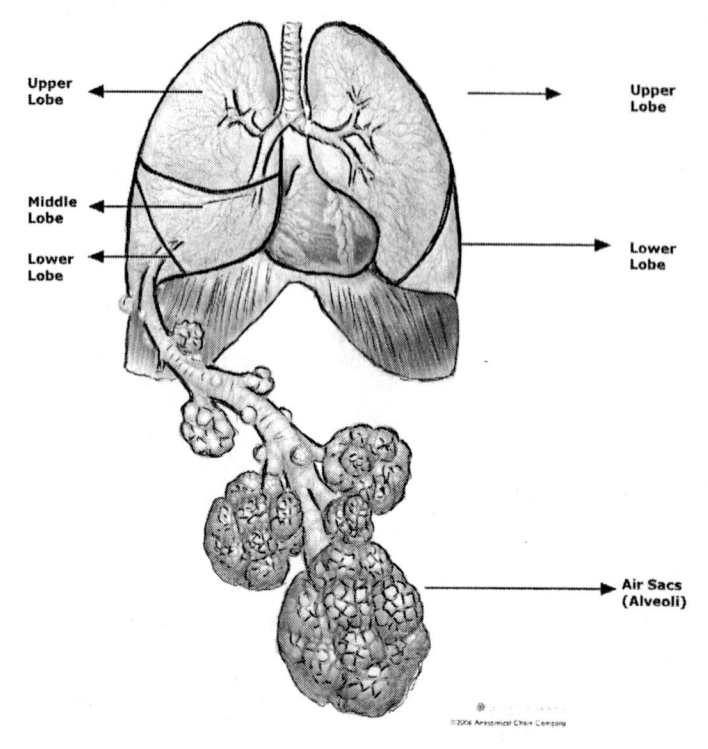

Upper Lobe

Upper Lobe

Middle Lobe

Lower Lobe

Lower Lobe

Air Sacs (Alveoli)

THE LUNGS

The importance of pneumonia, as compared to the rest of the airways, is that the lung has now become involved and this is a *vital* organ and, as such, demands more respect and attention. Germs (bacteria) can also reach the lungs through the blood stream. Infected blood from a tooth abscess or tonsillitis could also reach the lungs. The teeth and tonsils are practically neighbours to the lungs.

Any person with a cough may have an underlying pneumonia.

While it is usual to be ill with a high temperature and discoloured sputum these may not always be present. The patient may look well and there may be hardly any phlegm. A child with pneumonia may be running around and playing and have a normal appetite with no fever.

It is almost criminal to use a cough mixture at the first hint of a cough because it will suppress the only natural way the body has of getting phlegm out of the 'basements' of the lungs – and that is a long way up to the top. Once the infected 'pus' (phlegm) collects in the basement one has the beginnings of a 'pneumonia'.

Without listening to the chest with a stethoscope diagnosing a lung infection can be difficult. In the early stages of infection the chest X-ray may be normal. A cough that persists for longer than 3 – 4 weeks warrants a chest X-ray to exclude Tuberculosis (TB) or other pathology. Tuberculosis commonly affects the 'top floors' (upper lobes where the oxygen concentration is less); the TB germ prefers areas of low oxygen in which to survive. In the days before antibiotics patients were nursed flat to improve the oxygen to these areas to discourage the bacteria. The discovery of effective antibiotics has changed the management of tuberculosis. However, the emergence of HIV /AIDS and the appearance of TB that is resistant to available drugs have serious implications. 'Resistant TB' has become a deadly complication to a disease that does not yet have a vaccine for its eradication. Antibiotics for an uncomplicated pneumonia are usually prescribed for 5 to 10 days. Clues that the treatment is working are that the colour of the phlegm gradually becomes lighter/ clearer, the quantity of the phlegm becomes less, temperature returns to normal and the patient feels better within 48 to 72 hours.

The decision to change an antibiotic to a 'stronger' one is often tempting to the impatient when the expected improvement is not immediately forthcoming. However, this move should be guided by sound medical judgment and, perhaps, the support of other measures like laboratory examination of the sputum or chest X-ray to try and ascertain the reason for the failed response to the first antibiotic. A blocked bronchial tube (lift to the basement not working) is usually followed by collapse of the lobe to which that particular tube was supplying air. If a lobe or any part of the lung does not get air it will 'collapse' and this needs the expertise of a competent physiotherapist to get the tube 'unblocked' - not necessarily a more 'potent' antibiotic.

The presence or development of shortness of breath (dyspnoea) whether a history of asthma is present or not warrants review by a doctor and often a chest X-ray. Adequate hydration is important to make the phlegm less sticky and easier to cough up. This is safer and less expensive than a cough mixture. Laughing and crying also help to promote the cough reflex. A child that is crying is taking in deeper breaths and exhaling for longer during each 'cry'. This encourages more air into the 'basement' and this is often compromised when breathing is shallow.

Taking in a deep breath and forcing out all the air as though one was trying to laugh heartily without making the sound of laughter also helps to bring out phlegm. Breathe in as deeply as possible and let the air out slowly through pursed lips until there is no more breath left; this is a useful yoga exercise. It helps move air from the basements encouraging the use of the whole lung instead of the upper half to two thirds, as is normally done. Nature has also incorporated the 'sigh' into our normal breathing pattern to help take a deeper breath and clear the 'basements'.

Using a nebuliser with only warm water in the chamber (without the medication) will also help to loosen phlegm. If there is an element of tightness of the chest, especially in an asthmatic, the addition of a bronchodilator drug to open up the airways will be beneficial.

The role of nutrition must not be underestimated even though a temperature and nausea may dampen the appetite. Whatever the patient is happy to eat or drink – make it count for maximum benefit: ice cream and jelly, soup with added butter, eggs, peanut butter, fruit juices (freshly made) and with additional sugar.

The following supplements may help hasten the recovery phase

- Zinc tablet (15 mg) – 1 daily (for the infection)
- Vitamin C – slow release tablets – 1 daily (for the infection)
- multivitamins (Formula 4 Plus – also supplies the other 15 mg of zinc – the total requirement of which is about 30 mg daily)
- Omega 3 capsules – 3 daily (anti-inflammatory and tissue repair)
- Vitamin E – 200 I.U. – 1 capsule daily (antioxidant)

Bed rest is mandatory, especially if a fever is present.

If the right lower lobe (basement) is identified (by the doctor) to be the site of the infection then the patient should lie on the left side in order to keep the affected (right) side uppermost and allow gravity to help get the phlegm out of the right lung and into the bronchial tube on the affected side.

If the chest wall is gently thumped with the cupped palm it will help to loosen phlegm and make it easier to cough it out. Seat the patient in a chair. Place one hand over the chest wall in front (under the breast in a female) and the other behind the chest. Have the patient breathe in deeply and exhale slowly. As he or she exhales vibrate the chest gently between the two hands. This also helps to break up or loosen phlegm. It is often underestimated that one of the most important measures in the treatment of pneumonia is to cough the phlegm out of the lung – the latter should contain only air and not infected pus!

Cough mixtures have no place in this treatment and should not be encouraged. Nature designed the best 'remedy': the cough reflex - without it we would probably not survive. It helps to protect the airways and lungs from any foreign body (sputum / phlegm) and, therefore, needs to be encouraged - not labelled negatively as a "bad cough" – the cough is never 'bad'! The body needs the cough but not the phlegm and the latter may need an antibiotic especially if the sputum is persistently yellow or green in colour. If it is clear this may imply a viral infection for which antibiotics generally do nothing!

Sputum that is discolored *only* in the morning (on arising) and clears as the day progresses should not need an antibiotic. Mucus that accumulates overnight in the sinuses and chest may discolour itself. If the colour persists throughout the day it implies an ongoing infection and should be treated with an appropriate antibiotic.

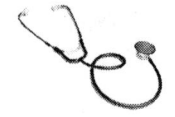

PREGNANCY

Intercourse has the risk of a pregnancy. The function of sperm, once it is introduced into or around the vagina, whether by penetration or foreplay, is to find its way to the egg. That is what it is programmed to do – like a robot.

One spermatozoon (of which there are millions) is all that is required to produce a pregnancy. The safest time in the menstrual cycle when pregnancy may not occur does not really exist. The only way of guaranteeing that pregnancy does not occur is to keep the sperm and egg apart. Masturbation may help deflate a tense situation and avoid the need for contraception when, on the spur of a romantic moment, no contraceptive is available. It is a useful alternative when a simple 'NO' is insufficient. Proficiency in the practice of masturbation may save both partners much heartache and an unwanted pregnancy.

A condom may help but is not guaranteed: incorrectly applied, slippage within the vagina or damage during intercourse will defeat the purpose. Using Vaseline or other oil based lubricants will also damage the latex. 'K-Y Jelly' is safe (and expensive). Saliva is not an option as its introduction in the vagina carries with it a risk of transmitting infection from the donor's mouth – this can hardly be a healthy source of lubricant. In the tragic event one is about to become a rape victim having the presence of mind to lubricate the vagina with one's own saliva may help lessen the trauma of forced intercourse as the vaginal walls are not prepared for such an onslaught. Furthermore, if the vagina is traumatized the risk of contracting an infection from the perpetrator is made easier. The use of a condom could prevent a pregnancy and, perhaps, save one's life – who would know what infections the perpetrator harbours. Always have a condom handy.

Pregnancy should ideally be planned. The nutritional status of both prospective parents should be improved before the expected mating of a sperm occurs with the egg. The qualities of the sperm and egg are directly dependent on the nutrition they receive. A reliable source of supplements containing multivitamins, zinc, omega 3 (salmon oil), vitamin E, calcium/magnesium and folic acid should be taken for at least two months before conception is planned. These should be continued throughout the pregnancy and for at least three to six months after the delivery as the confinement, breastfeeding, lack of sleep and coping with husband, other children, grandparents, the home and workplace, will take their toll on the unprepared mother.

However, the best supplements are doomed to fail without the benefit of satisfying sleep. Have the partner share the nappy changes at night. This skill is not inborn in the male sex and may have to be taught. Choose a time for the 'training' – preferably on a doll before the arrival of the baby and the 'green slimy stool'. The experience could put him off nappy changing forever.

It is not easily recommended that celebrations, after the pregnancy is confirmed, should take on a grandiose style. Nothing is guaranteed in life. Today's pregnancy can be next month's miscarriage and the undoing of the expectations that the news of pending parenthood will inevitably bring will be that much more difficult to overcome. Keep an open mind and a 'one-day-at-a-time' approach.

Weight gain is part of the pregnancy. The growing foetus and its (amniotic fluid) liqour and the increase in the circulatory fluid in the mother are normal. Additional gain from 'eating-for-two 'and unwise eating habits will add on unwelcome weight that will often stay, sometimes for life. Resist the temptation to stray from a sensible eating plan.

The foetus is a 'parasite' and will obtain whatever it needs from the mother at the latter's expense. It is essential for the mother to make certain her diet is providing the nutritional requirements of the foetus or it will 'leech' it from the mother.

Many pregnant women do not receive calcium as a supplement or their daily intake may be inadequate. Calcium is necessary for the development of the foetal bones. It will be removed from the bones of the unsuspecting mother and contribute to osteoporosis in her later life. Calcium, as with all other supplements, must first be absorbed from the gut before it can be made available to the body. The majority of the prescription calcium supplements are synthetic (laboratory made – calcium phosphates, gluconates and carbonates) and these have a poor absorption rate of about 8 to 13%. The rest is lost in the toilet. There are alternatives made from natural sources that have up to 76% absorption.

The first three months of the pregnancy are crucial in the development of the foetus as the vital organs are being formed. It is safer in this period to avoid all medication – even paracetamol – if possible. Taking medication during the rest of the pregnancy should be at the discretion of the doctor. Coffee, cigarettes (active and passive forms), all types of alcohol and any quantity of it should be avoided. Smoking during pregnancy may condemn the baby to a lifetime of asthma triggered by the toxins present in tobacco.

Bending the lower back for any purpose should be avoided as ligaments of the spine tend to soften and stretch in preparation for the delivery and can be easily damaged by injudicious strain to the spine. Tightening the pubococcygeus muscle (identified by attempting to stop the flow of urine in midstream) will strengthen it. This muscle assists in the control of the bladder, vagina, rectum, the lower spine and the abdominal wall. Learning to control this particular muscle will also help in childbirth. This muscle together with those of the front wall of the lower abdomen are the main role players in "Push, push, push now" "Don't push, don't push relax now" scenario of the delivery room. The pubococcygeus muscle also helps prevent the bladder and womb from sagging and also flattens the tummy. Childbirth may weaken the tone of this muscle and make the vagina very 'roomy' and less stimulating during future intercourse. Minor surgery immediately after childbirth can correct this – bearing in mind that a vagina fully primed for intercourse after adequate fore-play will dilate anyway.

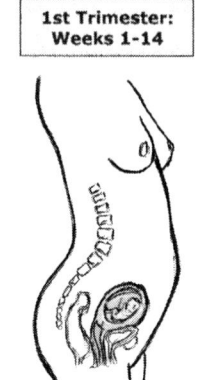

1st Trimester:
Weeks 1-14

Lateral view of the fetus
at the end of the first trimester
of pregnancy.

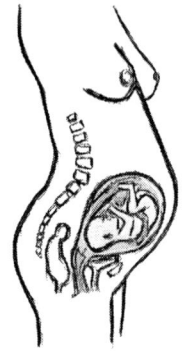

2nd Trimester:
Weeks 15-30

Lateral view of the fetus
at the end of the
second trimester of pregnancy.

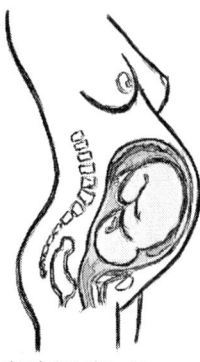

3rd Trimester:
Weeks 32-40

Lateral view of the fetus
during the ninth month
of the third trimester of pregnancy.

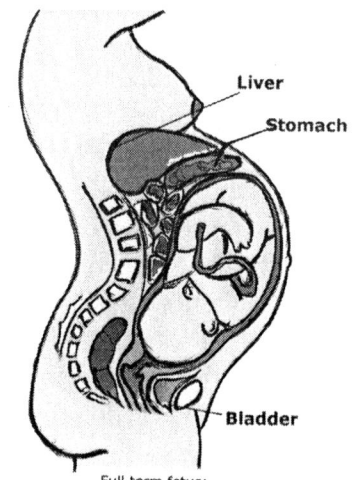

Liver

Stomach

Bladder

Full term fetus:
Crowding of abdominal contents late in pregnancy.

Approximate Fetal Growth		
Week of Pregnancy	Weight	Length (Head to Heel)
4	1/32 ounce	1/8 inch
12	5/8 ounce	1 to 3 inches
16	4 3/4 ounces	6 inches
20	12 ounces	10 inches
24	1 1/4 pounds	13 inches
28	2 pounds	14 1/2 inches
32	3 1/3 pound	16 inches
36	5 1/2 pounds	18 inches
40	7 1/2 pounds	20 inches

FOETAL GROWTH DURING PREGNANCY

Any vaginal bleeding during pregnancy requires urgent medical attention. An internal examination by a doctor or nurse is not advised unless it is done under sterile conditions to prevent possible infection within the womb or worsening of the bleeding. The latter may occur if the placenta is developing close to the opening in the cervix.

At any time between periods a sexually active female in her reproductive years could be pregnant. Such a person experiencing pain in the lower abdomen may be having an 'ectopic pregnancy' (pregnancy in one of the fallopian tubes) and this is a surgical emergency. Bleeding does not have to accompany this pain. The plot will thicken if a period has been missed or a pregnancy test is found to be positive.

Meals should be nutritious and not bulky to avoid the heartburn that can become troublesome as the womb grows upwards, pushing the stomach upwards as it does. Food and acid gastric juice from the stomach may find its way into the gullet (oesophagus) the lining of which cannot tolerate the acid and causes a burning sensation in the lower chest. Taking small meals more frequently, avoiding lying down after a meal, sleeping almost sitting up propped on pillows, using an antacid after meals or an extract of aloe vera (to avoid the use of drugs), avoiding foods known to precipitate or aggravate heartburn are some measures to control the symptoms.

A temperature (fever) during a pregnancy warrants early attention. There should be a working thermometer in the medicine cabinet. Asthma, eczema and migraine tend to become worse during pregnancy. Surgical stockings can become uncomfortable in hot weather but may help prevent the onset of varicose veins in the legs, especially if one is standing for long periods. These stockings may also prevent deep vein thromboses (DVTs of air travel notoriety) that are an added risk in pregnancy.

Wearing high heels and, alternatively, flat shoes will throw the back into a compromised position - begging for backache.

Some swelling of the feet is not unacceptable especially as the pregnancy progresses and puts pressure on the veins of the legs. However, this swelling will be aggravated by hot weather, sitting for long periods and the excessive intake of salt. Adequate daily intakes of fruit and vegetables will help avoid the constipation that often plagues pregnant women. Six to eight glasses of properly filtered water will help constipation and avoid exposing the foetus (from an early age) to the harmful chemicals in conventional drinking water that ordinary chlorination does not remove. Chlorine itself is a chemical the foetus could well do without.

Taking fibre (both soluble and insoluble) as a supplement gives the gut a 'bulking' effect that avoids the hunger pangs and prevents the sharp rises in blood sugars that will occur after a carbohydrate load. It also helps achieve better control of glucose levels, improving the management of diabetes in pregnancy that may have serious consequences for the foetus and the mother. Diabetic pregnant mothers need careful follow up and should start their antenatal check-ups early - they will require insulin for their diabetes as the oral agents are contra-indicated in pregnancy

As mentioned above any sexually active female can be pregnant at any time even if there appears to be a menstrual period. The bleeding could represent a miscarriage. Pregnancy can be confirmed by a urine or blood test. The former depends on the length of time of the pregnancy; if less than about ten days this method is not very reliable - the blood test becomes positive soon after conception has occurred. This becomes more relevant if the pregnancy has to be terminated.

Abortions are not normally performed after the twelfth week of pregnancy. Anybody can have an abortion (done in a hospital setting and not on a kitchen table), and the husband's consent or parents', if the mother is a minor, are not necessary. Pregnancy in the mentally retarded or victims of rape and incest, or women whose health both mental and physical would be compromised by the pregnancy are also legally entitled to have their pregnancies terminated.

Women who have a miscarriage and those having abortions for unwanted pregnancies should have individual counselling (in an ideal world) both before and after. Having a 'D & C' (dilatation and curettage) on a Friday and being back at school or work or home on Monday pays scant attention to the effects, both immediate and long term, that this 'death' or loss may have on the mother.

No matter how painful it may seem at the time, and how much better it might feel by not doing it, one should avoid not confiding in one's parents if an unwanted pregnancy should occur. These are the very people who have had you before and are therefore experienced in the ways of a pregnancy and can relate to it. Suffer the consequences like an adult rather than as a coward. Fathers, on the one hand, may see more red than sense, visualising the sexual onslaught on their poor defenseless darling ravaged by a nameless, faceless swine and, on the other hand - that slut of a daughter whose mother he has been warning for years will do exactly this kind of thing to bring the good name of the family into dire disrepute. If parents do not have the trust of their daughters by the time they reach the age of fertility then the moment of the colour change on the pregnancy test kit will not be the time to achieve it. Nonetheless, there is little to match the sense of isolation as may occur if parents are excluded. If the procedure has been shrouded in secrecy and if anything should go wrong (nothing is guaranteed in life – and doctors are not God) parents may then be introduced to a situation when little can undo the damage the lack of trust has caused. Credibility cannot easily be regained.

Where exactly do these pregnancies occur? There are few places that are 'sacrosanct'. If the opportunity presents itself and the venue is available it can happen. Parents work and the house is free for long hours before they get home. This is a common and most convenient site. Hoping and praying that such activities are not happening could be wishful thinking. Any teenager or adult with a penis can impregnate a female of childbearing age. Teaching sex education and safe sex has little meaning if the situation is ripe for a mating and no condom is available. The sexual drive is not a learned habit like blowing one's nose (this has its own problems!). It is an instinct almost as powerful as the stimulus of hunger for food. Both are designed to ensure the preservation of the species.

In the heat (sic!) of a passionate moment when the urgency, propelled by both the fear of discovery and the inexperience of self control, to copulate is so overpowering the best sex education and the fear of HIV/AIDS or an unwanted pregnancy are the thoughts furthest from the coupling minds. This urge to copulate is much stronger in the male sex. Ignoring this difference may well be an underlying factor that helps swell the ranks of unwanted pregnancies. Pushing for equal responsibilities between the sexes ignores this significant difference in the power of the sex drive between men and women.

Women and teenage girls need to be singled out in the relationship – they are the ones who become pregnant. If the mother of a teenager with Down's syndrome can recognise the need for contraception (and even a hysterectomy in this situation) mothers should empower their girls to avoid a pregnancy.

How parents themselves feel about sex, drawing from their own life's experiences, must play a role in shaping the sexual behaviour of their children. Respect for each other, the absence of abuse in any form, functioning as a family unit even when difficulties do arise - each plays a role. The underlying thread should be love. Without this ingredient few marriages and families will survive and the unwanted pregnancy often becoming an extension of these difficulties.

Living in a council flat with limited space and more occupants than can have the privacy for growing girls to escape the attention and advances of growing and grown males (brothers, cousins, uncles, boarders, stepfathers, fathers, grandfathers, sleep-over school friends) can make a mockery of sex education. The sex drive is a powerful instinct and experimentation is bound to take place. By their very physical nature boys have a stronger drive and become easily aroused and will become the 'hunter' stalking their 'prey'. The hunter (boyfriend) 'marks' out his quarry (girl) and pursues the object of his attentions (?love) until he has either made a 'conquest' – raped /had intercourse / married / divorced or has moved on to other 'quarries'.

While society has established rules and codes of conduct and even laws to control peoples' sexual urges the basic instinct for preservation (sex or intercourse) remains much as it has been for thousands of years. A parallel that comes to mind is a turbo-charged V 8 engine installed on a bicycle!

Unwanted pregnancies and requests for abortions will often remain a product of an impoverished economy that allows inadequate housing and unemployment. Parents, who do not know, do not have the time to know nor care enough to know of the whereabouts of their fertile children also pave the way for these disasters.

A male who will easily pass up the opportunity to have sex is the rare exception. Sex is the one preoccupation that is guaranteed to take precedence over almost any other thought that may occupy a male mind. This statement is the one that is the most underestimated. Rape experts will have us believe that the vast majority of these heinous assaults on females are fuelled by the wish to dominate, that sex and lust play an insignificant role. What 'domination' is being played out when a ninety year old great grandmother or two month old infant or injured road traffic accident victim are being sexually assaulted?

The person responsible for 'impregnating' a female should be present at the time of birth or during the abortion. How else will they ever associate the hot passion in a crowded back seat with the screaming, bleeding and general mayhem that appears to break loose at the time of delivery? Apprehended rapists and irresponsible males, with penises bigger than their brains should be present to witness the 'products of passion' when the gynaecologist scrapes out the living foetus through the vagina. This orifice can look quite different under the drapes of sterile green sheets and the glare of theatre lights and the gore of blood.

Most normal pregnancies 'deliver themselves' – if they are allowed to. The services of the gynaecoligist should be reserved for situations that are beyond the expertise of the midwife. Instead private enterprise has seen an excellent opportunity to turn what nature intended as a natural phenomenon into a thriving business. Where the experienced midwife applied her expertise to do home deliveries, we now have a situation where an over-qualified Ear, Nose and Throat specialist is being summoned to treat a sore throat.

Today's pregnant mother is working (almost to the day of delivery), often in stressful jobs, running a home and husband and, possibly, other children in addition to the demands that even a normal pregnancy will make upon her. Instill into the unsuspecting first-time mother the fears of others who have been through a pregnancy, and

'Doris' with her unsuccessful epidural and the hell she went through, and 'Beverley' with her botched caesarian section – and is it any surprise that the 'experts' are called in to do most of nature's work?

Human beings are possibly the only mammals who experience childbirth as 'A living hell', an event akin to dying, with the mother firmly proclaiming "Never again" and "All this pain for one moment's pleasure!" Nowadays the husband is also a first hand party to the blood and gore. Has this legacy of pain been handed down from mother to daughter, feeding off the insecurities and fears of ignorant young women who are brainwashed into believing that childbirth is a traumatic experience best smothered by an epidural or caesarian section?

Are there gynaecologists, both male and female, who, having witnessed the daily onslaught of the emerging foetus from the hapless mother, continually exposed to the nerve-wracking screams of women in labour, decide that this passage is, indeed, too traumatic to be borne by mortals without some kind of intervention? Television shows and movies that depict scenes of childbirth help propagate the view of the miracle of birth as a scene from 'The Poltergeist' - does watching horror movies make one tread more warily in the dark? Are impressionable pregnant young women similarly affected, perhaps from a very early age? In some countries pregnant women who deliver in rural areas, behind a bush, in time taken off from working the land and unexposed to these fears, do so without the fanfare and near-death trauma that 'modern' mothers are made to undergo.

The supine position, with both legs strung up in stirrups is probably not the position nature intended, considering that the erect stance is a fairly recent part of our evolution and that childbirth also missed out on the adjustment. Looking at nature's blueprint and guidance from the animal kingdom the squatting position must be the way to a more natural birth. This is not an unknown position in some cultures but, nevertheless, is not universally accepted.

It is possible that years of indoctrination has made the squatting position appear undignified – one more accustomed to being used for bowel and bladder evacuation. For generations the examining couch has been a familiar part of the physician's rooms. Its use extended itself admirably into the gynaecologist's domain –

- the working height can be adjusted
- once the legs are in the stirrups and the area draped in sterile towels the doctor can work undisturbed cut off from the patient's view
- the patient cannot see anything
- the emerging part is easily visible
- any instruments necessary to assist in the delivery are at hand and easily used
- the husband hiding at the head end of the bed is well protected

Ever tried using a bedpan in the supine position? The advantage of gravity and the use of the abdominal muscles and those of the floor of the pelvis are not utilised to their maximum advantage.

The issue of sex during pregnancy and after the delivery deserves special attention.

Provided adequate steps are taken during the pregnancy, especially closer to the expected date of delivery, sex need not be such a contentious issue. The rear entry position with the couple lying on their sides and the husband behind will avoid the deep penetration that can be problematic in the last weeks of the confinement. The missionary position is not recommended as lying on the mother's back puts enormous pressure of the weight of the heavy womb on the large vessels along the front of the spine. This compromises vital circulation to the foetus. For this reason the mother should not, as a rule, sleep on her back but rather on her side. Sex can become the last thing the recently delivered mother has on her mind, saddled with all the responsibility that comes after the birth. Whereas the sex starved husband may have the idea that the drought ends with the passage of the placenta! The pain and discomfort of an episiotomy (minor incision to the vagina sometimes necessary to widen the canal to make the delivery easier and less damaging to the birth canal) can also put a damper on sexual desire.

Sex should not be a matter of 'debate' and the husband is 'expected to be considerate'. The wife has gone through nine months of pregnancy and then the actual birth and any other procedures that were necessary for the delivery (perhaps a caesarian section) and the new baby and its attendant responsibilities and the eager visitors who travel from far and wide to view one's handiwork – there is no thought of sex. Yet this is the time to strengthen relationships that may have been taking strain in the last weeks of the confinement both for husband and wife.

Sex for the male can be a purely physical thing; there will be time later for five course sex. The deflating blow is often that the new arrival has taken precedence over everything and everybody and often the husband is 'neglected'. To get love one has to give it, often, first. Consideration for the spouse can pay dividends. It may help get a nappy changed at 3 am or the feed warmed at six.

Ignoring the need for sex and hoping the other partner will understand without discussion will not help the problem and often magnifies it out of proportion. The recently delivered wife on the one hand could be thinking "Surely he cannot want sex after all that I have just been through what with the baby being so demanding!" The husband, sulking to himself thinks "Can't she see we haven't had sex for months and now that the baby is born that prospect looks even more remote?", "Why the hell should I masturbate when I have a wife?" And "Why the hell should I take the garbage bin out when all she can do is attend to the baby's needs and ignores mine?" And "What happened to that sweet wonderful woman I married who swore that I would always be the only one in her life?" Look for the friend in one's partner and put oneself in the other partner's position and decide how one would prefer to be treated.

As mentioned earlier, do not underestimate the need for sleep, nutrition, exercise and love. Aim to have sleep spread out through the day and night in bite-size chunks instead of hoping to get a normal 'eight hour' sleep. Accept that until the infant settles into a sleeping pattern life will not be smooth sailing.

Meals should be supplemented with calcium, a multivitamin, Omega 3 and Vitamin E (200 I.U.). Exercise can be at a more sophisticated level at a gymnasium or walking outdoors away from exhaust fumes. Of course, all smoking should be banned within the house. In homes where children are exposed to cigarette smoke the incidence of chest and sinus or ear related problems are higher than smoke-free ones. Use the pregnancy, when the mother has avoided all cigarettes, to kick the addiction. Smoking even one cigarette a day during a pregnancy may increase the baby's chances of developing asthma. Smoke that is inhaled by the pregnant mother passes into the mother's blood and is then carried to the womb and into the blood of the foetus - robbing the growing brain and other organs of vital oxygen and 'suffocating' the baby.

Alcohol, as with all drugs, should be avoided. The first three months of the pregnancy are particularly important for such abstinences as the vital organs are being formed. Many drugs (cough mixtures and 'flu remedies') find their way to the baby through breast milk.

It is normal to have a discharge (bloody but not foul smelling) from the vagina for some days after the delivery. This should become less and less and eventually stop any time from about 10 to 20 days. The uterus, in the lower part of the belly, can be tender for about a week or so as it shrinks down (involutes) to it non-pregnant size (smaller than a small fist).

An episiotomy is an incision (cut) made under a local anaesthetic at the time the head of the baby is about to be delivered and the vagina is found to be not wide enough to allow the head to pass without tearing the vagina. Allowing the latter to happen is considered poor obstetric practice as the tear may extend itself into the rectum (back passage) with serious future complications for the control of the anal sphincter and possible incontinence of stool. A controlled incision limits the damage and the wound heals faster. The lax tissue around the vagina can be 'taken up' and sutured after the delivery to give the vagina a 'tighter' feel during intercourse.

An episiotomy wound usually heals quickly because of the rich blood supply but can be tender for up to 2 weeks. While the 'sitz bath' is often recommended to help in the healing this method exposes the bladder and vagina to bacteria from the wound and the back passage (rectum). A safer alternative is to shower normally, perhaps, twice a day directing the water toward the vagina. Zinc supplements and Vitamin C help promote faster wound healing. Adequate fluid intake (green/herbal tea without sugar) should be taken to help in the production of adequate breast milk and keep the bladder irrigated. The bladder and urethra (tube connecting the bladder to the outside) take some beating during the delivery and the extra fluid will help flush the bladder and prevent bacteria from causing infections (cystitis). Bacteria love stagnant urine and can proliferate from a single bacteria to millions within two hours!

All infants should be breast-fed. Mothers (and husbands) should be aware that breasts were designed not for looking perky in revealing swimsuits but for producing milk. Protective antibodies from the mother are passed to the baby through the milk for up to three to four months after the delivery. These antibodies protect the infant against many common infections. The incidence of gastroenteritis (diarrhoea), which often kills many infants, is much less when babies are breast fed. There are drugs without detrimental side effects that can stimulate breast milk so that mothers do not complain that "The milk dried up" or "was insufficient". Breast-feeding should be actively encouraged. Mothers should be allowed at least three months after the delivery to be with their children so breast-feeding and other motherly functions can be fulfilled.

Parents and in-laws should understand that the newly delivered mother and husband need to feel reassured that there is life after a pregnancy.

On the other hand the new parents should also understand that their baby is their own responsibility and not that of grandparents. Today's convenient 'babysitter' will soon be dictating what to feed the baby and how often they can indulge their grandchild with chocolates. Determine early how much 'interference' one would tolerate for once the green signal has been given grandparents have a habit of trying to get their own way. This is notwithstanding that they have had a lot of experience rearing their own children and their advice could save a lot of "I told you sos".

Grandparents should also bear in mind that the new parents , living on their own, wish to be their own bosses and can become very possessive of their new found joy and may wish to show that they are in control and can survive on their own. Allow them the freedom and offer advice as a friend, not as 'We know better'.

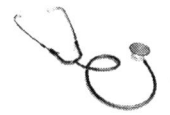

SEXUALLY TRANSMITTED DISEASES

Syphilis and gonorrhoea vie with each other for the title of the original 'sexually transmitted disease' or STD as they are called for reasons other than brevity – it lends a cloak of privacy to a sensitive subject.

The outbreak of AIDS has certainly highlighted an area that previously received scant attention viz., the consent to investigation and confidentiality of results and their role in the work place. If AIDs had been discovered 50 years ago it would probably have received as little attention as diphtheria or poliomyelitis had done. It is cold comfort to those who contract an STD but, as the name implies, these diseases can only be transmitted by a sexual encounter so the penis or vagina is usually involved one way or another. Any contact with the mouth, anus, blood, liquor (from the womb at the time of birth when the 'water breaks'), saliva, semen, urine or breast milk can transmit the Human Immunodeficiency Virus.

Sitting on a toilet seat can spread an STD if a person who is so infected has open sores on his or her buttocks and uses the toilet seat thereby contaminating it so that any other person who has an open skin lesion also on the buttocks using the same seat will also become infected. Using toilet paper to cover the toilet seat before sitting on it may help. A safer alternative may be to 'squat' over the toilet bowl without making any contact with the toilet seat.

The ideal would be disposable seat covers in all public toilets. Concerned users and women in particular should carry their own for such emergencies – like condoms! It may encourage the fairer sex to use public facilities especially in these times of heightened awareness of the AIDS spectre. It may also help to reduce the number of bladder problems this gender has that would rather have a bladder ready to burst than the prospect of using an unfamiliar toilet.

There are five infections that are commonly included in the STDs – syphilis, gonorrhoea, herpes, chlamydia and the HI virus. A person who has had unprotected intercourse may request a 'shot of penicillin' as a prophylactic measure against an STD infection. This should be strongly discouraged unless a diagnosis has first been established - even if it seems expedient at the time.

All of these infections require a blood sample in order to test for their presence. Done privately the tests are expensive and can make casual sex a costly (and dangerous) affair. Ideally, if a person has unprotected intercourse a blood sample should be taken as soon as possible and repeated within 2 weeks – which is how long it takes for infections like syphilis to become positive and to know if the levels of the test for chlamydia have risen to indicate an active infection. If HI virus antibodies are not detected the test should be repeated after 3 months. This is the 'window period' during which the test could become positive. Depending on how often one has unprotected sex and with how many different partners the tests could theoretically go on indefinitely, provided each previous test was negative.

The blood test for gonorrhoea is not very reliable. With this infection the male develops a burning sensation in the penis during the passage of urine. This is usually accompanied by a discharge from the penis (gleet) which, if present, should be presented to the doctor for a sample to be taken before the infected person passes urine, the best time being early morning. Gonorrhoea in the female is more difficult to detect as the symptoms described for the male partner are usually absent and the infected female may not be aware that she harbours the disease. Unfortunately, this makes it easier to spread around.

Any person with symptoms of burning urine must see the doctor early. It is important to confirm the diagnosis because bacteria other than Gonococci (which causes gonorrhoea) may produce the same symptoms. The implications for the partner also become very important. There is often the guilt and blame that goes with the suspicion of an STD that could have serious implications for a relationship. Undetected and untreated gonorrheal infections of the fallopian tubes (they carry the eggs from the ovaries to the womb) lead to 'adhesions' that block off the tube resulting in sterility. Treatment for gonorrhoea should be offered to both partners.

Any male or female in today's sexual climate who has had unprotected (and this protection is not guaranteed with the use of condoms) should be considered positive for an STD until the tests prove otherwise. There is little need to know the symptoms and signs of the different types of infections because there may be none, and neither the person who is infected, the person who he or she will spread it to nor the attending doctor may be any the wiser. The final arbiter is a blood test!

There may come a time in the not too distant future when marriage certificates will have an addendum: 'The above person is certified to have no evidence of an STD as of the. ...... (Date) and attested by the pathologist who performed the test.

To push this to its more complete extension it should also state whether there is a history of smoking, diabetes, hypertension, hypercholesterolemia, obesity and alcohol abuse with additional laboratory evidence to exclude inheritable genetic abnormalities.

If this information is of interest to insurance companies, whose sole concern is the financial risk to their investment, then what concern should a prospective bride or husband have before tying the wedding knot? Perhaps the future may also identify the individual who has the chromosome (genes) carrying the trait for wife or husband abuse. There already exists a chromosome for alcoholism. The woman or man who marries a smoker or alcoholic or other substance abuser should be aware in advance that such a person may die long before the expected date of departure that God intended.

Ideally, any person who has exposed him or herself to an STD must not have intercourse or preferably not without a condom with any other person until adequate blood tests exclude such a disease. This should include the incubation period of two weeks for certain of the infections and three months for the exclusion of the HI virus. The

HI virus test may be negative at the time and only become positive after the 3rd month from the time of exposure. During this 'window period' such a person may be infective and have no symptoms to warn the person carrying the infection or the one about to receive it.

Any contact between the mouth and the anus/vagina carries with it a risk of spreading infections like hepatitis (affecting the liver) and those affecting the gut – giardiasis, amoebiasis and salmonellosis (causing abdominal discomfort and diarrhoea) and E.coli infections of the bladder (cystitis). A finger introduced into the anus will harbour such organisms on the skin and under the nail and this will require cleaning, such as is practiced by a surgeon scrubbing up for an operation This is unlikely to happen in the back seat of a car in a clandestine romantic affair! Oral sex *after* anal intercourse carries an even greater risk of such infections.

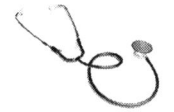

SEXUAL ABUSE

Rape has become the scourge of all females and males. The young and the elderly, mentally handicapped, the infirm, accident victims lying wounded at the roadside and in need of medical attention, children and adults in institutionalised care – no person is safe. Any mother who has a daughter runs the risk of her baby being ravaged; any mother who has a son could be rearing a future rapist.

Families that have known the trauma of rape committed by a trusted family member often deny or downplay the heinous deed to hide the shame and disgrace of exposure. Church elders who perpetrate this crime face the same agony. Mothers are often too trusting or find it easier to simply ignore the truth and hope it will go away. Wives may adopt a sympathetic stand defending their spouses even when they themselves are the victims of abuse. There may be a number of reasons for this among them fear of further abuse (both physical and sexual) aimed at them or the children, the withdrawal of monetary support and the perceived risk of losing a home or husband.

The perpetrator is usually known to the victim. Any male who has access to a female can be a potential abuser, given the opportunity or appropriate setting the deed is possible. Grandparents, uncles, cousins, nephews, teachers, drivers of lift clubs and school transport, wardens of hostels and other institutions are often placed in positions of trust and responsibility that offer ample opportunity to gain the confidence of their charges. The abuser marks out his quarry and stalks the victim in his own time and place. Parents often work; where do the children go after school or when they are ill and cannot be in school or the crèche? If a female offers to take care of them – are there any males about (either resident or visiting) that the parents of the intended victims do not know about? Because it is not suspected telltale signs are not looked for. Male ejaculate is not visible to the naked eye once it has dried though it does have an 'alkaline' odour – like 'Jik' (a bleaching agent).

Situations that encourage prolonged and unsupervised contact with potential victims e.g.

- Classroom
- Church
- Neighbour's house
- Workplace
- Internet
- Relatives – grandparents, uncles, nephews

In the classroom a student (quarry) is singled out for special attention. The predator is dealing with an unsuspecting, trusting, grateful-for-the-extra-attention young virgin. The adult has plenty of time and opportunity. A uniform lends itself to trust by association - whether it is a policeman, priest, paramedic, nurse or doctor.

The Internet has also created a haven for sex-offenders right under the noses of unsuspecting family members. Closed doors, late hours, computer illiterate parents and a whole world of seemingly innocent girls and boys are at the end of a mouse. The impressionable victim does not stand a chance pitted against the patience and cunning of the experienced stalker.

Children who do not receive the sympathy, understanding and attentive ear of their own family may appreciate the opportunity of receiving this from a seasoned paedophile. The movie 'Cape Fear' makes compelling viewing, illustrating how young people in need of emotional support can be manipulated by an unscrupulous adult.

Children with an unexplained discharge from the vagina or anal area or bladder infection should have the possibility of sexual abuse considered. Mood or behaviour changes or unexpected poor performances in school , recent reluctance to be left alone or to be in the company of certain people with whom the child was previously comfortable, a change in mood, mannerism or train of conversation with the arrival of a person into a room , changes in established sleep patterns or nightmares and bedwetting (enuresis) of recent onset, unusual friendliness or outward displays of inappropriate familiarity or affection towards a male friend or relative, a sudden reluctance to allow the genitalia (private parts) to be washed or touched should warrant further discreet investigation.

It may be sufficient to inform young children less than five years of age that the purpose of the genitalia is for the passage of urine and that nobody except their parents should show any interest in these parts of their bodies. Tact, gentleness and understanding are important so that unnecessary preoccupation with or unfounded fears about the genitalia are not generated. After this age the additional function of reproduction could be introduced as they may have already become explorative and know the pleasure of fondling their genitalia.

The fear of promiscuity in this education is unfounded. Trust should be developed at an early age and the advice to "Report all to mum – regardless" inculcated so that the child does not fear exposure. Children need to understand that there may be things that go wrong in their lives that they may not have total control over but that no matter how bad it looks, not confiding in parents will always be worse than the disclosure.

If the child is immediately reprimanded or, worse still, punished for any 'wrongdoing' this will seal the fate of future trust. The 'disclosure' should be done in private and confidentiality respected, away from other siblings and relatives but always inclusive of the other parent. Children must understand that there cannot be any secret that cannot be heard by both parents equally. Both parents should understand that, where a child feels more comfortable with one parent alone, as they often do, the child should be aware that the other parent will be privy to the secret without fail – sooner or later. It should also be understood that the confidence will be respected. This avoids alienating the other parent, often the father, and presents a picture of a united front and shared parenthood.

Females will always be vulnerable to the attention of men. Knowing this must make mothers and people in charge of females more wary and take men less for granted whoever they may be. Parents of children sleeping over at friends' homes must do some homework before they entrust others with their precious progeny. Similarly, parents must be seen to be concerned whenever their daughters (and sons) leave the house reinforcing the idea that somebody cares enough to ask questions. This should not be confused with a lack of trust and should be balanced with an adult's intuition and greater years of experience.

Peer pressure is a reality and children need to develop the skills necessary to cope with it. This begins at an early age – when they are starting at a crèche or preschool. Read between the lines when the teacher says "Everything is fine". Does it fit with the other clues that come home with the child each day? Ask questions: "Who was naughty in the class today?" "What did teacher say or do when so-and-so was naughty?" "Did anybody get into trouble today?" "What punishment was meted out?" "Do the teachers lose their tempers with any of the children?" "And what do they say when they are cross?" This 'interrogation' should be done casually and introduced as part of the general conversation about school rather than on the lines of an inquisition. If the situation is appropriate ask openly if alcohol is being served. Know what your child is likely to do if an illegal substance was offered. Parents who smoke and then turn a blind eye to their own children's smoking are hardly 'turning a blind eye'. To avoid the hypocrisy that must accompany any admonishment against this addiction parents must stop smoking themselves before they can cast the first stone.

If parents can be penalised for sexually abusing their child or depriving them of food/clothing the law should be equally harsh for allowing them to smoke or take drugs or rape other people's children. If parents can have children they must be made to be responsible for the mayhem their offspring can cause. When a twenty-five year old man hijacks a car and shoots the owner in cold blood do his parents stand trial with him? The weapon did not fall out the sky into the young man's hand! Did the parents play any role at all in the events that may have had their seeds when their offspring was five years old? The hijacker did not come slithering out of his mother brandishing an AK47. When did things start to go wrong and where were the parents when it was happening?

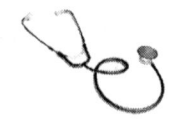

SINUSITIS

The bones of the face and skull contain fairly large air spaces to make the weight of the bones i.e. the skull – lighter. These 'air spaces' are called *sinuses* and are present in each cheek and on each side of the forehead and in the center - just above the bridge of the nose.

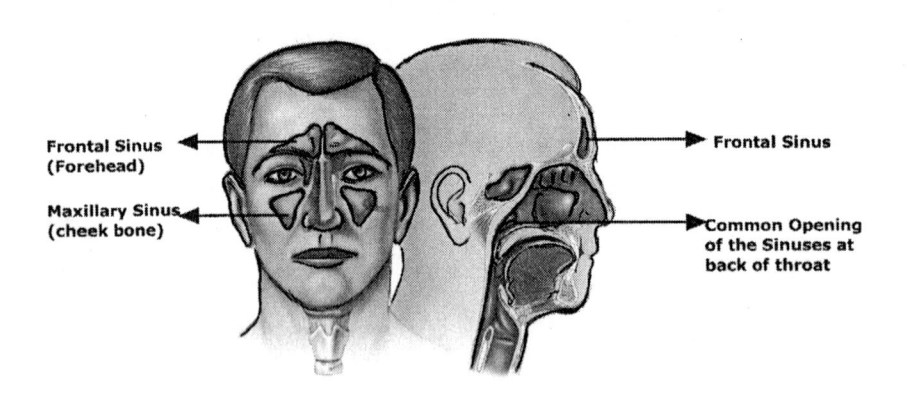

Frontal Sinus (Forehead)

Maxillary Sinus (cheek bone)

Frontal Sinus

Common Opening of the Sinuses at back of throat

SINUSES

There is another situated behind each eye The sphenoidal sinuses - one behind each eye are very close to the brain in the base of the skull. This position carries a potential risk of spreading an infection to the lining of the brain (meningitis).

If a sinus becomes infected pus drains out through an opening situated within the back of the nose and close to the adenoids. Enlarged adenoids may obstruct the common (single) opening of the sinuses on each side and lead to chronic sinusitis.

Generations of children have been admonished for sniffing when there is a nasal discharge – this is one of grandma's myths. Blowing the nostrils (under great pressure) may force infected mucus into the other sinuses and also into the middle ears. Each ear is connected by a thin tube (eustachian tube) that starts at the back of the nose and throat and their purpose is to equalise the outside atmospheric pressure with the pressure within the inner ear. It is safer to sniff the mucus backwards into the throat and then spit out. This avoids forcing every 'runny nose' into an infection of the sinuses!

These bony air-filled cavities have a lining (mucosa) similar to that of the nostrils. This mucosa may become inflamed and infected (sinusitis) and cause fever and severe throbbing pain depending on which particular sinus has been affected – frontal, cheeks, between the eyes or more deep seated behind the eyes. There may or may not be a post nasal discharge depending on whether the opening (ostium) of the sinuses is patent or not. If the mucus should become 'trapped' within a particular sinus or sinuses this may require drainage by the Ear, Nose and Throat surgeon if an adequate course of antibiotics does not first resolve the symptoms.

During the day the postnasal 'drip' is either brought out/coughed up or swallowed; but during the night (one cannot cough if one is asleep!) the patient is lying supine (on the back) and the mucus has no alternative but to drip down into the throat and, once there, behaves like a foreign body. The protective mechanism of coughing automatically kicks in and the foreign substance is evicted from the upper airways. Understandably, this cough will get worse at night!

Catchy advertising and dozens of over the counter preparations promise quick relief from these 'bad', 'irritating' coughs and a 'good night's sleep'! The truth is the body has developed the cough reflex to prevent any foreign substance (postnasal drip included) from entering the lungs. Using a cough suppressant may mask the cough but there is no longer the protection afforded by the cough reflex to prevent mucus/pus from entering the bronchial tubes and the lungs. Thanks to over-the-counter-remedies (O.T.C.) a simple 'sinusitis' could be converted into bronchitis or pneumonia, with often dire consequences. Without the *life saving* cough reflex mankind would have killed himself from lung complications aeons ago!

The pharmaceutical industry should desist from plugging ad nauseam every winter the merits of cough mixtures for the sake of profit. The main indication for a 'cough mixture' should be a cough that has no sputum i.e. 'dry and irritating'. Many patients who insist that their cough is dry are simply swallowing (!) the sputum as it is coughed up out of the lungs. Women are especially loathe to spit out phlegm! Would anybody cough out the sputum into a teacup and then deliberately swallow the spit? This illustrates *what the eye does not behold the brain does not bemoan!*

It is not well appreciated that though all the sinuses are interconnected they have a single exit opening and also that a connection exists to the ears through the Eustachian tubes (help equalize the pressure within the ear with the outside atmospheric pressure). Mothers who admonish young children, who become adults and continue the habit of blowing the nostrils, are 'helping' to spread under pressure, mucus to all the sinuses via the nose and possibly into the ears. Does this explain the very high incidence of sinusitis and ear infections? If blowing the nose is to be uncomplicated it should be done with both nostrils open i.e. unobstructed - without closing first one then the other nostril - as is the common practice.

A purulent discharge (yellow or green and all shades in between) from the nose or as a postnasal discharge (snorted backwards from the back of the nostrils and into the throat) requires an antibiotic and decongestant.

Side effects of many of the common remedies are often misinterpreted as being the symptoms of sinusitis itself and they include drowsiness and irritability. The least expensive and more effective single drug (as compared to the polypharmacy – multiple drugs – contained in almost every O.T.C preparation) is prednisolone 5mg usually in a dose of 2 tablets taken twice a day for 2 to 3 days. One precaution to be observed is that it should not be taken on an empty stomach (similar to the advice given when NSAIDs – non-steroidal anti-inflammatory drugs are used). Reluctance by the profession to use prednisolone stems from the side effects and complications that occur when this drug is used in large doses - 8 to 12 tablets daily for several months for certain conditions (usually quite serious ones).

Prednisolone, which is a steroid (not the type abused by athletes), can be life saving in an acute attack of asthma and is then used in a dose of 6-8 tablets daily for up to fourteen days. The dose suggested for sinusitis is smaller and is taken for up to 3 days. Steroids are anti-inflammatory in action; the underlying problem in asthma and sinus-itis is inflammation. In an acute allergic reaction steroids are given in large doses in injectable form. Some of the nasal sprays used in hay fever contain steroids in miniscule quantities. Many people are afraid to use steroids because of media exposure making it a 'bad-die'. This often includes doctors who would prefer to use other more 'user-friendly' drugs. One ingredient called 'phenylpropanolamine' (fee-nile-pro-pan-all-a-mean!) that is used in several OTC prepara-tions for sinusitis has been banned in the USA by the Federal Drug Administration (F.D.A.) – the watchdog of all drugs prescribed in America. This drug has been shown to cause brain haemorrhages yet in Britain and other countries the general public still receives it for 'colds, flu, sinusitis and coughs.

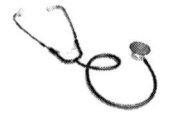

SORE THROAT

If swallowing is painful throughout the day this is strongly suggestive of an infection in the throat and this should be treated with a penicillin type of antibiotic unless there is an allergy to this class of drugs.

If the discomfort is present mainly in the morning and improves as the morning progresses the usual cause is mouth-breathing through the night because of blocked nostrils. Breathing through the mouth for prolonged periods dries out the throat causing discomfort. This habit also makes it easier to introduce an infection – no tissue in the body will tolerate 'drying out'. The blocked nostrils are invariably accompanied by a postnasal drip implicating the sinuses (sinusitis). This does not require an antibiotic but a decongestant to 'unblock' the sinuses. These episodes of 'sore throats 'are often mistakenly labelled as 'tonsillitis' and innocent tonsils are needlessly sacrificed.

If the colour of the postnasal drip is yellow or green anytime after midmorning an antibiotic should be prescribed as this implies that there is an ongoing presence of bacteria. The colour of the discharge is determined by the presence of specific bacteria that are yellow or green. Sometimes there may be a tinge or streak of blood in the mucus and provided this disappears within a day or two, is not cause for concern. If it persists for longer than a week or more, this will require the opinion of an Ear, Nose and Throat surgeon. This blood may have a more serious significance if it occurs in an older person (over 45 or so years) and probably more so if the person is a smoker. Mucus that lies within the upper airways and sinuses may become discoloured overnight but should *not* remain this colour for most of the day. The latter situation will need an antibiotic and not most of the 'junk' that is passed off as remedies for 'flu' and 'sinusitis'. One drug commonly used in these over-the-counter remedies – phenylpropanolamine – has been shown to cause strokes and has been banned in the United States.

A streptococci bacterium commonly causes sore throats or tonsillitis ('Strep. throat'). If it is not treated timeously with penicillin it could cause rheumatic fever that can in turn damage the heart valves. These particular bacteria can also affect the kidneys in a condition called glomerulonephritis – the 'glomerulus' is a part of the kidney through which the blood is filtered (like passing it through a tea strainer) and 'nephritis ' means inflammation or infection of the tubes through which urine passes within the kidney (nephron=tube).

Children and teenagers are especially prone to this potential damage to two vital organs – the heart and kidneys. Withholding a course of penicillin at the price of a few pence will not match the cost of replacing a heart valve damaged by rheumatic fever or the cost of dialysis for kidney failure as a result of glomerulonephritis. It is not the appearance of the throat (it does not matter what the throat looks like inside) that should determine whether the patient needs an antibiotic or not but the presence of pain on swallowing that persists after mid-morning or midday.

The tonsils acquire a notorious fame because they are often the seats of infection in the throat. They perform the very useful function of protecting the rest of the body by trapping bacteria within the tonsils if they should gain entry into the mouth. It is understandable that in the course of their duty the tonsils may become enlarged and painful when 'infected'. Lymph glands serve a similar protective function. However, if true tonsillitis should occur more than 4 –5 times in a year they should be removed (Tonsillectomy), as they are most likely harbouring the bacteria by becoming 'chronically infected' and defeating their purpose of being effective guardians.

The white patches that may occur on the tonsils in tonsillitis are caused by food/debris/bacteria that become trapped in the little crevices on the surfaces of the tonsils. Their presence does not mean the tonsils are infected – but imply that (because of pain in the throat) swallowing is restricted and not as effective in washing away 'debris' from the mouth. This accumulates on the tonsils. When diphtheria was rife this infection produced a distinctive whitish membrane-like discharge on the tonsils and throat. Diphtheria has been eradicated through immunisation in childhood. The 'DTP' vaccine affords protection against diphtheria, tetanus and poliomyelitis.

An important clue whether a fish/chicken bone is stuck in the throat is the patient is reluctant to swallow and saliva pools in the mouth. If the person can swallow saliva easily it is very unlikely that the 'foreign body' is still stuck in the throat and an urgent trip to the doctor /emergency unit can be postponed. If discomfort is present afterwards, as a result of minor irritation from a bone that has been successfully swallowed, an antacid may relieve the symptom.

A sore throat in an older person should not be taken lightly especially if it persists for longer than such an infection should ordinarily last (+/ – a week). Cancer of the throat would be a concern and an opinion from an Ear, Nose and Throat surgeon should be sought early instead of repeated prescriptions for more antibiotics and throat gargles.

A person who has had a recent general anaesthetic may have a sore throat afterwards. This is often caused by the endotracheal tube that was passed through the throat and used to connect the lungs to the ventilator. If the symptom persists for longer than 4 – 5 days an antibiotic maybe indicated, especially if the anaesthetist should disclose that the intubation (passage of the endotracheal tube) had been difficult for any reason.

If 'tonsillitis' has not improved within 48 hours on an antibiotic and the pain has become steadily worse in spite of analgesics the doctor should be seen *again* as the tonsil/s may have developed into an abscess (quinsy) and this would need the services of an ENT surgeon to drain the abscess and not, as is often prescribed, a 'stronger' antibiotic.

Asthmatics, who use steroid inhalers and do not rinse out their mouths after using the inhaler, are at risk for developing thrush in the mouth or throat. The presence of painful, white patches on the mouth or throat that bleed or leave a raw area when they are scraped off with a toothbrush should alert one to this infection. This is treated with antifungal drops or ointment.

Like a popular TV advertisement once proclaimed "It's not inside it's on top" one should be aware that *not every 'sore throat'* has to do with an infection inside the throat. The thyroid gland situated *outside* the front of the throat may become inflamed (thyroiditis) and cause pain/discomfort on swallowing as the gland moves up and down with deglutition (act of swallowing). Touching the gland in front of the neck will cause pain without swallowing. This will require blood tests and treatment for the thyroid gland but no antibiotics.

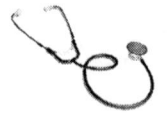

SOUNDING OFF

Knowledge has little value if it cannot be shared. A million sperm dutifully produced in the testicle will doom the species to extinction without the catalyst that sends them on their last journey. One lifetime is too short to disseminate the knowledge and experience that my patients have shared with me over the years.

Throughout my career I have found myself constantly trying to master the art of listening. Medical school shortchanged me in its acquisition. Listening is the catalyst that transforms the stethoscope into treatment. All the skills learned at university had one aim: the treatment of disease (and not always the patient). One did not need to listen that attentively in order to make a diagnosis and initiate therapy - "Sore throat?" "Say Ah!" "Take these capsules". "Next!" So what if the patient works night shift and his marriage is being threatened. What has this to do with the sore throat? Nothing!

This art of listening with a passion is what separates the men from the boys, the spouses from the abusers, the lovers from the users, the boys from the bullies, the politicians from the statesmen, the kings from the gods. The ability to listen to one's self is the first requisite: "Is that what you are saying?" Is that what you would wish the listener to hear? Getting it right the first time avoids the need to have to say "I'm sorry. I didn't mean that" or "Sorry I stepped on your toes", "Stole your wallet" or "Raped your daughter".

Listen to yourself with a passion: do you really want to do this or that? Make time stand still while you listen – banish the boredom; wipe out the wailing of the infant as you listen to the anxious mother.

Does the tummy ache mean a rogue teacher is terrorising the class, does the "I have a terrible headache" really mean it's payback time (no sex tonight) for standing one up a whole hour while cocktails were being shared with friends?

Attentive listening is a neglected necessity in today's times. In the days when grandpa and grandma ruled the roost they grasped better the art of it. Today's young mother, rushing home from a trying day's work, competing with men for jobs once the preserve of males, catches the train, her mind already 'closing down' the computer which served her at work and is now contemplating what she will cook for supper, hoping the corner store has not run out of milk.

As her foot crosses the front door "Mummy, mummy, Timothy threw sand all over the washing", and "Dad called to say he is playing squash tonight and can his supper be kept in the oven" and "Teacher said to bring money for the school play." Who has the time or the energy or the inclination to listen attentively? The 'tummy ache' receives 'paracetamol' and the class bully escapes. One cannot be listening, let alone attentively, if one is travelling through life on an express train. The pace has to be slowed down no matter what it takes to do it i.e. cooking meals in advance, cutting out the extra piano lessons, delegating household chores, hiring help for the heavier ones, getting husband to cook on two nights and getting organised. Successful people use a diary and understand that efficient use of their time is the equivalent of how they manage their money – time is money!

King Procrastination is the thief of time. I remember learning this in grammar school but its real significance escaped me until I was much older – Procrastination steals my time. It is difficult to keep track of the things one needs to do and one should not rely on memory to remember everything. This is unfair to the brain and a certain way to get less done.

A diary helps to see what one achieved with the limited time at our disposal. Be under no illusions: there can be only twenty-four hours in anybody's day. This, for a life span of 80 years, is the equivalent of 42,048,000 minutes. One has already used up so many of them to get to where one is at any given moment – how many remain? And, more importantly, how efficiently will one use what is left?

The person who knows the value of those remaining minutes is the one who has been diagnosed with cancer and has been told (and how this is calculated remains a mystery!) he or she has three months to live: this translates into 129,600 minutes. This person would cherish each waking moment, like a connoisseur swirling the last sip of a rare wine afraid to swallow for then it would be all gone, lost forever from the pleasure it gave the palate. We need to live as though we have cancer – and cherish each moment – for who knows when it will be the last. But I suspect that somewhere, between the last paycheque and the last account that demanded a slice of one's hard earned (but short lived) salary, the ability to savour the precious moment was lost. The lament is often that "Time goes so fast"! However, it is "going" no faster than it did last year or the one before that or the one a million years ago. Are we doing more than our grandparents and parents did with our time? Or is some of it an illusion of doing more?

If the TV breaks down for even a day presto! One has almost four extra hours. Ignore the TV for a month and suddenly one has 120 extra hours, which calculates to 5 whole days. For a year that equals 60 days i.e. 3 entire months! Simple arithmetic should dictate that one has access to only nine months of each year. Small wonder that time seemingly disappears so fast.

The seemingly faster passage is also linked to another phenomenon that has insidiously snaked its way into our lives, something that each successive generation has little knowledge about and innocently accepts what it sees as the norm. Worldwide, companies and businesses have come to realize that the prosperity of the past three decades following the recovery from the depression of the last world war was not going to sustain them into the twenty-first century. 'Downsize' has become the new description for shrinking businesses, merging with other companies and laying off staff. This has helped to produce more work for the remaining few, not necessarily more income.

The elusive salary disappears within the first week of its receipt. The brain is already planning for the following month's salary and in its expectation spends the following three weeks in a state of limbo with all things mental and physical put on hold until the arrival of the next paycheque. If one is living only for one week each month is it surprising that time does fly faster? The stress and unhappiness this creates in the work environment cannot be good for business. But then who cares? If one does not like the terms of employment then there are many others (already retrenched) to fill the vacancy. Is this the employee one is expecting should smile and care about the whims and fancies of customers and should go the proverbial extra mile?

The caring and concern must come from the top down. Let one late motorist into a busy lane and watch the goodwill spread itself as he or she lets another into the queue. One fifth of the wealth of the world belongs to 225 people. How many of the rest of the working population are employed simply to maintain this status quo, helping some executive's wife go overseas on holiday or some boss buy a new car? And for this the company pays the labour force. The job description should read, not 'bank clerk' or 'teller', but 'person employed to help Mr. Director to buy overseas oil shares'.

The job is not designed to make Joe rich but to keep his head just below the 'H.P.' (hire purchase) line. As long as his head remains below the H.P. line the TV that he purchased on terms with his first salary cheque will avoid being repossessed. Once this has been paid off then Joe will then make his next purchase – also on terms. This is the power of poverty. The TV cannot wait to be bought for cash when the interest saved could pay for two TV sets! The persuasion of advertising and the "I want it now" generation! This has become the accepted way of doing business. If every person refused to buy the car that has increased in cost from £150 in 1972 to over £14000 today to whom will the manufacturer sell its product?

Does anybody remember that the pocket of potatoes that not so long ago weighed 15 kg now weighs 10 kg but the cost remains the same? This marketing strategy deserves a special award for sheer business thievery. But then who remembers the difference in size between 10 and 15 kg?

Poor Joe has not a clue that as long as he is employed by Mr. Director he is never going to become rich. For this to happen, Joe must aim to become self-employed. But Mr. Director and Mr. Bank Manager must work hand in glove. The bank ensures that Joe will never get finance. This is the easy part: give him a cheque account and the hapless wit is bound to have at least one dishonoured cheque and that is the minimum requirement for never qualifying for a loan. Without the loan what private enterprise is Joe considering? Medical school equipped one to treat disease and improve health. Did anybody stop to inquire how health is to be acquired without wealth?

Poverty will remain the biggest obstacle in the way of improving the health of a nation. How can one improve the immune status of a school child without adequate nutrition (not food) so that common diseases do not undermine his or her health? Big business and misguided health officials will go a long way to foster the use of drugs to combat AIDS but little is made of the need to improve the immune status of the patient by using better nutrition and supplements.

How does one get good nutrition without money? Cheaper foods satiate the pangs of hunger but do not provide adequate nutrition. Tuberculosis is a reflection of a compromised immune status, be it from a breakdown following the Aids infection, diabetes, alcoholism or poverty. How can the scourge of tuberculosis be eradicated without improving the wealth, the economy, the buying power of Joe's salary? What medical practitioner worth his stethoscope is doing anything about improving the wealth of his patient? For without this, good health will remain but a dream.

The subject of Nutrition has remained an enigma all through my medical career. Prescribe an antibiotic for pneumonia, advise plenty of fluids and rest but nary a mention about nutrition. The illness itself impairs the patient's appetite. At a time when the body requires *better* nutrition than when the person was well this vital requirement is sadly lacking. How do the cells feed themselves without adequate nutrition when healing must take place with the help of blood cells? How does the adrenal gland produce hormones to help in a time of crisis?

The following cannot be produced by the body and, therefore, must be taken daily either in the food or, failing this, as a supplement:

- Vitamins
- Essential amino acids
- Fatty acids
- Proteins

The tiredness one feels at the end of a 'hard days work' is not always a result of 'working hard' but that the adrenal glands have inadequate supplies of four vitamins (A, B, C and E) used in the production of adrenaline and steroids which are secreted in the body's response to stress.

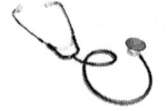

STRESS

The underlying causes of stress can be narrowed to a few important ones
- Work
- Sex
- Money
- Relationships
- Health

Sometimes all of them play a role and then chaos reigns. Of the five 'health' is the most important. If one is dead the others will not matter. Stress is often perceived as an affliction of the age we live in. Did the slave who helped push the stone to build the mighty pyramid suffer from any stress each time the taskmaster's whip cracked menacingly above his head? Did the soldier who helped Alexander the Great guide an elephant over the treacherous snow-clad Alps suffer from stress? Did any farmer suffer from stress each time a monstrous monsoon downpour threatened to wash away his precious crops? Stress has been with us for as long as we have been around though the guise may have been different. Sometimes we create stress for our own personal use. The teenager who cannot see that the dirty socks belong in the clothes basket is expected to learn now, after years of being allowed to get away with doing what he is still doing today, just because his mother cannot 'take it' anymore? The frustrated mother loses good adrenaline. The son cannot understand what the fuss is about and is certainly not going to see the lesson at that moment, which is something he should have learned a long time ago. Mum should recognise this and act accordingly to avoid the so-called 'stress'. Enlist the lad's help with a regular "John can you help me collect all the dirty clothes from the bathroom?" will lose a lot less adrenaline than "John, how many times have I told you not to leave your dirty socks in the bathroom?" However, one should not expect offspring to do the very things parents cannot or will not.

Each time one gets angry or upset the adrenal gland is stimulated to release adrenaline. This gland resembles a small 'Napoleon's cap' situated on top of each kidney. Adrenaline is the chemical that makes the heart beat faster and if produced often enough is one of the causes of stress, hypertension, heart attacks and strokes. During a heart attack morphine is given to relieve the pain because while this is present adrenaline will be produced and this in turn will make the heart beat faster. The faster the heart works the greater the demand for blood and oxygen and, given the nature of the problem, these cannot be supplied as there is a coronary arterial blockage. Pain relief can limit further damage to the heart muscle by cutting down on the release of adrenaline and cortisol (steroids).

In order for the adrenal glands to produce adrenaline and cortisol the appropriate building materials must be supplied. These include four vital vitamins – A, B, C and E.

The complaints often heard at the end of a day would imply that the person had worked very hard or had experienced a very stressful day. The truth is that these essential vitamins have been lacking and a regular supply will help improve the ability to cope with stresses. If food does not contain the above essential vitamins these will have to be outsourced from reliable supplements - the body cannot make or store them. Any 'stress management' programme that ignores the importance of improved nutrition is missing the petrol in the Ferrari!

Adrenaline and cortisol were designed to help the mammal to 'flee' in the face of danger. Without these the 100 metre sprint, with the heart rate pounding and respiration increasing to meet the demands of the physical challenge, the bladder that suddenly needs to be evacuated, the stools that become loose and the mouth that becomes dry – are all part of the picture of 'stress' produced by these two hormones. These short-lived bursts of hormones are vital to our existence. However, producing them continuously, as one tends to do in one's daily life, and the scene is set for the development of hypertension, cardiovascular disease, peptic ulcers and an early death.

People in general and housewives and the unemployed, in particular, often feel that their days are too unimportant or mundane to warrant the use of a diary. However, it could be an important start in the management of stress. Be under no illusions – it is the brain that controls every thought and action. A well planned diary helps the brain see the day as a planned event regardless of whether one is planning pot roast for supper, leaving a note for the gardener or planning a major directors' meeting. Putting the goals for the day on paper is the first step to achieving one's life ambitions. People who cannot do this on paper for one day will not easily succeed in planning for the year – let alone for longer. Anything that is not on paper is simply a dream waiting to become a reality. For many this step never materialises.

Live each day as though it were one's last. The tedium of a daily diary will change dramatically if one is diagnosed as having cancer and only a short time to live! Then every moment, in that hitherto 'boring' day, will take on a new meaning and value. Planning one's day will go a long way to reducing stress levels. The brain is presented with a dress rehearsal for the day to come so that the end product is predictable and, therefore, more polished.

Adequate, quality sleep is another prerequisite for reducing stress levels. Those working overtime and doing shift work often underestimate the importance of sleep. Sleep deprivation was used as a form of torture during the last world war. Its mental and physical effects are well known. Employers also need to understand this when they expect staff to work extra hours. Dangling overtime pay as the proverbial carrot often ignores the effects of the longer hours on the health and welfare of their employees and their families.

How many shift workers arrive home at unearthly hours and expect the, often working, wife to have supper warmed and sex afterwards. The sleep deprived and frustrated wife then carries her 'stressed' state to the workplace the following morning. How can this aid better productivity and at the end of the day have a mother that is free of stress and able to fulfill her obligations to her family (and the husband who will return again at midnight to make his own demands)?

Partying until the wee hours denies a responsibility to one's employer. Every employee should ensure that he or she is in the best possible condition, physically and mentally, to do the work to the best of his or her ability. This can hardly be possible if the employee has had insufficient sleep or nutrition, is being abused at home (or at work), has an ill child at the crèche, severe menstrual cramps or untreated hypertension.

Alcohol and other substances of abuse will rob the employee of the chance to produce his/her best whether this involves taking out an appendix or the garbage. Perhaps patients need to enquire from their caregivers whether they are in a fit state to be entrusted with their health or the garbage man their waste. Could this explain why bits of garbage happen to spill out of the bin onto the sidewalk? And why Mondays are not the best for car services! The stress generated from the abuse of alcohol and the lack of sleep, as a consequence, has little way of being detected and, therefore, prevented.

Management should be informed early, rather than later, when stress creeps in so that effective measures can be instituted before the problem becomes insurmountable. It could make the burden of stress more manageable. Employers are often in the dark about their employee's problems until symptoms start to show or work suffers to the detriment of colleagues or the company.

A recently married person opting to do night shift work is starting off on the wrong foot even though there could be pressing financial difficulties that make the overtime alluring. An unhappy sex life will not produce a happy employee and will generate its own stress and eventually backfire on the company that requested overtime work.

In the interests of reducing stress levels companies might gain more by subsidising the cost and attainment of better nutrition and vitamin supplementation. This could help increase productivity and at the same time promote healthier staff that will fall ill less frequently and have fewer life threatening diseases that, ultimately, lose much in the way of valuable skills and people that industry can ill afford.

Walking also relieves stress. To be beneficial it has to be performed at least three times a week for about an hour each time covering a distance of five kilometres or half hour daily doing three kilometres. Exercise improves the circulation to every part of one's body and releases endorphins responsible for lifting the mood and warding off depression and stress. Workplaces could invest in user friendly gymnasium equipment. Healthier staffs ensure more productive employees who will also welcome the concern for their welfare. Subsidising memberships to local gymnasiums by employers and medical aid schemes would be a step in the right direction towards a healthier population. A punching bag could be very useful for defusing tension.

Sex is an excellent stress reliever particularly within the environment of a loving relationship where the wife's feeling of "Why should I?" does not operate. Partners need to keep in touch with each other's needs. Sex in a good relationship should not be construed as a matter of 'consideration'. Wives would concern themselves no end about what to cook for dinner but not give sex a second thought because this is not regarded as a vital part of the day's activities.

Women may be blissfully unaware of the differing physiological needs that men have compared to themselves. Women could easily not have sex on their minds for days on end – quite the opposite to what their partners experience. To simply relieve stress and keep the wheels of good relationships well oiled sex does not always have to be a mind-blowing marathon affair. 'Quickie sex' is an excellent alternative and the wife does not have to feel cheated by it or feel used. Such feelings usually arise when there are problems within the marriage – when "Why should I?" feelings appear through the cracks. The old adage, that a family that 'prays together stays together', should have an addendum.

Whatever transpires within the confines and secrecy of the bedroom will not be accessible to the outside world. If the wife refuses to have sex with her partner who else will know of it? The husband may find that his pride and ego do not allow him to disclose this (embarrassing) problem to another living soul. How does a husband so denied of his sexual expression (marital right?) reconcile his frustration? Does he take a mistress? Does he engage the services of a sex worker? Does he rape somebody? Does he resort to sex on the Internet? His puritanical upbringing, religious beliefs and 'inability' to find alternative release, even in masturbation, may make these options difficult and, for many, impossible.

Society does not have easy solace for the sexually denied. Alcohol and the ears of a sympathetic barman may help to momentarily drown the problem. Alternatively, alcohol could then embolden the husband to take by force the sex denied him. Does the wife seek refuge in "Why should I when he comes home drunk?" - adding one more reason to withhold the sex that started the problem in the first instance.

Many quarrels and fights tend to occur at night or the early hours of the morning. If supper was taken at 6 o'clock and has long been digested and a marathon argument is being played out hours later this could reflect the effects of a low blood sugar level. If any alcohol has been imbibed the sugar levels can be further lowered as alcohol is known to depress blood glucose. And if the quarrel started earlier and *no supper* eaten the stage is further set for the effects of hypoglycemia (low blood glucose) – as occurs in diabetics who take insulin and do not eat adequately. The symptoms of hypoglycaemia include increasing irritability and restlessness, apprehension, trembling, emotional instability, aggressiveness or behaviour resembling drunkenness. Awareness of this physiological low blood sugar may avert related quarrels by offering a sugared drink for immediate relief and a more complex carbohydrate like pasta for a longer lasting source of energy. Oats make a useful night-time snack. Beware the alcoholic quarrelsome partner – a low blood sugar level may be contributing to the problem and correcting this may help defuse the situation.

In-laws, as potential sources of stress, may have a simple solution:- stay away from them. The husband or wife will never take your side against his or her parents and do not expect the partner to do this.

In-laws may find it difficult to accept one as their own 'daughter' or 'son'

Infidelity has no place in a marriage built on love and understanding and compromises. If it ever happens, and the decision is taken to remain in the marriage for whatever reason, get or insist on professional help *immediately* and not later. The intervening period until this is undertaken is often simply wasted time. The partner, devastated by the discovery, has no experience or skill in the handling of the 'disease' and the errant party would be heading for a separation by refusing to seek professional assistance.

The 'truth and reconciliation' that should follow the discovery must be seen and felt to be genuine and from the heart or else the future of the relationship may remain troubled and tenuous for up to a lifetime. It would be far better to make a fresh start early and suffer the pain at the time instead of waiting, perhaps, twenty years to learn the lesson that today's indiscretion has the potential for further infidelities. The stress that infidelity can generate will eat away at the relationship every day until the causes and solutions have been addressed.

If one is faced with a sudden stressful situation take a deep breath and hold it for as long as possible and then exhale slowly. This will help to relieve tension. Taking a sugared drink about twenty minutes before making a speech will help to dampen down the effects of adrenaline that accompanies such stressful undertakings. Massage therapy could be a useful adjunct to de-stressing – whether it happens as part of an aromatherapy session or through the loving hands of a caring spouse. There will be little resistance to a relaxing massage as a means of making up when things do not go right and one has caused pain or been party to a silly argument and this could be engineered into an erotic bit of foreplay.

A few precautions : –

* the room should not be cold
* hands should be warmed
* start with the back and sit astride the buttocks without putting one's dead weight on the partner

- avoid pressing directly upon the spine
- avoid applying excessive force – one is not expelling air from pizza dough!
- use the finger tips and thumbs
- use 'baby oil' or aromatherapy oil (more expensive?)
- avoid the belly and breasts – there are no important muscles there and pressure over the abdomen could generate an untimely visit to the toilet!
- steer carefully around the testicles
- avoid massaging over varicose veins in the legs
- avoid the anal area (risk of contaminating the hands)

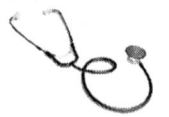

SWELLING OF THE FEET

Swelling of the feet is due to fluid (water) that has 'leaked' out of the veins of the legs into the soft tissues of the feet; this is called 'oedema' (pronounced without the 'o'). Depending on how much of fluid has leaked out the swelling may initially be below each 'knob' on either side of the ankle joint. If it progresses it will then come to lie over the front or top of the foot. It will not spread into the soles of the feet because the tissue here is thicker and more tightly bound, unlike the loose skin on the top of the feet. With the effect of gravity the fluid may collect under the skin up to the knees, thighs and, in extreme cases, into the lax skin of the scrotum (sac surrounding the testicles) and eventually in the abdominal wall.

There may be a number of causes for the swelling. The commonest is varicose veins, especially if the swelling occurs in one leg only or the amount of swelling is unequal - with one side more swollen than the other. Regardless of the cause, if the legs are kept elevated for several hours or overnight, the swelling often disappears back into the circulation where it came from in the first instance. Typically the swelling disappears overnight and is not present on waking up in the morning but reappears as the day progresses. The swelling, particularly if it is severe, may cause discomfort by stretching the tissues of the skin. Pain or discomfort disproportionate to the degree of swelling requires another explanation.

One cause of swelling of the feet can cause confusion if the swelling is not due to the presence of water but a thick mucinous 'jelly' that occurs in hypothyroidism. In this condition the thyroid gland is underactive and there is insufficient secretion of the thyroid hormone. If finger-pressure is applied over the leg against the shinbone or over the top of the foot and held so for a ½ minute or so there will be no indentation. However, if the swelling is due to *water* pressure from the finger, shoe or sock will leave an imprint in the skin.

If the swelling occurs in both feet more or less equally the causes that need to be excluded are failures of the following, independently or as complications of each other:- the heart, lungs, kidneys or liver. A medical examination and some investigations (urine testing, x rays and blood tests) become mandatory. Excessive intake of salt and heavily salted foods may also produce swelling – wherever salt goes water will follow! Certain drugs also cause retention of salt (and, therefore, water) within the body e.g. NSAIDs (non-steroidal anti-inflammatory drugs) used in arthritis. These drugs have become more easily available over the counter and this is bound to increase reports of side effects. While NSAIDs are also prescribed for period pains, part of the symptoms of premenstrual discomfort is due to fluid retention! The oral contraceptive may also cause swelling of the feet due to water retention.

A swelling over the front of one foot accompanied by pain and redness over the same area may be due to inflammation of the muscle that is situated on the upper part of the foot. In this condition (teno-synovitis – teno=tendon and synovitis=inflammation of the lining that surrounds the tendon) bending the toes and foot forward to its extreme will produce pain, as would the motion of walking. Bending the foot upwards relieves the pain. A short course of NSAIDs for 3 to 5 days, resting the foot in the elevated position and bearing weight on the *heel* (to avoid forward bending/ flexion of the foot) should relieve the problem. Sometimes the use of open sandals for the first time may precipitate the inflammation but more often no cause is established. Gout can also cause inflammation of this muscle and should be considered in the diagnosis, particularly when it occurs for the first time.

Swelling of the feet that is related to menstruation and occurring in a cyclical pattern (at the start of each period) is due to hormonal imbalances causing fluid retention and may be relieved by taking the oral contraceptive pill. If the swelling is pronounced a diuretic may be necessary for relief. This is a drug that helps the kidneys excrete salt (sodium) - and where salt goes water will follow.

If the swelling is due to varicose veins (even if they are not visible) treatment is more difficult. Stripping (removal of the veins by surgery) is not always successful. Injections designed to occlude them can be given into varicose veins. The use of compressive bandaging or 'varicose stockings' is a cumbersome option and irksome in warm weather. Nevertheless, they should be used when walking long distances to support the veins and prevent water from leaking out of them. Diuretics may also be required to reduce the swelling. Elevating the feet at every opportunity also helps; the person so afflicted with varicosities and swelling of the feet is very often overweight and inactive; correcting this will address the root of the problem. Treatment depends on the cause. To get the correct treatment a diagnosis (and this applies to every medical problem) must first be made. A diuretic ('water tablet') is often the mainstay of treatment especially if failure of one or more of the organs is responsible.

Patients who have swollen feet should be more concerned with what is causing the problem than the actual swelling itself even though the latter can cause discomfort, be unsightly and make shoes fit poorly. In this regard, new shoes should best be tried on in the afternoon rather than early in the day; a good fit in the morning may become no fit by the afternoon - when the feet have had a chance to swell.

Swelling of a leg/foot accompanied by redness of the area and pain is most likely due to an infection of the skin - cellulitis - requiring elevation of the part, antibiotics and an anti-inflammatory.

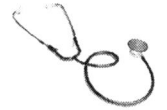

THE ANKLE JOINT

It is not often appreciated that the ankle joint is almost the last bastion that supports the entire body weight. Its role must surely be a far cry from that which nature intended considering that the original blue print was designed for '4 X 4' locomotion. By virtue of its distance from the mainstream of things (it is far easier to visualise the wrist than its counterpart the ankle) this joint is often neglected and yet, in collaboration with the foot, it helps to maintain balance and boost agility. Compound this with the added insult of kilogrammes of excess weight - in modern man's quest to eat him self into oblivion and allow the poor ankles suffer the consequences of over indulgence. That the joints perform so admirably, and often with less evidence of osteoarthritis than their next of kin, the lordly knees and their more proximal cousins – the hip joints, is a true credit to their Maker.

However, because of factors beyond control, like stumbling or falling when under the influence of alcohol, stepping into hidden holes or ditches, uneven pavements, missed steps in the dark or the foul plays in soccer - the towering erect body balanced (rather precariously in the above situations) will topple the person - with the ankle often twisting under the body. This may cause the 'housing' of the ankle joint to break the outer or inner parts of the ankle or, if the force is severe, both sides.

The two knobs, one on either side of the ankle joint, called the malleoli (pleural for malleolus) are the parts that are commonly involved in fractures of this joint. If during a stumble the foot turns inwards the outer knob (lateral malleolus) may fracture or if the foot turns outwards – the inner knob (medial malleolus) may break. Pain felt specifically on one or the other malleolus (knob) is strongly suspicious of a fracture. If this pain is absent one could put off the 'urgent' visit to the doctor until the following day on condition that no weight-bearing on the affected ankle is allowed.

It is difficult to distinguish a fracture from a sprain without an X-ray. If the ankle is *sprained* the pain is commonly felt in front of the ankle, usually on either the inside or outside of the top of the foot (forefoot). The treatment of the sprain (applicable to most joints) should include: –

- The immediate application of cold compresses over the injured joint for about 5 minutes at a time to reduce the swelling
- Supporting the ankle with firm strapping if this is tolerated
- Avoiding all weight bearing (that means using crutches or a friendly shoulder for support)
- Elevating the foot
- Taking an anti-inflammatory (if there are no contra-indications to their use – e.g. stomach ulcers or history of bleeding from them)
- Seeing the doctor within 24 hours – not a week later when the pain and swelling have not subsided

The decision to take an X-ray, if a fracture is not immediately suspected (i.e. a sprain), may be temporarily delayed on condition the affected ankle is not allowed to bear weight (Use crutches or observe strict bed rest). Beware hopping on the good leg as one could carelessly lose the other ankle!

The influence of obesity on ankle disorders should not be underestimated; if the joint should be replaced with an artificial one the aggravating weight factor is still present to torment the prosthesis. With the current trend towards heavier and heavier body masses the services of the medical fraternity – doctors, radiographers, radiologists, physiotherapists, sports-injury experts, occupational therapists, orthopaedic surgeons and dietitians are guaranteed.

Pain felt on pressing immediately in front of the ankle joint, where the leg meets the top of the foot (there is a crease in the skin marking the 'joint line') is also suspicious of a fracture of the ankle joint and warrants an X-ray.

Recurrent sprains of the ankle tend to stretch the ligaments around the joint making it more prone to future sprains and falls – especially on uneven ground (hiking on rocky paths). One simple preventative measure is wearing boots that go above the ankles and lacing them firmly to provide extra support to the ankles. A painful, hot and swollen ankle joint occurring suddenly without a history of trauma or after minor injury is very suspicious of gout. It can develop almost overnight and often during sleep. The diagnosis is more likely if there has been a past history of this condition, even if this particular joint was not affected before.

Pain in the joint, whether or not there is a history of swelling, occurring over a longer period of weeks or months suggests osteoarthritis or rheumatoid arthritis. In the latter condition there is often involvement of other joints especially the small ones of the hands and or feet and stiffness in the mornings.

Puffiness around the ankles may be mistaken for water/fluid. If the puffiness is confined to the malleoli only (knobs of the ankle) this is more likely due to swelling in the pad (bursa) that lies over the bony prominence (designed to protect it against injury). Similar pads or bursae are present over other bony prominences such as the points of the elbow or the front of the knees (housemaid's knees). Suspect fluid under the skin if it occurs below the malleoli and if pressure with a finger held for 30 seconds over the swelling causes a visible 'hollow' or indentation in the skin.

If both feet are swollen in the morning, before one has had time to be up and about, this may implicate the kidneys as the cause. Varicose veins of the lower limbs are the commonest cause of swelling of the ankles and feet, especially if one side only is swollen or one side more than the other. However this fluid is usually absent in the morning and becomes more prominent as the day progresses. If the heart fails as an effective pump a similar pattern of ankle swelling may occur except that the swelling occurs equally in both feet.

The following factors tend to precipitate or aggravate swelling of the feet and ankles: –

- Excessive salt in food (and drinks – so called 'sportsmen's drinks' are loaded with salt!)
- Hot weather
- Lack of exercise
- Sitting for long periods with the knees in the bent position (flying or driving long distances)
- The elderly and infirm – from lack of exercise
- Standing for prolonged periods (sales people)
- Obesity
- Pregnancy
- Oral contraceptives
- Steroids
- Non-steroidal anti-inflammatory drugs (NSAIDs)
- A swelling on the same side as a stroke.

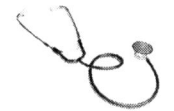

THE BABY

A 'baby' is an infant that has not yet started walking. The baby's clock starts ticking the moment the sperm penetrates the outer layer of the ovum (egg) and stops only when the heart finally ceases to beat.

The blueprint in the genetic code is survival, nutrition, reproduction and death – in that sequence. The foetus must survive the pregnancy and the birth and then receive nutrition, nurturing and protection to develop to adulthood in order to be able to find a mate and reproduce. That is the sum total of life. Anything extra man has added to the blueprint.

The 'additions' that he has made has produced changes such as nature never intended and in his continual search for instant gratification, pleasure seeking and an earlier death man has become his own worst enemy.

The baby is the innocent pawn in the giant chessboard of its life. Beginning from the introduction of the 'formula feeds', ready-made foods and fruit juices in jars with their reassuring labels that read 'no preservatives added' - the rot starts in the first year of the baby's life.

Breast milk is the closest the baby will get to what nature planned as a feed – the decline in its nutritional status begins as soon as it is weaned. Is it any surprise that Britain's statistics show that the incidence of cancer in children has doubled in the last 15 years? This should force parents and health authorities to sit up and take notice.

As soon as the baby leaves the breast parents, grandparents, uncles and aunts, crèches, nannies and other learned caregivers will ply the child with a whole host of junk foods, fancy breakfast cereals with phoney vitamins (that are poorly absorbed) and margarines that carry the disguised blessings of health authorities. These foods, in one way or another, may set up the unsuspecting child to contract some illness, whether it is an allergy, asthma, diabetes, obesity, heart disease or cancer.

To this will be added the brainwashing from thousands of hours of television advertising that will prime the child to regard all the 'foods' and 'drinks' mentioned above as the norm and necessary for normal life. This generation of babies, more than their forebears, will be relying heavily on science and medicine to keep them healthy and alive.

Until the age of 4 months babies cannot focus well enough with their eyes to identify faces and objects. It is important to identify a hearing disability early on because this special 'sense' is a vital link to the outside world (apart from touch) and is important in the mental development of the child. It is well known that a newborn infant that is denied human contact(or contact with another living creature) mayperish. This physical contact is a necessary part of healthy living throughout the life of the individual from the first minutes of its birth as it lies on the mother's belly or in the comforting crook of her elbow in the hours spent feeding it, to the physical contact and gentle Oohs! and Ahs! of admirers and well wishers, and the hugs and kisses that will pepper the life of the child as it grows.

The infant can read in the voice of its mother (since she spends more time with it than the father) whether she is at peace with herself – relaxed, happy and confident or stressed out, tired, unhappy, angry, abrupt, hurried, unsure of herself and worried. The visually impaired also have a keenly developed sense of hearing that will pick up these messages from the often subtle nuances of the tone, pitch, and loudness of peoples' voices.

Mothers need to be aware that their baby is 'watching' her every move through her voice. How often has it happened that a young mother, at her wits end with a 'problematic' infant that cries louder and louder no matter what she does, settles down within minutes of a grandparent picking up the child and speaking in a more relaxed, confident and soothing voice?

The mother may not be aware that the pressure she exerts with her hands when she is holding the infant (trying to pacify what appears to be the 'implacable') and the speed at which she is rocking the infant, may give her away and the infant cries louder.

Then there is the father who joins the fray and chastises the mother for not doing the job right and why does she not call his mother for advice or summon the doctor – "Maybe it's his tonsils" or "her appendix". The truth may be the father cannot bear to see the baby in such distress and why does mum not make it right – after all she's the *expert*, she spends all her time with the baby, and she should know what to do. Father is more accustomed to being away all day and arriving home after work to find baby well rested, washed, fed and smelling of 'Johnson's Baby Powder'. When he shouts at the mother and the mother screams back the infant is left confused and even more anxious. In these situations the person best qualified or experienced should be the one dealing with the baby and the others to leave the room.

Grandparents who succeed where daughter-in-law fails should avoid capitulating on their greater experience by making the young mother out to be 'totally incompetent' and "See how quickly baby settled down!" It will not inspire more confidence in the daughter-in-law and may add to the alienation between new mother and 'know-it-all' mother-in-law.

A crying baby is not testing the parents' patience. Crying is the only means of communication that the infant has to convey that something is amiss. We share this with animals and their young. With experience it is not difficult to recognize that there are 'different' cries for hunger, pain, being wet and uncomfortable, being just irritable and being ill. A child that has fallen out of the crib will have a different cry from that of a baby with a wet nappy; the screams of abdominal colic with legs doubled up are a far cry from hunger pains. The sound of the cry is unique to that infant and its mother can recognise her own baby's cry.

Parents should be wary of what is allowed into their babies' mouths because, for many years to come, even into high school, the children are at the mercy of adults who decide for them. The protection of the child from injury, exposure to the elements, sexual and physical abuse and neglect have become the concern of the powers that be but equal importance and attention should be paid to the nutrition the baby receives.

The Constitution protects the child in various ways but there is no law that prevents a parent from feeding a child sausages, crisp chips, chocolates, cakes and cool drinks.

It is easier to bribe the child with sweets and 'luxuries' to make them 'behave' better. What child can resist? And who cares if this sets the scene for obesity in their later years. The people causing the earlier dietary indiscretions will have long since died by the time it becomes the turn of the grandchildren to get diabetes and heart attacks. How often are caregivers equally guilty? The baby learns new things every moment of its life from the moment it is born. The stages in the acquisition of this knowledge culminate only in death. The first stage begins within the womb for 36 to 40 weeks. This is followed by the birth and until the baby is able to crawl and start walking independently. Most newborn animals must be able to walk and run almost from the moment of birth or perish in the jaws of predators or succumb to starvation, thirst or the elements

The next stage in its development is from the time it walks until it enters a crèche or preschool. The timing of the separation, in its journey to independence, has changed with the introduction of the working mother. It now occurs earlier, shortening the vital years of bonding with her child.

The next 20 years may be spent on education. This may even extend into their late 20s and by the time they are 30 may have found a mate and possibly have had children. The time between the ages of 30 and 50 time is spent working and preparing for retirement. The next 10 to 20 years may see chronic illness and death or old age and death later. Life is short. It is not surprising that it can 'all' flash by in a second in the mind's eye!

Modern parents may learn much too late that, in effect, the only close contact between child and mother may last as short as twelve months. Does this influence the development of the child, soon-to-be a schoolgoer, in a manner that sets the scene for difficulties for the child and later as an adult?

The less than twelve months spent with the child before it leaves the roost on its journey to becoming an independent adult version of its parents can hardly be adequate. Have mothers changed the rules because of trying to compete with men and finding more equitable roles for themselves? Has the power of economics driven the mother from her more natural role as nurturer to breadwinner and in so doing shortchanged the child from a development that is different from that which nature required for its progeny? What importance is given this brief contact between mother and child when later trying to explain the attention deficit disorder, substance abuser, hijacker, terrorist, rapist, robber, wife beater, divorcee or sacked employee?

And what of the role played by poor or inadequate nutrition in the development of the child? Does malnutrition explain some of the reasons why some children end up abusing drugs and others get on with their lives in a more successful manner? Do we owe our children more than we give them in trying to equip them to handle their peers, teachers, parents, grandparents, lecturers, employers, girl and boyfriends, partners in wedlock?

The child learns quickly that not all commands made by an adult require a response. It does not understand much of it anyway. Is this an underlying factor in the culture of 'not listening'? The baby is a miniature version of the adult but it is not, *and can never be*, an adult until it has grown and experienced the trials and tribulations of an adult. Yet how often has it been that an adult has addressed a baby as though it was also an adult even to the extent of expecting adult responses from it? Expecting it to understand complex issues of cause and effect – "I told you a dozen times not to do that", "Don't play with the matches – you will burn the house down", "Don't pull the cat's tail – it will scratch you", "You've just had your meal – you cannot still be hungry", "Stop crying like a baby", "Don't go onto the road or the cars will run you over", "I'm just going into the shop – stay in the car and don't open the door", "Don't eat those berries they are bad for you", – the list is long!

From the time the baby starts to crawl it is encouraged to walk. This is the milestone that will change the baby's life forever. If the child was aware of the trap that lies beyond this milestone it would do better not to walk for a time to come. The day it takes its first unassisted steps (to seeming freedom), and for the rest of its life thereafter, it will be hounded and smothered (almost to death) with "DON'T DO THAT", "DON'T DO THIS", "DON'T SPEAK WHILE I'M TALKING", "DON'T RUN", DON'T GO UP THERE", "DON'T GO DOWN THERE", "DON'T TALK THAT WAY", "YOU CAN'T DO THAT" and dozens of other "DON'TS".

These negatives may mar development forever and fortunate the child that extricates itself from this web of negativity, a web that will accompany it in almost every walk of life. This will be the future student who will cringe when the teacher asks "Who knows the answer?" Even if he or she does it may be difficult to overcome the years of inhibition. This reluctance may follow him or her through high school, varsity, work and marriage. He or she may hand down the same "Don'ts" to his or her own children. It will suppress the creative spark, that inquisitiveness that is so vital to a child yearning to learn as much as it can to prepare itself for his or her independence.

This is the child that will grow up believing "I can't do that!", "I won't be able to manage", "I'm sure it won't work" – two little words that will thwart its ambitions and shrink the size of its dreams – "I CAN'T". And where does it come from? - its own parents who handed it the same legacies of "DON'Ts" and "CAN'Ts".

The child also needs protection from harm. Little is to be gained if the child kills itself while learning to become independent. But growth may not be so free of pain that a thunderstorm, unknown in childhood and experienced for the first time in adulthood, does not leave the victim a whimpering wreck.

Trust and love are as vital to life and growth as food itself; nothing should be done to jeopardise this. Do not promise anything, no matter how convenient it may seem at that moment, if the honouring of it cannot be certain. The child has a poorly developed sense of time and what may appear 'not that long' to an adult may seem like an eternity to a child; the concept of "later" and "not now" and "just now" and "soon" and "tomorrow" is difficult for the young mind to comprehend.

The child has little idea of the meaning of "I'm busy now" and the culture of 'not listening' probably begins when the child has a need and cannot find an adult to take notice. The idea that it is okay not to listen and pay attention will infect the growing mind when it is faced with "Didn't I tell you a dozen times already?", "How many times have I told you not to do that?". This temporal development is too immature for adequate comprehension but it will follow the child into school, varsity, the workplace and marriage and the cycle will complete itself when the 'child' becomes a parent itself and does not listen to its own offspring.

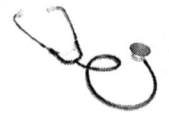

THE BLADDER

The bladder is a muscular bag for the collection of urine produced by the kidneys. From this storage site it is passed out through the urethra, the tube that carries the urine out of the body. The urge to pass urine is controlled by messages (nerve impulses) sent from the bladder (as it fills up with urine) to the brain to inform the person that it needs to be emptied. This urge can be voluntarily postponed if the moment is inconvenient. Women are often guilty of not responding to this 'call of nature' putting them at special risk for problems related to this organ.

From an early age the passage of urine (micturition) is more awkward for females, a swift tug on the zip and the male penis is exposed – ready for disposal of urine. Careful positioning of the right hand and a slight forward crouch helps to 'shield' the genitalia from prying eyes. A female, on the other hand, has to raise the skirt or dress or pull down the pants thereby exposing the buttocks and the genitalia.

Men may have ready access to a secluded corner, tree trunk or wall and can pass urine in the less conspicuous standing position whereas women have to sit or squat and would be reluctant to have their all and sundries displayed for public viewing. By virtue of their anatomy men can direct their stream well away from their feet. Furthermore, the fear of discovery may not allow women to completely evacuate their bladders leaving behind residual urine that encourages bacteria to multiply. The female may resort to using a public toilet only if she is desperate and the bladder allowed to fill to bursting point.

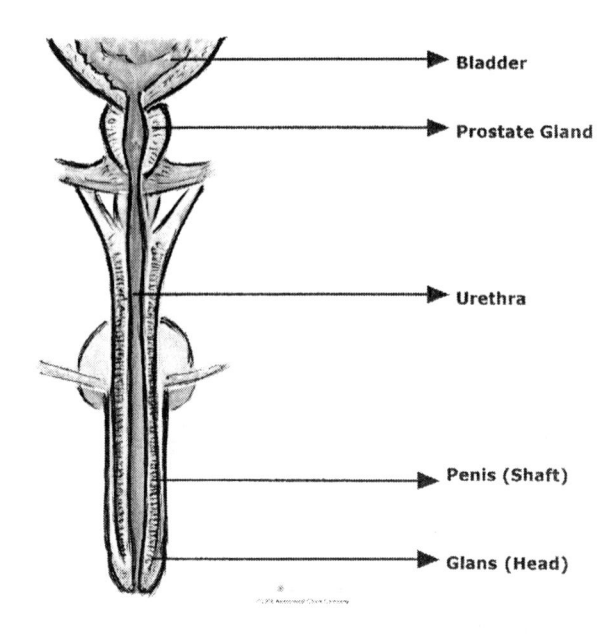

Bladder

Prostate Gland

Urethra

Penis (Shaft)

Glans (Head)

ANTERIOR (FRONT) VIEW OF PART OF THE
BLADDER & PENIS

The female urethra (4cm) is shorter than in males (8cm) and this would make it easier for bacteria to find their way into the female bladder to cause cystitis (infection of the bladder). The opening of the urethra is 'protected' by the foreskin in uncircumcised males whereas in the female the external opening of the urethra shares the exit with the vagina leaving it more exposed to menstrual blood and pathogens (bacteria) - the latter due to cross-contamination from the back passage (anus) and possibly during intercourse.

The penis helps to dispose urine away from the body avoiding the need for much toiletry save a few brisk shakes to dispose of the last few drops of urine. Women are less fortunate: the introitus (entrance into the vagina) is exposed to the urine and if cystitis is present may 'spread' the infection.

Toilets that have no seats, no toilet paper, doors that do not lock, no doors! No soap (as happens in so many public facilities and schools) - will discourage females from responding to the call of nature.

Furthermore, females use the effect of gravity to empty the bladder as different from males who make use of muscles (abdominal and pubococcygeus muscles) to control the stream of urine. They actively contract these muscles to maintain a stream to avoid wetting their feet! Men achieve better tone in their bladders and urethras. It is hardly surprising that the incidence of recurrent bladder infections, large bladders with poor muscle tone from being 'continually' stretched and incontinence of urine is higher in women.

E. coli bacteria normally live within the confines of the rectum (back passage) but introduce them into the bladder and one has the commonest cause of cystitis in females. How does this particular bacteria gain such easy access to the bladder?

- Close proximity of the anus to the vagina, less than 2 cm apart
- Water in the bathtub creates a bridge between the back and front passages carrying bacteria to the bladder
- Ability of the bacteria to travel between areas
- During sexual intercourse the vagina, urethra and bladder are being 'traumatised' by each thrust of the penis - allowing bacteria to gain a foothold

This begs the precaution that females of any age should never use a bathtub; a shower or, failing that, a bucket of water would be safer. Furthermore, the anal area should be washed in the squatting position to gain better access. This is more difficult to achieve in the erect position as the anus lies tucked away further backwards and hidden between the buttocks.

In females toiletry after a bowel action or micturition requires the toilet paper should be used from front to back (not in the reverse direction) to avoid the bacteria normally present around the anus. Washing the anal area with water, as is practiced in some cultures, is safer when the squatting position (eastern toilet pan) is adopted making it less likely for the water to contaminate the vaginal area. The use of water is a risk when the conventional western toilet pan is used because the vagina and the anus may lie almost horizontal making it easier for soiling to occur. Using a bidet can contaminate the entire perineum (back and front passages) with a misdirected jet of water. It is virtually impossible to accurately target the anus without simultaneously soiling the vagina. Filling the bidet with water as one would a wash basin has similar health hazards – how would one sterilize the bidet after each use? The use of the bidet could be compared to washing oneself in the toilet pan - albeit that the latter is also dutifully cleaned with disinfectants!

During intercourse the introduction of the penis into the vagina is not always done under visual guidance, especially in the missionary position (man on top) - any fumbling and the accidental contact of the penis with the anus will contaminate the glans (head) of the penis with bacteria. In the heat of the moment, the male ego is unlikely to admit he 'missed' the target and go off to wash himself!

This emphasizes the point that there must be no contact between anus and vagina whether accidental or otherwise. Anal intercourse must ensure the use of a condom before any contact is made with the anus to protect the male and the female from E.coli (or any other) infections. This condom must be changed before engaging in vaginal intercourse and, furthermore, the hands that removed the 'contaminated' condom must be washed thoroughly before a new condom is used or further genital contact made.

The rear entry position (woman on all fours) also exposes the shaft of the penis to the anal area, especially, if the male leans forward – bringing the penis in closer contact with the anal area. This exposure is made more likely if the female is lying prone (on her belly); using a condom in these two positions will not avoid the exposure of the vagina to anal bacteria. A precaution would be for the female to thoroughly wash off the anal area in anticipation of intercourse in any position. As mentioned above, such toiletry can only be properly achieved in the squatting position.

Underwear that has already been worn should not be put on back to front as the back passage would have contaminated the part making contact with it and will now be facing the vagina. Females should empty the bladder before intercourse to avoid trauma to the bladder especially at its base or floor, which is the area that makes intimate contact with the 'roof' of the vagina. The bladder should also be emptied as soon as possible after intercourse; urine is being produced continuously by the kidneys and this output is increased during the intense stimulation that occurs with intercourse, particularly during prolonged foreplay. Emptying the bladder timeously may flush out any bacteria introduced during intercourse.

One of the commonest causes of kidney failure is previous kidney infections (pyelonephritis) but many of the patients who develop these do not give clear histories of such previous infections (pyelonephritis). How did the kidneys become infected? And when did they occur? If bacteria have been silently tracking upwards from the bladder this makes a strong case for taking seriously every episode of cystitis bearing in mind that the kidney is but a hand's breadth distance away from the bladder.

The symptoms of a bladder infection (cystitis) are 'frequency' and 'dysuria'. Urine is passed almost every 10 to 15 minutes and though the quantity may only be a few drops each time the urge to pass it is accompanied by an over-powering, intense burning pain willing the victim to want to stay in the toilet.

Beware the elderly and the young for they may not have these symptoms. An elderly person who goes off his or her food for 24 to 48 hours for no apparent reason has a bladder infection until proven otherwise. Not every person with a fever or loss of appetite may have the flu! Always have the urine tested. Every home should have test strips (used in doctor's surgeries and hospitals) and conditions such as kidney and liver disorders and diabetes may be detected earlier. The same applies to stool testing for blood in the earlier detection of bowel cancer. The skill required in performing the tests is hardly at the rocket science level.

The base of the bladder is the most sensitive part of the organ. It contains a dense supply of nerve endings that send messages to the brain telling one when to pee – especially in the morning when the bladder is full with an overnight collection. Turning from the supine position onto the side temporarily takes the pressure off this area and buys some short relief. If the bladder is inflamed from an infection this irritation sends the same message as though the bladder was 'full' and must be emptied immediately - whereas only a few drops may be passed each time. Because urine is being formed continuously by the kidneys a small quantity each time will force the sufferer to go to the toilet in expectation of passing a large quantity.

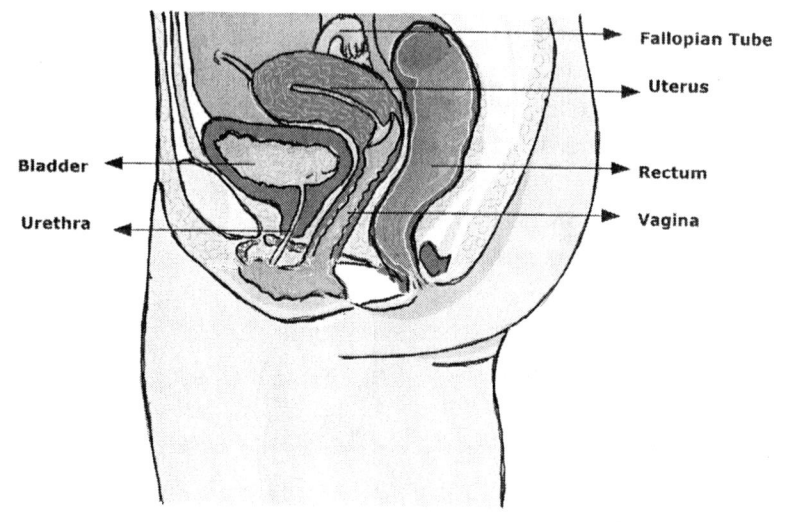

THE BLADDER & RELATED STRUCTURES

There may or may not be fever, nausea and vomiting. Pain may be felt over the lowest part of the belly where the bladder lies – in the middle of the lowest three squares. If it occurs under the ribs at the right or left outer square of the upper three this would imply that the infection has spread to the kidney/s (pyelonephritis). This is always a serious complication of cystitis (it now involves a vital organ) and makes it mandatory, with *every* bout of cystitis, to have a sample of urine sent to the laboratory for identification of the bacteria and the correct antibiotic to which the bacteria are susceptible. Ignoring this paves the way for future bladder or kidney problems.

Cystitis is common and visiting the doctor for every episode and receiving the 'same' treatment each time has many a female sufferer taking the short cut and self medicating with 'Citro Soda' to relieve the symptoms. This is prescribed to change the pH of the urine from acidic to alkaline because bacteria love acid urine in which to multiply. However, it does not address the infection. It may be that patients, who seemingly respond to 'Citro Soda' alone, are probably not true cases of cystitis.

It is not uncommon for women, as they approach, or are already in, their menopause to experience a dryness of the lining of the vagina due to lack of oestrogen from the ovaries. This can make intercourse 'dry' and uncomfortable and cause further 'trauma' to the lining of the urethra and bladder base - mimicking the symptoms of cystitis. Once laboratory-tested urine excludes an infection an oestrogen cream ('Premarin' vaginal cream) maybe applied *once a week* to replace the missing hormone; this relieves the symptoms fairly quickly

Ideally, 3 to 4 weeks after cystitis has been treated, another specimen of urine should be tested to exclude the continued presence of bacteria. The latter not produce symptoms but have the potential to set off another infection, setting the scene for 'recurrent cystitis' and, possibly, undetected spread to the kidneys. The average cost of dialysis for kidney failure runs into the thousands whereas the cost of a urine analysis is a pittance by comparison.

Collecting a sample of urine from a female requires special precautions: it should be passed into a sterile container immediately on arising in the morning. A shower is taken or, alternatively, the patient is instructed to wash the introitus carefully with soap and water before any urine is passed. The first half cup or so is passed normally in the toilet pan and the next bit into the sterile container (opened just before use to prevent contamination). The collection is best done in the squatting position – allowing the introitus (vaginal area) to be opened widely so that urine does not make contact with the sides of the vagina. This 'clean catch' specimen is important to ensure the laboratory does not culture bacteria that normally inhabit the vagina (called commensals). These do not play a role in cystitis but will contribute to costly laboratory fees and, possibly, unwarranted antibiotics. As an emergency guide if newsprint can be read clearly through a see-through container of urine it is very unlikely that the sample came from an infected bladder.

Supplementation with

- Vitamin C (slow release) – 1 tablet daily,
- Zinc tablets – 1 daily
- Formula 4 Plus – 1 sachet daily

may help in earlier recovery from cystitis and, indeed, infection anywhere in the body. Taken long term for chronic or recurrent cystitis they could help in its eradication when combined with an appropriate antibiotic.

A vaginal infection (vaginitis) may also produce symptoms suggestive of cystitis. This invariably requires a pus swab taken from the vagina to establish the true nature of the discharge. Not every vaginal discharge is due to thrush and the over-the-counter availability of antifungal medication is open to serious abuse.

Cystitis occurring in an adult male requires a rectal examination to exclude an infection of the prostrate gland (prostatitis) which can mimic the symptoms of a bladder infection. If the prostate is innocent, an intravenous pyelogram (IVP – X-rays) or ultrasound examination of the kidneys is mandatory once the cystitis has been adequately treated.

Any child presenting with cystitis will also need this test to exclude (as in the adult) a structural abnormality any where along the urinary tract from the kidneys to the urethra. An adult female is 'allowed' to have one episode of an uncomplicated cystitis without the need for an IVP. If it recurs within a short time (two to three weeks) this X-ray becomes necessary.

A stone (calculus) situated anywhere along the urinary tract will be a constant source of infection and can be demonstrated by IVP or ultrasound examination – the latter is less invasive. An IVP is a series of X-rays taken after a radio-opaque dye (visible on X-ray) is injected into a vein. The dye follows the same course as in the formation of urine and is excreted through the kidneys and into the bladder. Any abnormalities of the urinary tract such as stones (calculi), structural abnormalities like 'double kidneys', tumours and kinks in the ureter may be detected. However, there is quite a heavy exposure to irradiation and this investigation should not be undertaken lightly; prevention of cystitis is safer – as with all other preventative medicine.

Drinking 6 to 8 glasses of properly filtered water will help flush out toxins from the kidneys; the body views all medication as 'toxins'. Women who are out of their homes or offices and unwilling to use a public or unfamiliar toilet may be reluctant to take this quantity of fluid. This further encourages bladder infections.

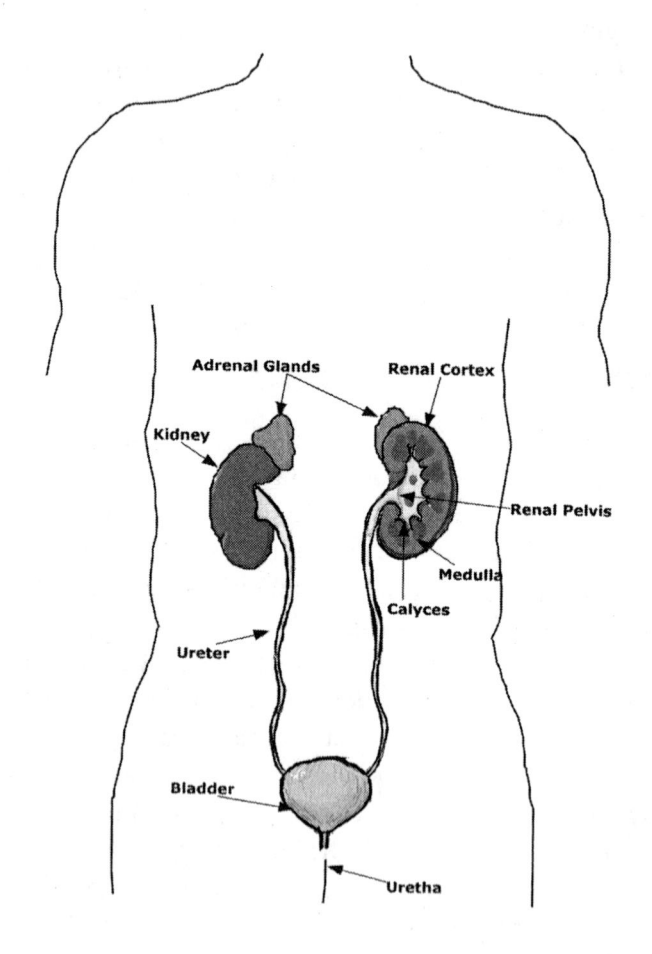

URINARY SYSTEM

During sleep the amount of urine produced by the kidneys usually decreases because there is no further intake of fluids. This is not ideal, especially if antibiotics, analgesics and other drugs are taken before retiring at night. This reduced output of urine may expose the kidneys to these 'toxins' and cause damage to them. This may be prevented by taking extra fluid just before retiring to bed and getting up at least once during the night to empty the bladder and drinking more water again.

It is unwise to allow the bladder to remain distended for long periods. Given that it is a muscular bag it can become stretched and thickened over time causing problems later in life. Furthermore, the longer urine remains within the bladder the easier it is for bacteria to multiply.

Unless it is deliberate, as outlined above, the passage of urine at night (nocturia) as a recent symptom may be the first sign that all is not well with the kidneys and warrants a visit to the doctor. Diabetics pass excessive quantities of urine because of the extra sugar in the blood that is being passed out through the kidneys. In an attempt to get rid of the extra glucose the kidneys produce more urine – hence the 'polyuria' (frequent passage of large quantities of urine) and 'polydipsia' (excessive thirst).

Any person who
- starts to drink a lot of water (or cool drinks or tea)
- passes lots of urine
- feels more thirsty than usual
- loses weight

may have diabetes and should be investigated.

A gradually increasing difficulty in passing urine suggests an enlarging prostate gland (in men only) that is pressing upon and obstructing the passage of urine through the urethra as this tube passes through the prostate. Nowadays, drugs are available that may shrink down the prostate. Failure to achieve this will require surgery. If this difficulty in passing urine should happen suddenly and for the first time, over a matter of hours, the usual cause is medication that has been taken e.g. certain eye drops used for glaucoma of the eyes (increased pressure within the eyes).

If the obstruction develops over a few days it may be that the prostate has become infected and swollen; a course of antibiotics usually resolves the problem. Urine is passed at regular intervals to prevent it from accumulating within the bladder. If a stone (calculus) blocks the exit of urine at any level after it leaves the kidneys, the dammed up urine may cause the kidneys to swell (hydronephrosis) and, if left unrelieved, will eventually damage the affected kidney.

The pain that accompanies a stone in the 'urinary tract' is one of the most severe known to man. Characteristically, it radiates from the kidney (under the side of the ribs) down to the groin on the affected side. The person so afflicted is unable to lie still – tossing and turning trying to find a comfortable position. This is in stark contrast to the patient with an inflamed appendix who will shun any movement and lies motionless to avoid aggravating the pain.

Drinking excessive quantities of full cream cow's milk – more than a litre per day – and the regular abuse of antacids may lead to the formation of stones in the urinary tract (kidneys, ureters, bladder and urethra) because of the high concentration of calcium.

Gout sufferers are also at risk for uric acid stones as they produce excessive amounts of this acid, which filters out through the kidneys. Taking extra fluids helps to flush out the rogue acid and Citro Soda maintains the acid in a soluble state, making it easier for it to be passed out in the urine.

Incontinence of urine is the involuntary leakage of urine and this may occur for several reasons. The incontinence that occurs when the pressure within the abdomen is increased (suddenly), as in sneezing, coughing and laughing, is called 'stress incontinence'. This is more common in women and is due to poor tone in the urethral sphincters (valves) and surrounding vaginal muscles that allow the sudden leakage of urine. This poor control and weakness may be due to, or be aggravated by: –

- multiple pregnancies
- difficult labours
- obesity

- previous operations – like hysterectomy (removal of the uterus) and prostatectomy (removal of the prostate in men)

Urine that escapes without the person being aware of its passage may also occur in conditions where the nerve supply to the bladder may be damaged as in diabetes, lower spinal cord injuries and operations on the prostate – called 'neurogenic bladder'.

Incontinence occurs when the bladder is full and cannot 'contain' itself. This is called 'overflow incontinence'. It may be avoided by preventing the bladder from distending itself and regulating bladder emptying at frequent intervals instead of waiting for the urge to micturate (pass urine).

The tone in the urethra can be improved by learning to strengthen the muscle that controls these sphincters – the Pubococcygeus. This muscle extends from the pubic bone - immediately behind the base (root) of the penis or just above the vagina - and extends to the tail bone (coccyx). This muscle controls the anterior (front) abdominal wall, bladder, vagina, penis, rectum and the lower spine.

Exercising this muscle will help to

- keep the tummy flat
- improve control of the bladder
- improve one's sex life
- brace the lower spinal muscles and ligaments employed in bending and
- prevent faecal incontinence (losing control of the bowel)

The pubococcygeus muscle can be identified by imaginarily stopping the flow of urine in midstream.

In stress incontinence this muscle can be 'tightened' to help close off the urethra especially before a sneeze or cough.

To reduce the problem of a neurogenic bladder avoid allowing it to fill up and, with some experimentation, it is not difficult to predict how often to 'empty' the bladder. Though there is no sensation of the organ filling up and there is no voluntary control over the release of the urine, the bladder can be squeezed and 'emptied' manually by pressing over the lower abdomen at regular intervals.

The conventional alternative is a permanent catheter placed within the bladder and the outlet is connected to a plastic bag that is pinned on the inside of the trouser leg; this bag is emptied as necessary. However, these catheters are potential sources of infection and can become life threatening to such patients. An important precaution with these plastic bags is that they should not be placed or raised above the level of the bladder as the urine may then flow retrograde (backwards) into the bladder. Where the tubing enters the bag there may be no valve to prevent this – a point manufacturers need to address.

A safer but more cumbersome method is to attach a special condom onto the penis (called Paul's tubing). The condom has tubing at its end that connects to a collection bag. It avoids the risk of infection being introduced when a catheter is inserted into the bladder; obviously this applies only to males and, of necessity, requires a sizeable tumescent penis as the condom has to be secured to the organ.

Recent surgical techniques to alleviate incontinence show good promise. A sling is fashioned to cradle the urethra – picture a string lifting a loop of hose pipe.

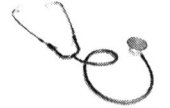

THE EAR

An infant's hearing should be evaluated when noises fail to startle the baby or it does not turn the head towards the source of a sound.

Ear wax is produced by glands in the skin of the ear canal and its purpose is to protect the ear from dust, insects (it is poisonous to them) and other foreign particles. The wax is carried along the surface of the canal as the cells of the skin move outwards from deep within to the outside of the ear. If the production of wax is greater than can be handled, or the canal is narrow or crooked, wax may accumulate and impair one's hearing. This will require removal either with special drops that loosen the wax or manually with syringing or suctioning; the latter options requiring medical expertise. A safe way to clean the ear is to put into it a few drops of olive oil and (overnight) plug the ear with some cotton wool. The oil may be warmed slightly to make it comfortable to the touch. Regular use of the oil helps to soften wax and may avoid the need for ear-syringing.

The use of 'earbuds 'is not easily recommended because of the risk of injury. The lining of the ear is easily traumatised and this may set the scene for an infection. It may be preferable to moisten the bud with clean water first. Children who watch adults use them run the risk of perforating their own eardrums as they are unable to gauge the depth of entry. Grip the earbud midway between the two ends between index finger and thumb and place the ring finger in front of the ear to support the hand. This controls the depth of entry which should be the *entrance* to the outer ear canal only - there is no need to go beyond this hunting for wax. The latter lies mainly on the floor of the canal (which should be the target area) avoiding the need to twirl the earbud round and round.

Leaving the ear buds exposed to steam in the bathroom will cause the cotton tips to swell. This will also make them softer and less abrasive to the delicate lining of the canal

Pain in the ear could be 'referred' pain coming from the jaw joint or teeth. It would need an examination by a doctor. The same applies to any discharge from the ear or hearing difficulty - especially if accompanied by pain. Wax in the ear does not ordinarily cause pain.

An infant that continues to cry/be in pain without an obvious cause could be troubled with an ear infection. To exclude this will, again, require an examination with an auriscope (special torch with a speculum to view the ear canal and ear drum – it will *not* reach the other ear!) Such an infection, in which fluid builds up behind the eardrum, can lead to a ruptured drum and possible future hearing difficulties. In this situation a 'grommet' (a tiny little tube) is inserted through the eardrum to help drain the accumulated pus. This prevents rupture of the drum as the grommet is positioned well away from the tiny bones attached behind the drum so that hearing is preserved. These little bones help to transmit sound,

The ear passage helps to 'dilute' sound before it reaches the eardrum. Using a 'Walkman', mobile phone hands-free ear pieces, mp3 players and similar devices may damage hearing because the sound is concentrated and channelled to the eardrum as a constant bombardment. This is not what nature intended. Listening to loud music in a car with the windows closed has a similar devastating effect on hearing and will lead to premature deafness. This damage is magnified if the music has the 'bass' turned up. Exposure to noise, any noise or sound that exceeds 90 decibels may result in damage to the ear.

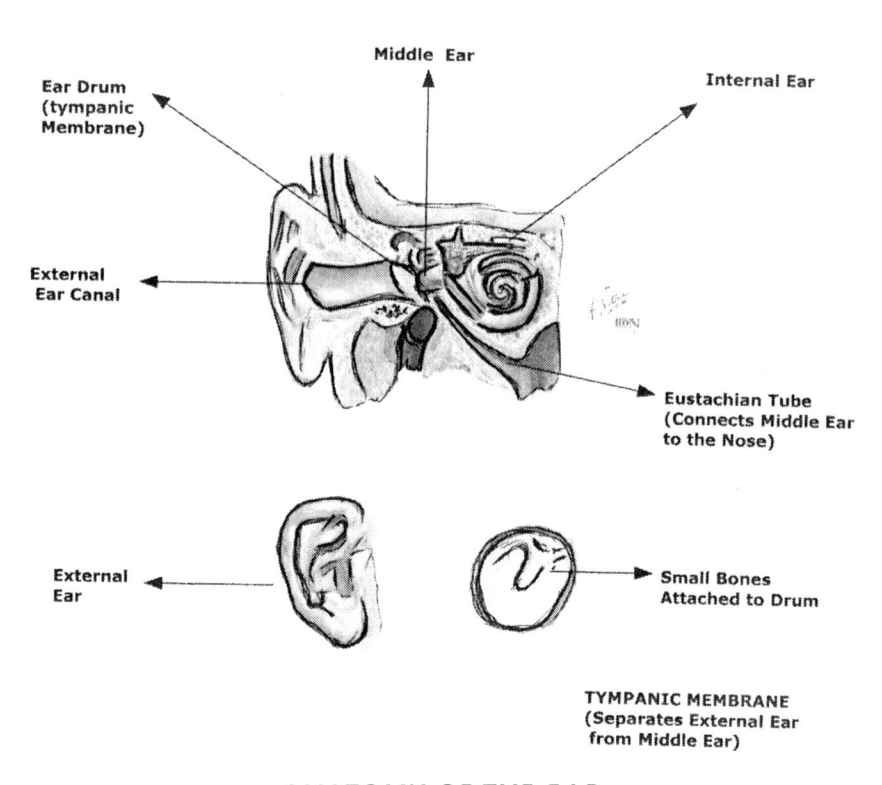

ANATOMY OF THE EAR

To draw some perspective into noise levels (measured in decibels): –

- Normal conversation produces sound measured as 50 to 60 decibels
- Loud music measures 100 decibels
- A pneumatic drill at one metre measures 120 decibels
- A jet engine at 30 metres measures 130 decibels

Sudden loud noise e.g. firework or gunfire causes greater damage to hearing because the ears (tiny muscles on the ear drum) have no time to adjust to the sound.

- At 55 to 60 decibels noise causes irritation
- Between 60 and 65 decibels irritation levels increase considerably

- Greater than 60 decibels may result in serious damage
- Greater than 90 decibels will result in certain injury to the ears
- 90 to 120 decibels will cause deafness and pain which may be temporary
- A ringing sound (tinnitus) that persists after the insult or assault upon the ears may imply permanent damage.

Exposure to constant noise has been shown to:

- cause stress
- raise blood pressures
- increase heart rates and
- be linked to premature death.

Regular disco-goers and rock concert enthusiasts be warned! Noise levels as low as 30 decibels can disturb sleep. Restaurants that rely on a fast turnover of customers discourage long stays by playing loud and fast rock or rap-style music. Clothing stores that benefit from having customers linger longer play soft, soothing music.

"Excuse me. What did you say?" is the indictment one will be risking when hearing is impaired. It is a subtle loss. There are no symptoms except that sounds become more difficult to make out. Loud sounds to which babies, young children and teenagers are exposed because adults are unaware of the inherent potential risk of damage should fall under the category of 'child abuse'. Invest in good quality earmuffs and use them whenever one is exposed to noise whether from seemingly innocent vacuum cleaners or the din created by the washing-up of dishes. The simple message is - 'noise kills'.

Hyperacusis is a condition in which ordinary sounds appear louder than normal and can lead to irritability. It may account for why the elderly do not tolerate loud music more than the generally accepted reason – the 'generation gap'. Spare a thought for them and make a conscious effort to prevent noise from being generated. Simple measures like playing the TV less loudly and washing up dishes more gently will lead to a happier environment and fewer chipped crockery!

Swimming pools with dirty water and sewage-polluted beaches can cause ear infections. These may be reduced by using earplugs coated with Vaseline to avoid creating a moist environment within the ear making it easier for bacteria to grow. Instilling a few drops of olive oil with also help flush out water from the ear canal. Any discharge from the ear – smelly, bloody or watery needs professional advice. Reddish wax can mimic blood.

Motion sickness is caused by upsetting the equilibrium of a thick fluid within a set of semicircular tubes present within the ear. The persistent rocking movement of a boat will disturb this fluid and cause vomiting and an unsteady balance. The childhood game of turning round and round and then losing balance has the same effect.

Sudden onset of true vertigo, in which the room and surrounding objects spin around, often associated with uncontrollable vomiting, can be quite alarming and severely debilitating but is not a life threatening situation. This is called acute labyrinthitis and can be precipitated by a viral infection affecting the nerve that supplies the semicircular tubes within the ear. These are the tubes that control balance. An injection or (less painfully) a suppository into the rectum (back passage) may be necessary to stop the dizziness and vomiting. The condition is usually short lived and settles down within two to three days - or longer if one is unlucky. Taking a tablet to prevent motion sickness about an hour before travelling will avoid the vomiting but beware of drowsiness as a side effect or the rest of one's pleasure cruise or flight will be spent in slumber-land! Caught without medication, concentrating very hard on an object that is stationary (on land) may help avoid having to vomit into the 'paper bag'.

A narrow tube (Eustachian tube - see diagram) connects the nose to the middle ear. Its function is to balance the pressure within the ear with outside atmospheric pressure. Blockage of this tube with mucus from a cold or sinusitis will allow pressure at high altitude to build up within the affected ear and cause severe pain. Taking a young child or infant by plane should warrant unblocking this tube with medication before the departure or face the prospect of a screaming child during the journey. It can be effectively treated in the older person by pinching both nostrils tightly and blowing through the closed nose. A popping sound signals release of the pressure after blowing the obstruction out the tube into the middle ear, bringing immediate relief.

Admonishing young children, (and adults), to "Stop sniffing and blow your nose" as countless generations have coaxed, cajoled, threatened and even punished, may not have been sound advice. Blowing the nose sends the offending mucus shooting up through this tube and into the middle ear leading to possible ear infections. The mucus is also blown into the sinuses setting up infection in them as well. The alternative: it is safer to sniff the mucus upwards into the back of the nose and out the mouth or swallow if necessary! Gastric acid will take care of it.

Infants should be fed with the head held high up in the crook of the mother's elbow to prevent regurgitation (vomiting) through the nose. The milk may find its way into the middle ear via the (Eustachian) tube setting the scene for an ear infection. Furthermore, this tube is more horizontal at this age making it easier for the milk to reach the ear. Milk makes an excellent medium for bacteria (germs) to be cultivated.

Slapping a person over the ear can rupture the eardrum. Pressure from the blow is transmitted via the air within the ear canal forcing the eardrum inwards. Blood or clear fluid within the canal following a head injury is likely to be due to a fracture of the base of the skull (the part of the skull the brain rests on). This is serious and warrants immediate medical attention and a CT Scan of the brain.

Piercing the ear lobe for earrings with contaminated needles can transmit diseases like HIV/AIDS, Hepatitis and syphilis. Changing the needle may not be adequate precaution as the base of the needle holder can be soiled with the blood of a previous client.

An allergic reaction to an earring is not excluded if this does not occur initially. With continued use the outer metal coating may wear out or oxidation (discolouration) may take place resulting in an allergy. Any infection following a piercing will require the earring to be removed before the infection can resolve and the same to be sterilised or replaced if bacteria are not to be reintroduced. A persistently wet or itchy area behind, on or around the ears may be due to eczema. A cut to the ear lobe usually requires stitches as bleeding will not easily stop. The skin here is very thin and the underlying cartilage (which makes up the ear) will not allow the cut edges to seal as the skin would in other parts of the body.

Not every deaf person will benefit from hearing aids. This decision should be made by the Ear, Nose &Throat (ENT) specialist before expensive (often imported) equipment is bought. Persons with long-standing gout (inflammation of joints caused by uric acid crystals) may have small bead-to pea-sized swellings along the upper border of the ear lobe. These do not require special treatment apart from better control of the gout.

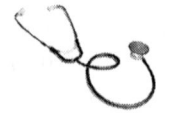

THE EYE

Any pain in the eye requires a medical opinion as soon as possible. Redness without pain may look more worrying but can wait until the following morning.

If the eyelids are sticky on waking and have to be parted with the fingers—the cause is usually due to an infection (conjunctivitis).

This requires an antibiotic in ointment or droplet form – *not* 'Eye Gene' or 'Safer Blue' or other OTC (over-the-counter) preparations that promise to make the eyes 'brighter'! This is physically impossible – but good for business.

Conjunctivitis is a common eye condition and often treated casually with OTC Sulphur-containing antibiotics. Invariably the condition does not respond as the organisms have become resistant to sulphurs due to their indiscriminate use.

Any eye infection in the newborn warrants immediate medical attention. Any eye infection developing after sexual intercourse, where the possibility of a venereal infection cannot be excluded, also requires urgent attention.

The antibiotic ointment/drops should be applied 3-4 times a day for up to 10 days. Discontinuing it as soon as the symptoms start to subside is a mistake, as the infection often recurs. The entire eye does not need to be smothered with the ointment! A half centimeter bead should be applied to the *outer* corner of the eye. The blinking action of the eyelids will carry the medication to the inner corner of the lower eyelid to two tiny openings that carry the tears into a larger passage, the tear-duct. This duct carries the tears from the inner corner of the eye to the nostril on that side and explains why crying is followed by 'sniffling'!

If the opening of the tear duct (punctum) becomes blocked the tears will flow over the eyelid and spill onto the cheek. In the short term this may be due to an infection and an antibiotic, as for conjunctivitis, may resolve the problem. If it persists for a length of time, weeks on end, the tear duct may need to be 'reopened'. This is a minor procedure in which a thin probe is introduced into the duct to unblock it – much like a plumber unblocking a drain! Having it done may resolve the inconvenience of a dripping eye!

If children (and some adults!) are loathe to have medication instilled into their eyes the ointment or drops can be applied on to the *closed* eyelids (outer corner) and with the blinking action of the eyelids the medication will spread itself across the eyeball. Avoid touching the eyelids with the nozzle of the container, as this will contaminate the latter.

The use of towels and facecloths should be avoided in conjunctivitis as they will harbour the infection and spread it to the other uninfected side and also to others who may use the same. A safer alternative is to use a 'tissue' that is then discarded. Touching the infected eye directly may contaminate the fingers and disseminate the bacteria – as would kissing, embracing or shaking hands.

Rubbing the eyes for any reason – itchiness, tiredness or simply getting up in the morning – is not recommended. It could damage the cornea if done repeatedly. Avoid using the pads of the finger tips to rub the eye to relieve an itch – the fingers are not sterile. As a compromise use the back of the knuckle of the index finger instead.

It is well known that cataracts are the leading cause of 'curable' blindness. The point that is missed is that this blindness is not as a result of a diseased eye, such as occurs in diabetes, but is due to a mechanical problem.

The lens gradually becomes more and more opaque allowing less and less light to enter the affected eye. When the cataract becomes 'mature' no further vision is possible. However, no physical harm will come to the eye if this cataract were not removed (immediately). If the window in a room was considered to be the lens and the room itself the rest of the eye then misting up the window (lens) with steam will gradually reduce the amount of light entering the room (retina – part of the eye that does the 'seeing'). But this does not affect the contents of the room; the window (lens) can be changed at any time (cataract operation). An artificial lens can be used to replace the original. This obviates the need for the familiar thick lens in spectacles. A cataract can be a complication of diabetes and better control of sugar levels could prevent it.

Cataract extraction is done under local anaesthetic, is a relatively minor procedure and advanced years is not a major setback. In countries like India where so many are done it is virtually a 'lunch hour' procedure – like their vasectomies! One important requirement for the operation – considering that it is done while the patient is wide-awake – is that he or she must lie absolutely still. A person with a persistent cough cannot lie still! Complications from the procedure are rare.

Ultraviolet radiation can also cause premature cataract formation as well as injury to the retina. Investing in good quality sunglasses specially designed to keep out this form of light can prevent this as cheaper ones are ineffective. Sun glare reflected off water surfaces and snow is another hazard facing the growing numbers of sports enthusiasts.

Motorists are also at risk, especially long distance drivers of cars and trucks. The sun visor should be in the lowered position at all times during the day to avoid exposure to UV light – it also reduces the glare from the field of vision; whether there is bright sunshine or overcast sky the visor should be in the lowered position. Without the visor the eyes are screwed up trying to avoid the glare. This will result in headache from continually contracting the muscles around the eyes.

Any blow to the eye requires the urgent opinion of an eye specialist. The eye may appear normal on the outside but may have internal damage like bleeding. Though the eyes are tucked away in protective bony sockets the following impact injuries carry a high risk of injury

- Balls of all makes and sizes cricket, soccer, tennis, table-tennis
- Contact injuries with fists and elbows
- Pellet guns and rubber bullets and
- Snapping branches on hikes as the leader releases them after passing through a thicket!
- Children running or playing with sharp objects in their hands (pens, pencils, scissors, knives, forks, sticks)
- Exploding champagne and soft drink bottles (always cover the cork or bottle top with a heavy towel while it is gently removed *with a twisting action*)
- Fireworks and crackers
- Catapults are deadly missiles for eyes
- Stone throwing has similar hazards

Ageing brings on a form of degeneration involving the macula. The latter is a tiny speck in the retina (like the blood spot in the yolk of an egg) that is responsible for actual vision. Such degeneration currently has no definitive treatment. 'Carotenoid Complex' – one capsule 3 times daily could be a preventative measure or it could reduce the rate of further degeneration. While the medical profession dithers seeking 'more evidence' of the merits of taking carotenoid supplements more affected elderly patients will have lost their eyesight to this crippling disease. Stronger spectacles for failing vision from macular degeneration are useless and misguided as they will not improve it.

In diabetics new blood vessels tend to grow in the retina, especially around the macula. Bleeding under the retina is a serious complication of diabetes mimicking the accumulation of blood behind the lining of the shell within a hen's egg. Laser treatment uses heat to coagulate the blood vessels and stop the bleeding. It can also prevent new vessels forming around the macula.

Regular examination of the urine and eyes forms an integral part of the management of diabetes and are as important as checking blood sugar levels. Diabetics who test positive for protein in the urine invariably have changes within the eyes. Keeping the blood glucose levels as close as possible to normal, i.e. between 4 and 6 mmol/L help to reduce the complications of diabetes.

Glaucoma is a condition in which there is increased pressure within the eye and, left untreated, will compromise the blood supply to the retina and result in blindness. This pressure can be measured with a special instrument (tonometer). Clues that point to an elevated pressure are halos seen around electric lights (street lamps) and pain in the eyes. As mentioned earlier any pain in the eye warrants a visit to the doctor.

Television should not be viewed in total darkness; the lighting should be from behind the viewer. Sitting close to the screen does not 'damage' the eyes but children who do this should have their vision tested.

Omega 3 is recognized as important in the development of the brain and the retina and should be taken throughout the pregnancy. To this end manufacturers of formula feeds are adding it to their products but the medical profession has yet to see the light. The company manufacturing Omega 3 is important - *not all* products are equal in quality.

In the following situations the eyelids cannot be closed completely

- Bell's Palsy (in which there is a 'paralysis' – (usually temporary – of one half of the face)
- Grave's Disease of the hyperactive thyroid gland – in which the eyeballs become prominent. There is a risk of the cornea (brown/blue/green part of the eye) drying out during sleep as the lids do not meet to protect the eyeball with secretions intended to keep the tissues moist. This can lead to the formation of ulcers on the cornea, which heal and leave scars that would obstruct vision. This is more limiting when the scars lie close to the pupil – the aperture through which light enters the eye. At night the eyelids may be kept closed with an adhesive tape (Cellotape) and artificial tears instilled into the eyes as often as is necessary to prevent them from drying out.

- Naturally prominent eyeballs.

While these precautions may become tedious and then neglected they are vital to the preservation of vision; corneal transplantation is not an option because the cause would remain unchanged!

In a condition called Sjogren's syndrome there is deficient production of tears and saliva resulting in dry eyes and mouth. Keeping gum in the mouth (without chewing continuously - risk of setting up inflammation/arthritis in the jaw-joint!) may help to keep saliva flowing. The Bushmen of the Kalahari keep a pebble in the mouth to keep their mouths dry in desert conditions.

'Squinting of the eyes' in trying to see clearly, especially in children, often implies difficulty with vision and requires optical assessment. There may be headaches associated with reading or watching television. Teachers should rotate their pupils so that those moved to the back rows that have difficulty reading off the blackboard can be referred for visual testing. They would otherwise remain undetected in the front benches! Regular eye testing in schools will help detect abnormalities earlier.

Infants under the age of three months cannot focus upon objects and are relying on sound to follow with their eyes though they give the appearance that they can, indeed, see. After this period they should be able to follow moving objects. Failure to do so should be mentioned at the baby clinic.

Contact lenses should not be used

- In the presence of an eye infection until it is adequately treated
- If there is any hint of discomfort or pain. The lens itself may harbour the infection and will need to be discarded; disposable lenses are a blessing in this situation.

Sharp objects like pens, pencils, knitting needles, chopsticks, skewers, knives, forks and sticks have no place in the hands of children if their use cannot be supervised. *Running* around with these objects has the potential for turning 'play' into tragedy!

Catapults are weapons designed to cause injury; many an eye or defenceless bird have seen the darker side of these seemingly innocent 'toys'! Pellet guns are guns and have no place in the house unless they are stored in a gun-cupboard under lock and key.

The lead from pencils can damage the cornea causing staining and scarring. Sanding machines and angle grinders send off fragments of metal at high speed that can lodge in the cornea or the eye itself. This will cause immediate pain that is aggravated by movement of the eyelid over the cornea – as in blinking. To prevent it a clean folded handkerchief should be taped over the affected eye in the closed position and medical attention sought as early as possible. Metal particles cause a ring of rust in the cornea, and the longer the foreign metal remains the greater the risk of necessitating excision of the rust with serious implications for future vision.

Ultraviolet burns of the cornea, commonly caused by exposure to the sun (snow-skiing) or arc welding (arc eyes) do not usually have any symptoms until about 12 hours later when the patient experiences severe photophobia (intolerance of light) and agonising pain in the eyes. All such 'burns' should be seen by a doctor or ophthalmologist immediately because of the risk of damage to the cornea.

A greenish/orange dye (flourescein) is instilled into the eye to exclude or confirm the presence of foreign bodies, ulcers or burns of the cornea – only damaged areas of the cornea will take up the dye. This green discoloration can be seen through an ophthalmoscope (instrument that illuminates and magnifies). The dye is harmless but objects will appear orange in colour until the tears have naturally washed it out of the cornea.

If a person has suffered a stroke the eyes may not move towards one side. Avoid placing the bed or chair in such a position that the person cannot take in the surroundings through the good side otherwise he or she is faced with a blank wall, the loss compounded if there is an additional inability to communicate.

Staring at a computer screen for long periods will place a strain on the eyes and the muscles that help to move them in different directions. One should regularly look away as a matter of habit and move the eyes up, down and side to side for exercise. Make a conscious effort to blink frequently. Squeezing the muscles around the eyes as tightly as possible and then opening them widely will help to 'stretch' them and relieve tension. This is safer than rubbing the eyes!

Any laceration of the eyelids should be sutured by an eye-specialist to avoid the risk of them healing with scars that will leave the eyelashes growing askew/inward. This has the potential for abrading the delicate cornea with the eyelashes and being a source of constant irritation each time the eyes blink.

A stye is a little pimple situated on the margin of the eyelid and represents an infected root of an eyelash; removing the latter with a pair of tweezers may help to drain the pus. It invariably requires antibiotic ointment/drops applied to the eyelid as for conjunctivitis.

A meibomian cyst is often mistaken for a stye. In this condition one of the glands in the eyelid *away from the margin* becomes infected. It is seen and felt as a red, button-like swelling on the inside of the lid (conjunctival side) – usually the upper one. It causes pain/discomfort and in the acute (early) stages the application of heat (warm compresses or a gently warmed spoon) will provide considerable relief. If these simple measures fail to resolve the pain an antibiotic ointment should be used for a minimum period of a week. This should preferably *not* be a sulphur-containing one as this has become ineffective through over-prescription. The swelling usually settles down but can reappear.

Ophthalmologists should be reluctant to remove the cyst unless it has recurred about 3 to 4 times in succession. This is done under local anaesthetic and does not require hospitalisation. The procedure is timed for when the acute inflammation has subsided.

If the whites of the eyes (conjunctivae) become darker or take on a tea-stain discoloration this is of no medical significance and it does not imply the person is abusing drugs! If jaundice occurs due to problems with the liver or gall bladder the increased bile in the blood causes the whites of the eyes to become yellow. The degree of yellowness often reflects the severity of the blockage of the bile. Jaundice requires urgent medical attention.

Drinking large quantities of carrot juice may also give the whites of the eyes and the skin in general a yellow tinge - more easily seen in the palms of the hands. This is due to excessive quantities of carotene present in carrots - cut down on the juice!

Doctors examine the colour of the lower eyelid looking for pallor of the conjunctiva (inner aspect of the lid) – pink is healthy. A pale colour is usually due to anaemia which may be the result of deficiency of iron, folic acid or vitamin B12. Blood tests would be necessary to confirm the diagnosis.

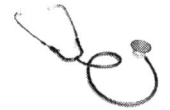

THE HANDS

The hands are the most frequent point of physical contact between people yet they hardly receive a passing glance. They closely resemble the feet; not too long ago they were organs of locomotion.

One could read 'pages' into a handshake.

- The long grip – the length of time the hands stay in contact often reflects the intimacy of the relationship.
- The firm gripper holds the hand with the correct amount of pressure without crunching them, sending a message of confidence, of being at peace with oneself and with one's fellow man.
- The vise-gripper is doing it deliberately to dominate and cause pain. The person upon whom the pain is being inflicted is unlikely to complain since this may be tantamount to declaring the recipient is a sissy and a wimp who 'could not take' the jousting of the 'stronger/ more dominant' male. Animals do this when they meet for the first time and may actually attack the newcomer! The relationship being struck up by such a handshake can hardly be construed as a happy one. Close friends do not indulge in this type of handshake. Vise-grippers have little consideration for the feelings of others. Big, burly men who pump iron to boost muscle to bolster insecurities in other areas of their personalities have a penchant for this type of handshake.

- The limp grip – highlights insecurities and feelings of intimidation in the recipient set off by the owner of the more prominent grip and, often, the world at large.
- The short grip – common when the meeting is mainly of a business nature where intimacy is not an issue and the association is not intended to be protracted. This form of greeting may also occur when the meeting is likely to be unfriendly and the handshake becomes perfunctory, being offered more as a courtesy. The extension of this form of hostility may well be 'no handshake'.
- If the handshake is cradled by the left hand. An extension of this very warm connection would be when all four hands are used – with the intimacy being reciprocated by both parties.

There is very little one can do without the hands and yet the amount of care and attention these work-horses command is only realised when they are unable to serve.

The thumb is the equivalent of the other four fingers – without it the hand is useless. If a choice had to be made – better the thumb saved and the rest of the hand sacrificed! This should emphasize the point that any problem involving the thumb deserves priority attention and not a 'wait and see' approach. This includes infections behind the nail (paronychia) and any injury to this digit, whether crushed by a door, struck by a cricket ball or basket ball, falling on the outstretched hand / wrist and experiencing pain either in the digit itself or in the 'hollow' behind the thumb.

Stretching the thumb away from the index finger will bring out this 'hollow' between the two tendons of the thumb. Pain occurring in this hollow (called the 'snuffbox' - because users of snuff used to position the powder in this hollow before sniffing it) may be due to a fracture of the scaphoid bone which lies in it. It may only become apparent when it is X-rayed after 2-3 weeks when it has started to show signs of healing or an MRI Scan (more sensitive than an X-ray) is done early. If the X-rays at the time of injury are normal and pain persists longer than a week a fracture of this bone may have been missed.

Pain occurring in any joint of the finger needs an explanation. One of the earliest symptoms of rheumatoid arthritis is early morning stiffness lasting for periods from 5 to 30 minutes or longer. The joints commonly involved early in this progressive condition are the small ones of the hands starting in the knuckles of the fist followed by those next in line down the fingers.

Small hard swellings /nodules – called Heberden's nodes – may occur at the sides of the joints located at the ends of the fingers. They are caused by osteoarthritis and in the active phase are painful but later become quiescent ('burnt out'). They occur more commonly in women, cause much deformity and look unsightly - making the unfortunate ladies embarrassed to show off their once beautiful hands. Rheumatoid arthritis, as a rule, does not occur in these end/ terminal joints of the fingers.

Injuries to the nail often result in a subungual haematoma (blood under the nail) that causes a blue discolouration. The pressure of the blood under the nail causes severe, throbbing pain that may easily be relieved by making a tiny escape route - allowing the blood to be evacuated. Normal nail is 'dead' and as such cannot feel pain; it is the tissue under the nail that is very sensitive. As an emergency measure a tiny hole can be made through the nail to allow the blood to escape. This would bring instant relief and for this reason alone is worthy of the attempt. The procedure is simple and painless though the idea of it can be quite daunting!

Wash the finger to 'sterilise' the nail and use a clean needle - preferably not a sharp one (sewing needle) – an 'office pin' would do. Choose a spot in the middle of the haematoma and, with a gentle rotatory motion (shaft of the pin gripped between the tips of the thumb and index finger), using the point of the needle - carefully 'drill' a hole through the nail. It requires gentleness and almost no pressure on the nail (this will cause more pain). It can take up to 15 to 30 minutes – to get through the less than 1 mm of hard nail. As soon as the blood pool under the nail is reached it will start to ooze out of the opening. Do not expect it to gush out like a fountain! The drilling is stopped once oil is struck!

The opening may quickly become blocked with blood but a few twirls of the tip of the needle will reopen it. This is repeated until no further blood or pink fluid appears through the pinhole opening or the pain has eased.

A fishing hook that has pierced a finger must not be pulled back because the barbs on the hook will cause more and unnecessary damage to the tissues. The secret is to remove the 'eye' of the hook with cutting pliers and push the hook in deeper until the pointed end extrudes through the skin and then have the hook pulled out. This is not for the faint hearted. Expect to have this done in the Emergency Unit under a local anaesthetic.

The hands are often exposed to chemicals (washing up liquid, detergents, and a whole range of other toxins) that may affect the skin and cause allergic reactions – dermatitis. The treatment (not always obvious or observed!) is to *avoid contact* with the offending agent! Failing this, appropriate gloves should be worn or products used that do not have the nasty side effects of common cleaning preparations. 'Super 10' and 'LDC' are two cleaning agents that can do the job of over ten separate products. They reduce the quantity of garbage, can degrease an engine and be safe enough to drink – accidentally that is! They can be used without gloves and after the job is done leave the hands feeling as though a moisturiser has been applied! They are safe to clean the leaves of indoor plants and are eco-friendly enough to be discarded into the drain.

Tingling or numbness in the fingers implies that a nerve is being compromised somewhere along its course from the neck (cervical spinal cord) down to the fingers. One quite common condition is 'carpal tunnel syndrome'; comparison is made with a 'watchstrap' around the wrist that is compressing the nerves that pass under the strap en route to supply sensation to the fingers. Pregnancy, an underfunctioning thyroid gland (hypothyroidism), working with vibrating machinery and rheumatoid arthritis may also cause this condition. The pain or pins and needles sensation in the fingers typically gets worse at night and may move upwards into the forearm. The abnormal sensations are felt in the thumb, index, middle and half the ring fingers. If they persist or worsen an operation, in which the 'strap' (ligament that surrounds the wrist) is cut and the pressure released, relieving the symptoms.

Any injury involving a joint (any where in the body) often needs an X-ray to exclude a fracture – missing it may compromise the future function of the joint and lead to osteoarthritis. This is too big a price to pay for ignoring the initial injury – as trivial as it may appear at the time.

An infection or swelling of the fingertip (pulp of the fingers) demands early medical attention. The blood supply to the tips of the fingers depends on arteries that lie on the sides of the fingers and if there is swelling in this area the blood supply may be compromised, and this is never a good thing (anywhere in the body). Fingers have been amputated for such negligence!

The hands are prone to being pricked with foreign objects like the barbs of fish fins, spicules of bone from animal carcasses and chicken bones. Some fish like the 'catfish' or 'barbel' have poisonous barbs and many a finger has ended under the surgeon's knife due to allergic reactions and subsequent infection following injuries with these barbs. Butchers are at risk of being pricked by spicules of bone from a carcass and this should be treated early with an antibiotic even though the injury may appear trivial.

A splinter in the hand or finger, if it is fairly superficial, may be seen as a line of discolouration beneath the surface of the skin and can be removed without too much fuss. The secret is to use a rather 'blunt' (not sewing needle sharp!) needle like an office pin and the 'track' opened up in layers starting very superficially and avoiding direct pressure on the splinter, as this will cause pain. Begin the 'excavation' slightly away from the surface of the splinter. A 'tweezer' may be used after sufficient exposure of the foreign body. Left for long periods (weeks to months) a firm swelling may form around the splinter or other foreign object. This is the body's defence mechanism against the intruder – producing fibrous tissue around it, similar to that found in a scar. If there is a low-grade infection it will continue to discharge (fester) until the foreign body has been expelled either naturally or with minor surgery. A person with a splinter injury,(regardless of how trivial it may appear), in the setting of exposure to manure or garden dirt should receive an anti-tetanus injection within 12 hours of the injury. Tetanus is a life threatening infection. A booster vaccination should be received every ten years, especially, if one is at risk for such infection.

Using the hands as instruments of combat as in karate training may cause damage to the small joints of the hands resulting in arthritis; today's 'black belt' may well be tomorrow's osteoarthritis requiring anti-inflammatory drugs and possibly surgery!

Hammer drills, jackhammers and other vibratory tools, used over prolonged periods may cause damage to the soft tissues of the hands. This can result in contractures that tie down the fingers in scar tissue making movement of the affected fingers painful and restricted – invariably requiring surgical release.

If from the bent position (fist) one or two fingers cannot be straightened without the assistance of the other hand this condition is called 'trigger finger'. The tendon of the affected finger is being trapped in the palm of the hand. A steroid injection combined with a local anaesthetic given into the palm close to the base of the affected finger may resolve the problem. Failing this minor surgery will be required. If the trigger finger is a result of recent repetitive injury (gripping the steering wheel for protracted periods) avoiding this may be all that is required.

Should a ring get 'stuck' on a finger because of swelling of the tissue or obesity (!) and applying soap fails to facilitate its removal the following manoeuvre may be more successful:

- First apply soap to the part of the finger away from the ring and
- Elevate the hand above the head for about 30 minutes
- Use a length of string, and allowing a few centimeters of the beginning to be secured by the thumb, wind it around the finger – beginning immediately past the ring and working away from it in the direction of the fingertip. This is done slowly and precisely and as tightly as is comfortable so that

each completed turn of the string is placed one behind the other until just past the first knuckle of the finger.

- Wait 3-5 minutes to allow the 'fluid' in the finger to be 'drained' away from the ring and then
- Quickly unwind the string from the end closest to the ring;
- As the string is being unwound the ring is pulled off. This may avoid having to cut (and ruin) – the ring!

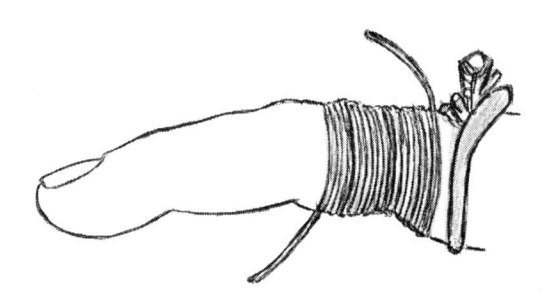

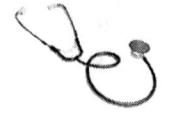

THE HIP JOINT

The hip joint is not easily examined (unlike the knee and ankle) because it is hidden under large muscles and soft tissue. Pain that occurs in this joint in *any age* group warrants an early visit to the doctor and an X-ray.

There are two important areas of the skeleton that are commonly affected in osteoporosis: the spine and the hip joints. This condition of 'holes in bones' predispose these areas to fractures. Postmenopausal women who do not take calcium supplements and do not walk for exercise are very vulnerable. Figures from the USA quote more than 200.000 fractures each year of the hip joint alone.

Of these, 30.000 die either as a direct result of the break or from complications that occur afterwards. The hip is a large joint and during a fracture air or blood clots can enter the damaged veins of the bones. These emboli may reach the lungs and result in blood clots (pulmonary emboli) which could be fatal.

The patient is often elderly (usually female) who may have spent a time waiting for the operation and then convalescing after the hip replacement. This period in bed makes them susceptible to lung infections (pneumonia) and bedsores. Inactivity/immobilisation will lead to muscle wasting and further loss of calcium from already depleted bones.

Lying in bed for protracted periods also places them at risk for blood clots in the leg veins (venous thromboses). Small segments of clot may break away from the main thrombus and travel up the veins causing emboli in the lungs.

The inherent risk of fractures of the hip joint (and men are not exempt!) makes it mandatory to prevent osteoporosis. The structure of bone in osteoporosis in which calcium is missing looks like 'Crunchie' or 'Aero' chocolates – except the holes where calcium is missing are bigger! It is hardly surprising that it breaks so easily! Unfortunately, osteoporosis does not enjoy the media-grabbing attention of cancer and heart attacks and the elderly will continue to pay the price.

Supplementation with calcium and Vitamin C can prevent osteoporosis. One woman in four will at some time in her life break the hip. If they survive the immediate dangers and, later, the secondary complications, they may never be as mobile as they were before the hip got replaced!

Then there is the small but ever-present risk of the artificial joint becoming infected. This could entail a lengthy stay in hospital on antibiotics and or, worse still, the prosthesis being replaced. This will only be possible when the infection has cleared.

The theory behind the fracture has always been that the victim of a hip fracture first fell and then broke the bone. However, research shows the fall is often the result of the fracture sustained in the first instance by a minor stumble. This may happen getting out of the shower or chair. Furthermore, the elderly are often taking medication to lower their blood pressures. This is compounded by a side effect common to most blood pressure drugs – i.e. dropping the blood pressure on assuming the erect position (called postural hypotension).

After prolonged periods of inactivity, such as after a night's sleep or a spell in front of the television, assuming the erect position suddenly may also drop the pressure and cause a stumble or fall. Standing on a chair to hang up a curtain or reach for a shelf may be the last chore one may perform independently before leaving for the emergency unit!

Fractures of the femur (thigh bone) commonly occur at their upper ends – where they enter the hip joint. The femur is the longest and strongest bone in the body. It angles upwards and outwards and, as it gets closer to the hip, turns inwards (neck of the femur). This short piece (neck) that bends inwards to enter the hip joint is often where the bone breaks.

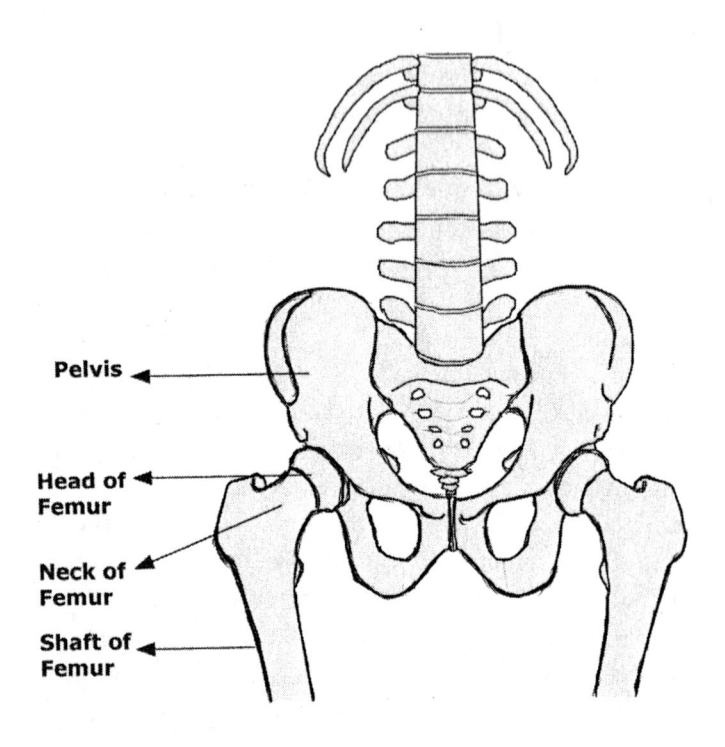

THE HIP JOINT

Is enough being done to prevent these and other fractures? Health schemes and government agencies have no qualms about paying thousands for a total hip replacement but often refuse to pay for supplements of calcium and vitamin C and Omega 3 – supplements that could help prevent osteoporosis. This does not even consider that the victim may require a second hip replacement if the first one should fail for whatever reason and that the patient with the prosthesis may never walk or run normally again.

Any elderly person who falls should have a fracture of the hip excluded because it happens with a minimum of force (stumble). Suspect a fracture of the hip if there is a history of a fall along with: –

- Inability or reluctance to move the hip or leg
- Pain in the hip or groin when the straightened leg is gently rolled from side to side and
  Any shortening of the affected limb.

An elderly person (who may have Alzheimer's disease and a poor memory) with such a fracture may not recall the minor stumble or attach little importance to the latter.

If a fracture is suspected medical attention must be sought immediately because of the risks attached to this particular joint injury. The victim may rapidly become shocked from losses of large amounts of blood within the fracture area. The large vessels that run along the neck of the femur often tear and bleed heavily and not all of the bleeding may be visible, given that this joint is well hidden from view.

If a hip fracture is suspected: –

- Avoid moving the patient – as far as is practical make the person comfortable where he or she fell
- Immobilise the affected side with rolls of blanket and strap the suspect leg to the good one
- Keep the patient warm with blankets (they are often shocked) – do not give them anything to drink - should they need an anaesthetic
- Reassure the patient until the paramedics arrive.

Perthes' disease of the hip occurs most commonly between the ages of 4 to 8 years and boys are affected more than girls. It presents with pain and limping and is believed to be caused by interruption of the blood supply to the rounded end of the top of the femur (thigh bone) – where it lies within the hip joint. It emphasizes the point stressed earlier – any pain in a joint requires a timely orthopaedic opinion.

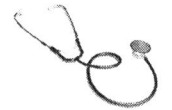

THE IMMUNE SYSTEM

Since the detection of the Human Immunodeficiency Virus and AIDS the immune system has become a household term. However, its importance remains shrouded in mystery and ignorance.

Whereas it is understood that, without the vital organs, the functions of the body would come to a standstill, the role of the immune system has been relegated to a lesser status. Little can be further from the truth – the most expensive car in the world is useless with a flat tyre!

The immune system is responsible for the defence of the body against foreign invaders. In certain situations it may also turn the body against its own organs. In organ transplants the immune system determines whether the body will accept or reject the new organ. Drugs are used to suppress the immune system in order to ensure the body accepts the donated organ.

The protection of the body begins with the skin and linings that cover the mouth and other orifices. This may be compared with the moat and wall surrounding a castle. Within the castle are the soldiers – the cells of the immune system – the B cells (B lymphocytes) and the T cells (T lymphocytes), which are part of the white group of cells.

The castle walls need protection and for this the following nutrients play an important role in maintaining their integrity: –

- Fatty acids (Omega 3 and Omega 6)
- Vitamin A
- Niacin and

- Zinc

Vitamin A deficiency results in infections of the eye. The gut may be described as an important 'passage' within the castle. Its integrity in protecting the rest of the castle from invaders requires *antibodies* which in turn requires vitamin A, sufficient protein intake, folic acid, vitamins B-6, B-12 and C, copper and zinc.

Treating patients with AIDS and the HI Virus with anti-viral agents without properly improving and supporting the immune system is ignoring the very basis of the disease! and, as has been mentioned elsewhere, simply stating "Eat healthily" to the victim is like wishing the bungee jumper who has no rope around the ankle "Good luck!" The advice to eat healthily is too vague and does not address the cost of doing so or the deficiencies of over-cultivated farmlands.

A failing immune system has no specific symptoms to warn the person. There may be recurrent infections (skin boils, bladder infections, common colds and influenza) and a feeling of constantly being run down and tired.

The past 100 years have seen a gradual decline in our immune system. It can be traced to the discovery that food can be cooked and eaten. Heat damages many of the nutrients in vegetables and fruits and alters the structures of proteins, fats and oils.

Mediterranean cultures that use olive and other oils in their natural state (unheated) do not share the cardiovascular diseases of others who use the same oils for cooking. Research into the dietary habits of Eskimos/ Inuits has clearly shown that heat damages the Omega 3 fatty acids in fish. But how popular or safe is raw fish?

With the introduction of cow's milk as a convenience food (on tap as it was!) man is the only mammal that drinks the milk of another mammal and nature did not intend this! Milk has the dubious title of the original 'fast food' – pleasant tasting (even 'addictive'), a virginal colour equated with purity and the producer venerated with a status next to godliness in countries like India. Milk became an established part of our food chain for the following reasons: –

- It was easily available once the cow was domesticated

- Relatively inexpensive even free, if one owned a cow and a patch of grass,
- Versatile in its uses and facile in the advertising – 'milk builds strong teeth and bones' and indeed it is the 'perfect meal' – *but for the calf* – for which it was designed! The quantity of fat and salt present in cow's milk was never intended for human beings. Furthermore, the hapless cow is pumped with antibiotics and hormones to help it produce the massive quantities of milk that help to swell the coffers of the dairy industry and supply an ignorant population that has been reared on mamma's words of wisdom - that extolled the virtues of milk.

The 1890's – just over a hundred years ago – saw the introduction of steel rollers to crush wheat to produce 'refined' white flour. The most important component – the germ or growing part – of the wheat is removed and fed to cattle as fodder! If it was retained the shelf life would be shortened and the flour spoiled.

To obtain a single dose of vitamin E one would have to eat about 250 slices of white bread or 4 ½ loaves of wholewheat bread! The vitamins added to bread are synthetic and, therefore, poorly absorbed from the gut! If better quality vitamins were added it would price the bread out of pocket!

Similarly, rice and maize have been stripped of their nutrition – all in the interest of longer shelf lives and bigger profits. Mealie/maize meal will rot on the supermarket shelves if the germ or growing part of the maize seed was not removed. This 'germ' maintains the health of the walls of the cells in the body and this in turn protects the cells against toxins and foreign invaders. 'Refined' wheat, maize and sugar should be redefined as 'Sidelined' – for all the nutritional value they have left compared to what Nature provided in the original product!

With the invention of the car and television levels of activity and exercise have fallen far below what are essential for good health. Motorists in shopping malls frustrate themselves trying to find a parking space as close as possible to the entrance. The introduction of the term 'couch potato' bears testimony to the statistic that 85% of the American population borders between overweight and outright obesity. It is predicted that the next 15 to 20 years will see 50% of the UK population labelled as 'obese'. There are prices to be paid for this and the mortality rate of AIDS will blur in the not too distant future when death from hypertension, diabetes, cancer, cardiovascular disease and obesity will continue to kill humans long after a vaccine is discovered for the HI Virus.

The average television viewer, including those that "Watch only the news and National Geographic", spends about 3 – 4 hours a day engaged in this *inactivity*, losing about 60 days per year. This is a staggering loss of 2 months of valuable time each year! This inactivity contributes to obesity. In addition, television advertising primes the viewer to buy food and drinks that further encourage obesity.

The constant bombardment of advertising sinks indelibly into the subconscious minds of both young and old, only to resurface in the supermarket. Picking products off the shelves becomes almost a reflex action. Manufacturers and advertisers have a finger in the golden pie.

The situation has been made even more heinous with the advent of 'Internet' shopping. The 'mouse' and the clatter of the keyboard are replacing the short walk from the car to the lifts and the long searches for goods on supermarket shelves that spelt some 'exercise' for shoppers!

There was a time when the corner store supplied most of the needs of the home. This was not a social outing but a shopping of necessity. With the arrival of the convenience stores and supermarkets we have changed the way we shop or, more precisely, 'gather food'.

Where once the weekend was the time for leisure and recharging batteries shopping at the mall has become a social event in which the whole family participates in the 'forage for food'.

From an early age children are able to match television advertising with the real thing at the supermarket. And what are there in the plastic packets (now thankfully banned – at least in some countries) that swell the trolley to overflowing? Cheese, chocolate, cream, cake, chips, cool drinks, polony, sausages, fruit juices, biscuits, sugar, jam, margarine, liver paste, pate, pastry – all of which will one way or another impair the immune system!

The hunting fields have been reduced to orderly rows upon rows of brightly lit shelves all ripe for the picking and placed at convenient levels so that no muscles are unnecessarily strained reaching for the 'fast movers'. The once elusive and thrashing prey can now be studied at length to make quite certain that the sell-by date has not expired and the ingredients checked! Once blood and bruises and, sometimes, life itself were risked for the hunter's prize - now the plastic card is all the weaponry that is required. Food manufacturers and retailers have made significant changes that affect our immune systems.

Farmers use more and more potent fertilisers but these mainly replace nitrogen, potassium and phosphorus in the soil; trace elements like selenium, molybdenum and zinc are not put back and become deficient in the fruit and vegetables that are cultivated. This rape of the farmlands has been continuing ever since demand began to outstrip supply. The vegetables look the same as they did 50 years ago but the nutrition that was meant to be drawn from the earth – is missing. The oft quoted advice from people of learning to "Eat healthily" is laughable!

Mentioned above and reiterated now: cooking food damages the vitamins, proteins and other nutrients. The Eskimos (also called Inuits) do not have heart disease as it is known to the rest of the world because of their high consumption of fish, much of it in its natural (unprocessed) state. Heat destroys the precious Omega 3 fatty acid present in the fat of fish. Canned fish is healthier than meat or chicken but much of the benefits are lost through the heat used in its manufacture. The same applies to the effect of heat in the canning of fruit and vegetables.

Food colourants (to make the appearance mimic or better the natural thing!), preservatives, sugar, salt and other additives intended to improve taste and appearance undermine the nutritional value of food. Cells in our bodies are deprived of this nutrition - compromising their function.

Braaing (South African) or barbecuing meat allows the fat to drip onto the fire and in burning releases toxic fumes that rise up to settle onto the food. This conjures up the image of spraying food with a hose connected to the exhaust fumes of a car! The blackened bits of barbecued meat (burnt toast included) have been shown to cause cancer!

Refined sugar must take pride of place in man's ingenuity to rob a natural food of every single vitamin, trace element and anti-oxidant and leave only the glucose or 'sugar'. This is the pure white sweet crystal that finds its way into almost every food and drink. Media advertising has been responsible, in no small measure, for inculcating into an unsophisticated population that relies heavily on 'sugar', to reinforce time after time that 'sugar gives you go'!

A can a day of any popular soft drink taken for a year contains an average total amount of a staggering 17 kilogrammes of sugar. How many school children are drinking more than this in tuck shops every school day? How many dinner tables carry the soft drink as part of the meal? And how many schools bear any responsibility for teaching our children that it is not okay to be indulging in foods and drinks of poor or almost non-existent nutritional value? Manufacturers of the crystalline substance extol the virtues of their product and 'research' appears to support mainly that excessive intakes lead to 'caries of the teeth'! This is not borne out by the alarming increase in obesity that is drowning our bodies in fat. For years the tobacco manufacturers had us believe a similar hogwash!

How does 'refined sugar' influence the immune system?

It has been estimated that a normal white cell has the ability to destroy up to 13 bacteria within about 45 minutes; take 6 teaspoons of sugar and in the same time span the same white cell can destroy only 6 bacteria. If the subject is fed a pie or other pastry the number of bacteria destroyed is reduced to 3!

Diabetics have a depressed immune system and are more prone than non-diabetics to infections in general, and of the bladder and skin in particular. The incidence of tuberculosis is also higher in diabetics than the general population. Tuberculosis poses a special threat for those who have their immune systems depressed by the HI virus. These infections result in swifter deaths due to the emergence of virulent strains of tubercle bacilli (the germ that causes TB) that do not respond to conventional anti-tuberculosis therapy. Alcoholics and socio-economically disadvantaged communities also have compromised immune systems that make them more susceptible to TB and other infections. The poor and the ignorant rely heavily on convenience foods.

Regular exercise boosts the immune system by producing endorphins and stimulating white cells. Patients infected with the HI virus should be advised to exercise with more conviction.

The positive effects of exercise in relation to the immune system are closely related to whether the activity is perceived as having a calming or stressful effect on the person. Marathons, big walks and periods of intense training tend to generate stress which, far from stimulating healthy white cells, may have the reverse effect of depressing them.

Exercise should be moderate and done on a regular basis. Weekend hikes share similar pitfalls as binge drinking – too much in too short a time!

Age also plays an important role in the immune system. Its peak efficiency is during childhood and the years leading up to young adulthood. With ageing the cells of the immune system (white cells) are less able to recognise and destroy foreign intruders that enter the body. This may explain why the elderly are more prone to contracting infections and cancers. Inadequate food intake and, more specifically, insufficient protein because of financial constraints, chewing difficulties, the appetite-suppressing effects of medication – all conspire to impair the health of the elderly. Recurrent illness and poor wound healing are warning signs of dietary deficiencies – especially of zinc and protein.

Inadequate dietary protein will compromise the function of the immune system. A malnourished child is more likely to succumb to an infection like measles. One of the cells of the immune system, the beta lymphocyte, produces antibodies that are themselves proteins. While it is well known that being overweight is fraught with medical problems it is less well appreciated that being underweight also compromises the immune system, lowering one's resistance to disease and infection.

Colostrum is the first fluid made by the mother's breast when infants are breastfed. It is rich in antibodies and cells that make up the immune system, helping to protect the infant until it is able to fend for itself in its defence against infection, particularly in the gut. Gastroenteritis is more common in formula fed infants

Bacteria utilise iron in order to proliferate. Iron supplements are, therefore, not recommended in the presence of infection. Breast milk contains proteins that bind iron making it less available to bacteria. Iron-containing multivitamins and tonics that are often used indiscriminately at the first hint of a sneeze may do more harm during an infection.

Inadequate sleep also plays a role in compromising the immune system. More young children and infants are being placed in crèches and in the care of minders because more mothers are working. This invariably means the child is awakened at an earlier (ungodly!) hour. The long distances between home and crèche, trying to avoid the early morning rush hour traffic and then leaving other older children in school - often in another part of the town or suburb – all contribute to earlier rising and aborted sleep.

Television encourages staying up till later because homework has been put off "Till after this programme" and the neglected assignment is either being done later the evening or night or early the following morning. One way or the other total sleep time is being eroded and this is often made up by cat napping for a few seconds at a time in the classroom. Concentration is compromised – the teacher may not even be aware that the student has stolen a few moments of shut eye. The desk may support the arm that supports the head; in a moving vehicle this may cause serious accidents – the traffic fine is not listing 'dozed off for a few seconds' as the offence! At higher speeds this could spell death for pedestrians and sleep-deprived motorists. What test do we have that will detect 'lack of sleep' – a "Sleepalyser"?

Stress is another factor that undermines the immune system. Stress uses up adrenaline and steroids and to replenish the supply of these important hormones from the adrenal glands four important vitamins are required – Vitamin A, Vitamin B, Vitamin C and Vitamin E.

While the medical profession still seeks *more proof* that supplements do any good – many of us will have succumbed to one ailment or another. The British Navy dithered for 30 years while it looked for "more proof" that the humble lemon/lime could prevent scurvy. While they debated more than 100,000 sailors died needlessly of this simple deficiency disease – all it required was Vitamin C from the lowly lemon!

The immune system can be improved upon by taking daily supplements of

- Omega 3 – 3 capsules daily
- Vitamin E – 200 IU units – 1 capsule daily
- Formula IV Plus – 1 sachet daily taken in the morning
- Carotenoid Complex – 1 twice daily and
- Nutrishake – 2 scoops daily.

Deficiencies of nutrients such as vitamin E, vitamin B6, zinc and proteins will compromise immune function and this becomes more important in the elderly or infirm.

Nutrition is not the medical profession's major forte. How can it be when pregnant women are being prescribed supplements containing 20 mg of calcium/day when their daily requirements are 1500 mg per day? Why do not the fruit and vegetables that are part of the "Eat healthily" programme contain the essential minerals and salts?

If the farmer is not adding the missing minerals and nutrients that mass production and poor crop rotation are leeching out of the soil how will the produce contain them? The current price being paid for these omissions is the high incidence of cardiovascular disease, cancer, asthma, diabetes, infertility and AIDS.

'Preventative medicine' will always be a thorn in the side of the pharmaceutical and medical industries – who will need their products or services if illnesses were to be *prevented?*

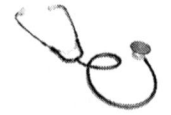

THE MEDICINE CABINET

The medicine cabinet or cupboard should be lockable and the key kept out of reach of inquisitive fingers – children are not to be trusted with medicines. Accidental overdoses in infants and children can have tragic consequences. Medicine cabinets, like gun cabinets, that cannot be locked should constitute grounds for child 'abuse' or 'neglect'. Children are curious creatures and love to explore. Taste is not always a deterrent. The pretty colours that drug manufacturers use in their tablets and capsules should question their safety where this age group is concerned.

Paracetamol is widely used as an antipyretic (for bringing down fever) and pain relief. 100ml of it contains 2400 mg of the drug. For a child weighing 10 kg. - The maximum dose in any one day should not exceed about 900 mg. Therefore, accidentally ingesting 100 ml. of paracetamol could be fatal. Fortunately, an antidote is available but it has to be administered within 8 to 24 hours of taking the drug.

Paracetamol is highly toxic to the liver, especially in a child - whose liver has not reached maturity. If this organ has been previously affected by diseases such as chronic alcoholic abuse or hepatitis (a viral infection) the damage from the drug may be greater.

Every medicine cabinet should have a thermometer. There is a wide range of different types available which are a far cry from the old mercury thermometers. With the newer heat sensitive single use strips there is no risk of accidental breakage and, more importantly, avoids transmission of infection from one user to the next.

Any recording above 37 degrees centigrade (previously measured as 'fahrenheit) implies an infection *until proven otherwise*. Feeling the forehead with the hand and guessing the temperature to be 'high' is inaccurate and could be misleading. If it goes beyond 39 degrees centigrade there is a risk of developing a 'febrile convulsion' (fit/seizure) from the fever. This may necessitate a lumbar puncture (using a needle to withdraw fluid from the spine) to exclude meningitis which is an infection of the lining of the brain and spinal cord – all this simply because the temperature was not accurately recorded and appropriate steps not taken to bring it down timeously.

Other 'must haves' in the cabinet should include: –

* pair of scissors
* pair of tweezers
* measuring spoon
* torchlight that works
* disposable gloves
* Bandages and cotton gauze
* 'Elastoplast' in a few different sizes
* Antiseptic solution e.g. Betadine or Savlon

Useful medicines to have in the cabinet (watch the expiry dates when buying them):

- Paracetamol (syrup or tablet as indicated by the ages of the family members), an anti-inflammatory (this may be used in addition to paracetamol or in place of the latter to bring down fever when it is ineffective on its own). Both these drugs are also available as suppositories (rectal use) if vomiting is a problem.
- Eye and ear drops are better avoided: a diagnosis is necessary should the need for these arise.
- An antacid that also contains an antispasmodic is useful for unexplained tummy aches and pains that are short lived (less than 48 hours)
- Drugs used in the treatment of diarrhoea may seem appropriate for the person making frequent trips to the

toilet but are not readily recommended. Treatment of diarrhoea is based on replacing that which are being lost – precious water and salt – using rehydration fluid. This is easily and inexpensively made with 8 teaspoons sugar and ½ teaspoon salt added to 1 litre water or 'Fanta' (may use less sugar).

- A cough suppressant is only useful for relieving a cough that is *irritating the airways* without producing much sputum. If mucus (sputum/spit) is present make use of the cough that nature provided to empty the airways – taking *a cough-suppressant* is misguided and irresponsible.

Adults and parents of children with coughs, perhaps, feel a sense of achievement when they queue up to buy cough mixtures and throat lozenges to pander to a childhood fantasy of playing 'doctor-doctor'. These products sold in winter make more income for the pharmac euticals than their regular drugs for the whole year! Our hankering to pip the doctor may have similarities to the DIY enthusiast who feels he or she can fix the leak in the bathroom tap!

- Antihistamine preparations in oral and topical (ointment) forms are useful for minor stings and insect bites or other allergies (food).
- Time-honoured antiseptic ointments like 'mercurochrome' used to paint a wound (and everything around it) red makes it very difficult to observe its progress or deterioration and should have no place in the medicine cabinet

If the public can be taught and encouraged to administer CPR (cardio-pulmonary resuscitation) there is no reason why the use of pre-filled adrenaline syringes should not be available in the home setting - diabetics are taught how to give themselves an injection of insulin.

Medicines that have expired (the chemist's or prescribing doctor's sticker often obscures the expiry date on the containers!) and bottles with unused medicines that are being saved for an 'emergency' should be discarded and replaced as necessary. Antibiotics that are reconstituted (mixed) with water cannot be used after the period for which they were prescribed. These do not have to be refrigerated. The practice of keeping medicines in the refrigerator is to be discouraged as it provides dangerous access to tiny fingers. Drugs like insulin (that must be refrigerated) should be kept in tamperproof containers - children have access to the refrigerator.

Child proof containers should be made mandatory for all medicines.

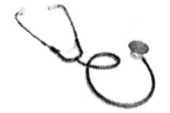

THE MENOPAUSE

The menopause marks the end of the fertile period in a woman's life. The onset varies from one person to the next; generally it seems to follow the timing of the mother's age at her menopause – on average around 50.

Menstruation does not end abruptly but often staggers itself over a period of about six months to a year. The amount of bleeding may gradually diminish with each successive month. The periods could disappear for one or two cycles, return and then disappear again only to return after a short period and then one month they are gone. It marks a turning point in a woman's life almost coinciding with the husband's time for retirement from gainful employment!

Human beings have an innate desire to feel needed and appreciated. Various factors may determine how the female adjusts to this milestone in her life. Her relationship with her husband plays an important role. By this time the children would have flown the roost to set up their own nests. Ironically, if procreation and successful parenthood have played important roles in the rearing of the children, especially for the mother, then menopause is the stage in her life that is likely to make her feel the least needed.

The ovaries make eggs (ova) and oestrogen; the placenta produces this hormone during pregnancy, and the testicles do the same for the male. Oestrogen stimulates the development of secondary sexual characteristics (breasts, pubic and axillary [armpit] hair) and growth and maturation of the long bones. As menopause approaches the production of oestrogen gradually wanes. This may occur before the periods disappear altogether and the symptoms of menopause i.e. the 'missing oestrogen state' may be confusing to the person concerned and her family. Initially, they may both be unaware of the reason for the changes that begin to appear. Blood tests are available that measure the level of hormones to confirm the diagnosis of menopause.

An 'early menopause' can be artificially created if both ovaries are removed at an age before the true menopause. In order to prevent osteoporosis and a higher risk of ischemic heart disease (angina) due to the missing oestrogen hormone - replacement therapy (HRT) should be considered. Research has shown that the incidence of ischemic heart disease or heart attacks after the menopause is the same as for men i.e. oestrogen protects the female until this time in her life. For this reason if a hysterectomy-ovariectomy is planned one ovary only should be removed. The remaining would be quite capable of supplying all the oestrogen the woman needs until menopause is reached.

The preferred ovary to be removed should be the right-sided one for the following reasons:

- The appendix could be removed at the same operation
- Pain arising later in the right lower quadrant of the abdomen will not have the ovary on this side to confuse matters for the surgeon if the appendix has already been removed!

The 'hot flush' is a prominent symptom of menopause. The severity may vary from one woman to another and not every female experiences it. The flush is followed after a few minutes by a cold sensation. Only the upper half of the body is so affected. It is often accompanied by perspiration, especially at night – soaking the hair and clothing to the point of intolerability. This can be embarrassing in company when, without any warning; the face suddenly takes on the appearance of a ripe tomato. A feeling of intense heat may occur without the hot flush, disappearing within minutes, almost as quickly as it appeared. It may be a blessing in cold weather but murder in the heat.

Other symptoms are

- Dizziness or lightheadedness
- Insomnia
- Irritability – little things may lead to heated arguments – all out of character for the affected person
- Changes in libido – sex maybe the furthest thought on her mind. These changes are ridden with guilt and sometimes with apprehension because she knows she is turning into a personality that she is unhappy and unfamiliar with and yet, no matter how hard she tries to control matters, an unseen force seems to take charge. If the spouse is ignorant of the condition or intolerant, impatient and unsupportive the depressed sex drive may well add to the unhappiness of the oestrogen-deficient wife
- Mood swings, weepiness and depression
- Appetite changes – usually ending up with more weight gain
- Fatigue, headaches, palpitations and shortness of breath

Treatment is aimed at replacing the missing hormone (HRT) and this may be taken as a tablet, patch or implant. The tablet is taken every day for three weeks and then the uterus is allowed a week to recover from the effects of the hormone. In this last week bleeding will occur as in a 'normal' period. If a hysterectomy has been performed this precaution does not apply and the hormone can be taken throughout the year – the risk of cancer removed by the gynaecologist's scalpel.

Bleeding should not be suppressed continuously because it increases the risk of cancer of the uterus. For women (and men!), who have grown to appreciate the absence of the menses after the menopause, the 'return' of her periods may not be welcome!

The fertile period for an average female is about 40 years spanning the ages from 10 to 50 during which time she would have used about 8000 sanitary pads for a total bleeding time of 7 years and almost 7 years of 'forced' celibacy - if sexual activity is suspended during the periods!

The hormonal patch applied to the skin of the abdomen twice a week may be more convenient than having to take a tablet every day. The patch may cause an allergic reaction at the site of application – presenting with itch and/ redness.

The implant method avoids the daily or weekly need for taking medication but requires a visit to the doctor each time it has to be replaced every 4 to 8 months. The medication (implant) is a slow-release 'capsule' that is placed under the skin (under sterile conditions) usually in the upper arm. For obvious reasons once it is implanted its effects can only be terminated by its surgical removal. This method may be too 'invasive' for many women and there is a small risk of infection.

One of the risks of HRT is a small to moderately high incidence of cancer of the breast and the uterus. It can also raise the blood pressure. This should be monitored if therapy is started.

Apart from controlling the menopausal symptoms the two main reasons for using HRT are: –

- reducing the risk of heart attacks and
- preventing osteoporosis – oestrogen helps bone utilise calcium more effectively.

However, the benefits of HRT are better understood only up to five years of use in menopause; after this period the advantages become blurred.

There is a significant risk of developing venous thromboses (DVTs) with the use of HRT. Smoking and HRT make dangerous bedfellows.

HRT does not give protection as a contraceptive and it should be known that women who are under 50 years of age can still fall pregnant for up to two years after the last period. For those over 50 the risk of pregnancy extends to about one year after the last period has ended. Alternative protection is necessary during this time.

Are there alternative ways of achieving the same ends without using HRT?

Exercise should be the number one priority and this should be an 'anti-gravity'-type activity like walking. Swimming may not be beneficial in the prevention of osteoporosis because it is not an 'anti-gravity' activity. Jogging is ill advised because of its inherent risk of damaging the hips, knees, ankles and the feet – which is defeating the purpose since this abuse itself may lead to damaged joints and osteoarthritis! Walking fits the bill more admirably.

The following supplements can be positive steps towards preventing cardiovascular disease and osteoporosis

- Omega 3 - (3 capsules daily)
- Vitamin E 200 I.U. - (1 capsule daily)
- Vitamin C slow release - 1 tablet daily
- Calmag - 3 tablets daily
- Lipotropic Adjunct - (2 tablets daily)

Oestrogen alone may not prevent osteoporosis without the building block that is calcium. Most of the calcium supplements sold in retail stores and health shops are synthetic (laboratory made) and, therefore, are poorly absorbed from the gut. At best about 13 % of the ingested amount is absorbed. If it is not adequately absorbed from the gut how will it ever reach the bone? 'Calmag' (manufactured by GNLD International) is reputed to have an intestinal absorption of 76 %. Furthermore, it is combined with magnesium, which helps to improve the absorption from the gut and the calcium is chelated (sandwiched between two proteins) to further increase absorption through the intestinal wall into the blood stream.

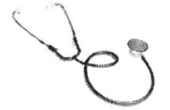

THE MISSED PERIOD

Any fertile female of reproductive age who is sexually active and misses a period is deemed pregnant until proven otherwise with a pregnancy test. If the period returns pregnancy is excluded provided this is a normal menstruation and not the bleed of an abortion. The true nature of the bleeding may be established with a pregnancy (blood) test.

If the female is not sexually active one or two missed periods are not significant. Often there is some underlying factor to account for this. Strenuous physical training could cause the periods to become scanty or disappear completely. Similarly, sudden stress or a debilitating illness can cause a missed period. The periods may also be disrupted if the thyroid gland becomes overactive (hyperthyroid).

If periods are missing for three consecutive months a visit to the doctor is warranted.

Females who have reached menarche (the first period) and then miss a period, and pregnancy has been excluded or is unlikely, this should not be immediate cause for concern as the pattern may be erratic at first. The periods may disappear for several months and then return. This start-stop sequence may continue for a while. If the periods remain absent after about a year of reaching menarche professional advice should be sought.

If an adolescent has not developed breasts or menstruated for the first time (menarche) by age 14 – medical advice should be sought.

With the injectable contraceptive 'Depo Provera' - periods are initially scanty and irregular for a variable time up to a year and thereafter may disappear.

As a woman approaches menopause, usually about age 50, the periods tend to taper off until they stop completely. Here again, a stop-start pattern maybe noted as the ovaries gradually cease producing oestrogen. However, if the periods have disappeared for up to a year and bleeding recurs, a gynaecologist should be consulted to exclude 'dysfunctional uterine bleeding' – a common, benign condition or a more sinister cancer of the uterus.

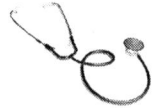

THE ORAL CONTRACEPTIVE

During pregnancy there are very high levels of oestrogen and progestogen in the blood and this prevents ovulation (further production of eggs) from taking place while the woman is pregnant. The oral contraceptives contain synthetic oestrogens and progestogens and, similarly, prevent ovulation by mimicking the pregnant state. Many of the changes in the blood chemistry during pregnancy are, therefore, also found in some women taking the pill! This explains the similarity in some of the side effects of both.

For the present the 'pill' is the closest we have to the most effective contraceptive. Unfortunately, it places upon the female (and unfairly so) the responsibility for ensuring it is religiously taken – along with the risks that may accompany their use and the side effects that occur with oral contraceptives. Certain factors concerning them should be considered: –

a) Do not smoke (period!) while taking the pill – there is a small but real risk of problems with blood clots occurring in those who smoke. Having a stroke at the age of twenty is a reality often ignored.

b) It must be taken every single day and preferably at the same time each day. Keep it near the toothbrush and take it with the last rinse of the mouth.

c) If diarrhoea and /vomiting occur a second tablet should be taken to reduce the risk of inadequate contraceptive cover. Antibiotics such as tetracycline should be avoided. Certain drugs that are used to hasten the transit time of stomach contents may make absorption of the oral contraceptive inadequate, especially medication used to alleviate nausea and gastric bloating. Similarly, the use of laxatives should be avoided.

d) If there is doubt about a pregnancy – as when a period has been missed – it is safer to have a pregnancy test (blood and not urine test as the latter may be negative in the early stages of pregnancy). This is important because the oral contraceptive can harm the foetus.

e) If the pill is forgotten for a day and intercourse took place it is safer to take the 'morning after' pill – if conception had occurred on that day the pill would be continued and nobody would be any the wiser.

f) An alternative form of contraception (injectable 'Depo Provera') should be used if one cannot be relied upon to take the pill regularly. How many pregnancies occur because the partner "Forgot to take the pill"?

g) Blood pressure and urine should be checked at least every six months because the pill can cause hypertension (high blood pressure) and should not be used in diabetes.

h) It should not be used if there is a history of deep vein thromboses – (clots in the leg veins), strokes, varicose veins, liver disorders (jaundice), severe migraine, hypertension or obesity.

i) The pill does not prevent sexually transmitted diseases as does the condom.

The freely distributed contraceptive pills used by family planning clinics may be those with higher doses of the hormones (because they are cheaper?). Those with smaller concentrations are safer and have fewer side effects but may be more expensive.

Strokes occur more frequently in women who are on the pill and this risk increases if they use them for longer than 10 years. Migraine appears to be a predisposing factor. As more and more teenagers are encouraged to use the pill for contraception rather than practice abstinence from intercourse the number of years they are exposed to the pill will increase and what this bodes for their future health remains to be seen. An average time on the contraceptive pill could span the ages 16 to 50 making it a *total of 34 years!*

While it has been shown that the pill is 'quite safe', the total number of 'pill years' should be kept as low as possible and aimed primarily at spacing children and *not* long term contraception. Once the family size has been established the aim should be a sterilisation procedure – tubal ligation (tying off the fallopian tubes) or vasectomy – the latter has advantages over female sterilisation.

The oral contraceptive may also be successfully used to regulate periods that are irregular, very heavy or painful. In these situations it may be taken for 2 to 3 months and then, hopefully, discontinued.

If teenagers will have sex anyway and likely fall pregnant in the act what has been gained by resisting the use of a contraceptive? The penalty may then be an abortion or unwanted pregnancy that will certainly change the lives of more than just the immediate couple in question. The promising academic career may come to an abrupt halt or be changed in midcourse! Common sense and all the advice given by mentors and parents may have no bearing when male and female sex hormones are riding high, the lights are low and the pants are down!

If the pill has been forgotten or unprotected intercourse (without any form of contraceptive) has taken place the 'morning after' pill ('Ovral' or 'Levonelle') obtainable at chemists should be taken for up to three days after the possible event (pregnancy) or on a preventative basis. For 'Ovral' take two pills as soon as possible followed by another two twelve hours later – (total of four pills) may prevent conception from progressing by sloughing off the lining of the womb. With 'Levonelle' a single tablet is taken within twelve hours of unprotected intercourse and not later than seventy-two hours after the event. Common side effects of the morning-after pill are severe nausea and vomiting.

The seven red tablets in the calendar pack of contraceptive pills are 'dummies' – they contain no hormones and result in break-through bleeding when they are taken. During this time the lining of the womb (endometrium) regenerates itself. If bleeding was to be suppressed for *long periods* it would increase the risk of malignancy of the uterus.

In any particular month if having a period were to be 'inconvenient' (going on honeymoon or holiday, writing an examination) the red pills may be omitted for one or two cycles (months) to prevent the breakthrough bleeding that normally occurs and then menstruation induced by simply taking the tablets as indicated on the calendar pack. If contraception is to coincide with a honeymoon, first-time users should start taking the pill for at least 2 months (2 cycles) before as ovulation (egg release) may still occur in the first month on the pill.

Side effects of oral contraceptives are less frequent with the low dose pills and as they vary from one pill to another it may be worth experimenting with a few before writing them all off. Nausea, weight gain, bloatedness and headaches are common but usually subside with continued use. For those afflicted with acne the use of the pill has been shown to be beneficial but the advantage is often lost once the hormone is discontinued.

Greater experience and added patient years have allayed much of the anxiety behind oral contraceptives and malignancy, and they have been shown to reduce the incidence of breast cancer.

In the meantime men wait with bated breath in the wings while an effective male contraceptive pill is perfected so that the burden of contraception is distributed more equitably between the sexes. However, the fairer sex should *not* hold their breaths for, if the onus of birth control lies solely with the men in their lives, many more women may find themselves with a pregnancy they did not plan – simply because "Honey, I forgot to take the pill!"

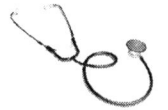

THE PAP SMEAR

The pap (short for 'Papinocolou') smear is a test for early detection of cancer of the vagina, cervix and the uterus (womb). The prognosis (outcome) in malignancy is far better in terms of effecting a 'cure' if the condition is detected at a stage *before* the cells become malignant i.e. the 'pre-malignant phase'.

The cervix is the lowest part of the uterus before it opens into the vagina. Picture a pear placed over the upper end of a short cylindrical tube with the tapered end of the pear lying a short distance into the tube. The tube represents the vagina, the tapered end of the pear – the cervix and the dumpy upper end of the pear being the 'body' of the uterus.

In this test a gentle scraping is made of the sides of the vagina and the cervix (tapered end of pear). The cells or 'mucus', that are part of this scrape, are then 'smeared' onto a glass slide and sent to the pathologist. Microscopic examination can show changes suggestive of cancer in the cells.

To exclude a malignancy in the vaginal walls the pap/smear test may be done once every five years.

The procedure is not painful but the person will be aware of being 'touched/ examined' within the vagina. It has similarities to using a wooden tongue depressor and gently scraping the inside lining of the mouth. No anaesthetic is necessary. The patient wears a gown, the underwear is removed and a sheet used to cover the lower half of the body. The female lies on her back with the knees bent and with a gloved hand the examining doctor or gynaecologist, without using any lubrication (this may damage the cells taken during the 'scrape') will insert first one and then two fingers into the vagina. Tensing the latter or keeping the legs together will make the examination difficult for the doctor and uncomfortable for the patient.

This part of the examination is to determine the position and size of the uterus, to feel the cervix, the ovaries that lie on either side of the uterus and any swellings related to the uterus. The bladder and the rectum may also be felt through the vagina. The rectum or back passage is situated immediately behind the vagina and the bladder immediately in front of it.

The smear is done under direct vision. This is achieved by introducing an (icy cold – and there is no reason it cannot be warmed first!) stainless steel speculum that resembles the beak of a large duck. The 'beak' of the instrument is introduced into the vagina with the speculum in the 'closed' position. The walls of the vagina are exposed by opening the beak at the top of the vagina – like a 'widely yawning mouth'. With the help of a light shone into the vagina (tube) – the cervix (tapered end of the pear) and the walls of the vagina are visualised and any abnormalities noted. A spatula is then used to gently scrape off the cells. Another type (that resembles a brush for cleaning babys' feeding bottles) with soft bristles at its tip is used to gently 'sweep' the opening of the cervix to obtain cells that have been shed from the body of the uterus (inside of the pear).

Any female who becomes sexually active should ideally have a pap-smear done yearly for life. As mentioned above the purpose of the test is to detect cancer at an early treatable stage. If the cells are suspicious but not definite for cancer the test will be repeated after three months. An infection in the cervix (cervicitis) can alter the cells and make them resemble the early changes of cancer. This infection is treated, usually with an ointment applied into the vagina/ cervix, and the test repeated after three months to confirm that the cells have normalised.

Vaginal infections may also be detected by the pap smear and appropriate treatment instituted.

A woman who has reached menopause and starts to bleed again after a year or so of not having periods needs an examination. Such bleeding is viewed seriously as the cause may be cancer though a more common finding is dysfunctional uterine bleeding (meaning the cause is unclear!). In a hysterectomy the entire womb is removed i.e. the entire 'pear' including the tapered end (cervix). Without the womb the risk of cancer in this organ is removed, making it unnecessary for a pap-test *each* year - once every 5 years may be adequate to exclude a malignancy in the vagina.

During the hysterectomy the ovaries in a *postmenopausal* woman are also removed as they serve no further purpose and are at risk of developing cancer. If the hysterectomy is performed in a pre-menopausal woman (who still gets her periods every month) one ovary is usually left behind to continue producing oestrogen. The patient should be informed whether the left or right ovary has been retained so that if pain should develop in it the side so affected may help establish whether the problem originates from this organ.

It is prudent to have the appendix removed at the same operation along with the right ovary.

After the procedure a trace of blood on the underwear/ sanitary pad is not cause for concern as the bleeding (spotting) usually settles after a day or two.

If a discharge is present for more than a few days after the pap-smear this may be due to an infection picked up during the procedure. This is not common but warrants a call to the doctor. It may be wise to postpone sexual activity for a few days.

The 'elderly' female or widow or those who are not sexually active anymore erroneously believe the pap-smears are not necessary. Many are too shy to have a doctor 'fiddling with their private parts' - especially when they have not 'been with a man' for a number of years. These women run the risk of developing cancer and often present when the disease has spread itself beyond the womb, making treatment difficult and often impossible. Disease and death cannot be worth avoiding a simple test that takes a few minutes. The cost of the procedure can never match the expense of trying to treat the disease once it has established itself.

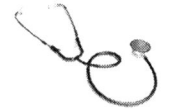

THE PROSTATE GLAND

This gland essentially occurs in males only and is situated under the bladder. The urethra, which is the tube carrying urine from the bladder through the penis to the outside, passes through the prostate gland. In women the prostate gland is very poorly developed – and exists as rudimentary glands on either side of the urethra.

Picture an inflated balloon with a longish nozzle/neck and a fist surrounding the neck close to the body of the balloon: the balloon representing the bladder, the neck the urethra and the fist the prostate gland. In the standing position the rectal tube (rectum) sits under the bladder and opens to the exterior via the anus.

It is, therefore, understandable that many of the symptoms of prostatic disease will also involve the urethra and sometimes the rectum.

Progressive enlargement of the prostate gland puts pressure on the urethra and causes increasing difficulty in passing urine (making the fist tighter). Initially there may be a delay in starting the stream when micturating (passing urine). As the gland gets bigger over time this difficulty will increase and may eventually make the obstruction complete so that no urine can be passed no matter how much pressure was exerted. This retention of urine requires urgent medical attention.

Certain drugs can cause a similar difficulty in passing urine e.g. some commonly prescribed antidepressants and eye drops used in the treatment of glaucoma (a condition of increased pressure within the eyes). *Any* new symptom that appears when medication has been recently started may be due to the drug itself and a doctor's advice sought.

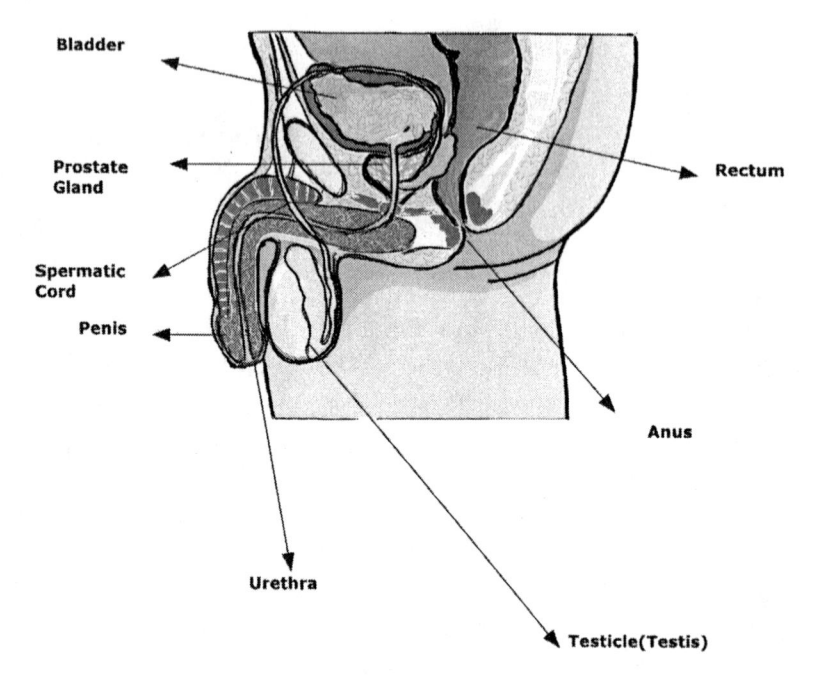

THE PROSTATE GLAND & RELATED STRUCTURES

Problems with the prostate gland usually begin after age 50. At first there may only be nocturia – getting up at night to pass urine. With time this may become more and more frequent. The straining to pass urine comes later and, as the urethra becomes narrowed, the once proud curved stream – that could stop a cockroach from a metre - now falls flatly at the feet!

Unfortunately, these symptoms *do not* differentiate an innocently enlarged prostate (benign prostatic hypertrophy) from one that is becoming cancerous. During the examination the doctor inserts a gloved finger into the rectum to reach the prostate gland to ascertain whether it feels hard or if small swellings or nodules can be felt in the gland. In benign prostatic hypertrophy the gland is enlarged but soft to the feel.

A firm prostate is suspicious of cancer.

A significantly elevated blood test for levels of PSA (prostatic serum antigen) will add to the suspicion. However, the levels may also be elevated if there has been a recent or current history of a bacterial infection of the prostate (prostatitis). If the evidence suggests cancer the next step is to biopsy the gland under ultra sound (X-ray) guide. The urologist, working through a narrow tube passed through the anus and using a special needle, takes tiny pieces of tissue from the prostate gland for laboratory examination. The biopsy is done under a local anaesthetic injected into the gland and the patient is discharged after it is completed – within 10 to 15 minutes. The procedure is more frightening in the imagination than is the reality. Admission into hospital for this is not necessary.

Other symptoms that may suggest a malignancy are loss of appetite, weight loss and backache. The latter may imply that the cancer has spread to the bones of the pelvis and lower spine. Cancer of the prostate is usually a very slow growing tumour and, accordingly, urologists may not be inclined to get overly concerned about it. However, this may not be how the *patient* views the diagnosis!

Surgery for benign prostatic hypertrophy is determined by the severity of the symptoms. However, research has produced drug therapy to try and shrink the size of the gland in benign prostatic hypertrophy – obviating the need for surgery in most cases.

'Masculine Herbal' tablets (one tablet twice daily) may help avoid the need for medication and, perhaps, even surgery. This is a combination of several herbs that may be an alternative to conventional treatment for problems ranging from impotence, premature ejaculation and benign prostatic enlargement.

A bacterial infection of the prostate (prostatitis) may present with discomfort during the passage of urine. However, the symptoms may not be as severe as the dysuria (burning urine) of an infection of the bladder (cystitis) or of the urethra (urethritis). Urine may be passed more frequently and there may also be discomfort during defaecation (passage of stool). As mentioned above the back passage is closely related to the base of the bladder and the prostate gland. There may also be a fever and a general feeling of being unwell.

Any adult male who experiences dysuria (discomfort or pain on passing urine) should have a rectal examination to exclude prostatitis. Urine should be sent to the laboratory for identification of the infecting germ/pathogen and the correct antibiotic identified. Ideally, about two weeks after the course of antibiotics is completed a second sample of urine should be sent to confirm that the bacteria have been eradicated.

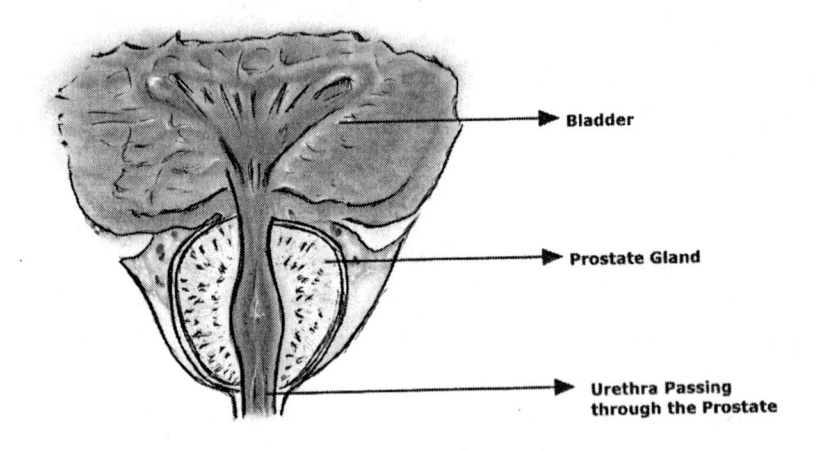

THE PROSTATE

Every male after age 50 should have a rectal examination of the prostate gland and PSA levels checked annually to exclude cancer.

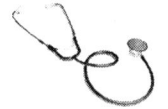

THE SHOULDER JOINT

The wide range of movements performed at this joint and the absence of weight bearing has both advantages and disadvantages over other joints. This versatility has no doubt been acquired through evolution as man became biped (walking on two legs) and used the hands and arms for more and more sophisticated and complex movements and manouvres. These may not have been possible if the upper limbs were being used solely for locomotion.

The price one pays for this ease and diversity of movement is the number of muscles one can injure and these are lumped together as the 'rotator cuff' muscles. Injury to one or more of these muscles is called 'rotator cuff syndrome'. This may come on suddenly, after a bout of unaccustomed activity such as: –

- Sawing or chopping wood,
- Using a hammer,
- Digging in the garden,
- Painting walls – especially ceilings
- Cleaning windows

A few days of rest (not using the shoulder) with the addition of an anti-inflammatory drug may be tried, provided there are no contraindications to the use of the drug e.g.

- History of ulcers in the stomach
- Kidney disorders
- Allergies to them

If the pain has not resolved after a week a doctor should be consulted.

An injection containing a steroid and local anaesthetic may be given into the shoulder joint if the underlying cause is 'bursitis' (inflammation of a pad /cushion within the joint). Relief often occurs within 24 to 48 hours. Sometimes the pain may worsen before it starts to improve! This is not unusual as the steroid acts as a foreign irritant to the joint. However, if the pain does not settle the doctor needs to be seen.

If a temperature develops after any injection into a joint the possibility of an infection introduced at the time of the injection must always be considered.

If the shoulder joint should become gradually painful over weeks (and sometimes ignored for months!) it may be necessary to have the joint X-rayed. While the shoulder joint is not prone to osteoarthritis this investigation may look for this and calcium deposits in tendons within the joint. If the response to the steroid injection is inadequate it may be repeated, up to a total of about three in a year, at intervals of a month or so.

In addition, physiotherapy and NSAIDs (non-steroidal anti-inflammatory drugs) may be prescribed. If these measures fail an orthopaedic surgeon may request an MRI Scan (magnetic resonance imaging which is a highly sophisticated X-ray) to identify the problem. If surgery becomes necessary this may be performed through an arthroscope (lighted tube) introduced into the joint through a small incision. Structures within the joint can be visualised through this instrument. Such an approach to surgery is less invasive (less cutting) and the recovery period and complications are reduced compared to open surgery.

Peculiar to the shoulder joint is the capsule surrounding it – every joint has one. It is very loose/ lax at the under-surface of the joint (in the armpit) and if the movements of the shoulder are restricted because of pain the capsule make become 'stiff'. If allowed to continue 'immobilised' the joint may eventually feel as though it has been set in concrete. At such an advanced stage hardly any movement of the shoulder may be possible.

Simple chores like dressing, brushing or washing the hair, reaching for shelves above shoulder level may become difficult or impossible. This is a physiotherapist's nightmare because of the months and months of treatment required to break down the adhesions (concrete!) within the capsule. The 'frozen shoulder' may be avoided by preventing the arm from being immobilised at the side of the chest wall. The assistance of the physiotherapist should be sought early.

Any pain occurring in the shoulder after a fall needs an X-ray to exclude a fracture or dislocation. If these are suspected expose the shoulders and sit in front of a mirror: both shoulders should be symmetrical – the gentle roundness of the joints as the curve leaves the side of the neck and drops onto the upper arm should be maintained. If the rounded appearance is not the same on both sides something is amiss.

A crackling sound when the joint (any) is moved generates much anxiety but has no worrying significance.

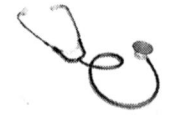

THE TESTICLES

The testicles (testes) are the two (aptly described) 'balls' that hang between the legs. Only males have them and their function is to produce sperm.

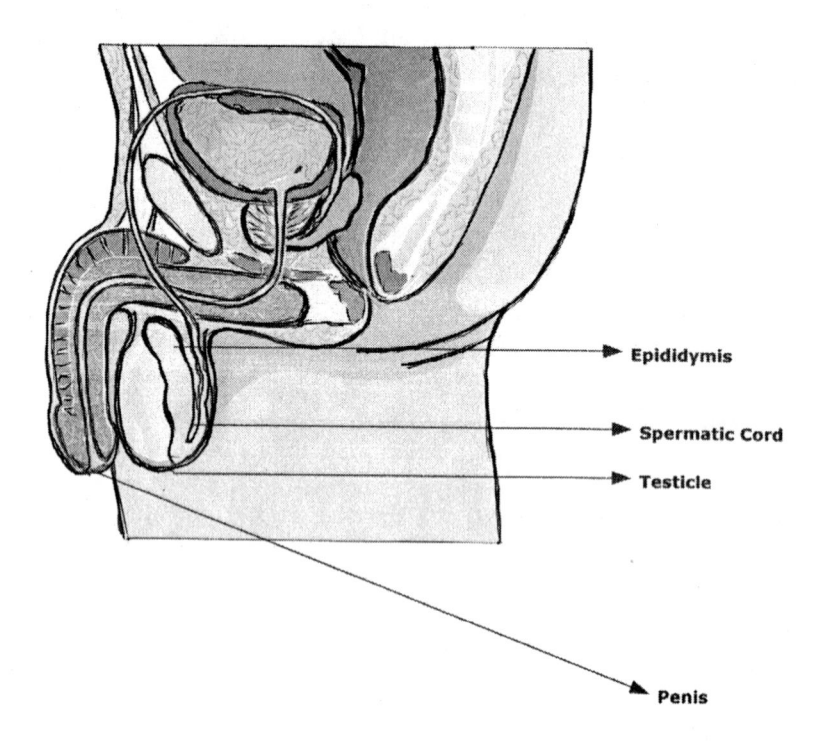

MALE REPRODUCTIVE SYSTEM

When they first develop in the foetus they are situated within the abdomen close to the kidneys, one on either side. As the foetus grows they 'descend' from that position down to the groin and then through a ready-made opening in the lower abdominal wall to lie in the testicular sac (scrotum). Sometimes one or both testicles may not come down completely if the descent is obstructed for any reason and they could remain within the abdomen.

In a child the testicles may move up into the groin and even 'disappear' at times and, when not easily visible, cause concern to the parents. It is not unusual for it to do this but by the age of 5 or 6 years they should remain permanently within the scrotum. If this has not happened by that age they will need to be brought down and stitched to the scrotum to keep it in place. This is a minor procedure requiring the services of a surgeon.

If this is not done timeously there is a risk of permanent damage to the testicle and possible sterility later in life. In an adult a testicle that remains within the abdomen has a risk of becoming cancerous.

The reason the testicles are housed outside the body is that heat (body heat) can damage sperm. To achieve good quality and numbers of sperm avoid hot baths as these would be the equivalent of literally 'boiling' the testicles in the tub – showering is safer. Other practices that may also damage sperm are: –

- tight underpants
- thigh-hugging jeans
- skin-tight cycling pants ('Lycra')
- wearing underwear to bed - young children should not be encouraged to wear underwear at all. The testicles are still developing (they do not make sperm until they reach puberty) and the heat generated from constricting 'Jockey-style' underwear may well be contributing to the higher incidence of infertility
- 'Boxer-style' underwear is less constricting and therefore safer
- working with a 'lap-top' computer on the thighs (and over the testicles) generates significant heat from the machine

- using an electric blanket in bed
- Shaving pubic hair - Nature intended this hair to act as a cushion to protect the organs from injury, prevent direct contact with the legs, and avoid sweat and heat conducted from the adjacent thighs and ambient temperature.

The message is clear - *do not expose the testicles to heat.*

The testicles are very sensitive to pain and, given their exposed position outside the body, trauma of any kind may produce such excruciating agony as to render the victim 'paralysed'. This could be an important Achilles' heel in a life-threatening situation. Confronted by an assailant from the front – take one step to the left of the person to position the right foot between theattacker's legs and bringing the right knee upwards into his groin with great force will strike the testicles and perhaps save one's life.

To this end every female should be taught the skills of self defence and this subject should be made compulsory at school level. As long as there are men about women may not be safe from physical harm. The namby-pamby physical education dished out as a tokenism by so many school curriculae could be put to better use in equipping women. Let the men know that women have been trained to protect themselves and wear an identification badge 'advertising' the skill – just as homes have signs claiming which security company is protecting their property! Some homes have only the sign as a deterrent!

On a different note, women tend to underestimate the very low threshold for pain in the testicles – a point worth remembering during foreplay and body massage.

Any swelling in the testicle – painful or not – warrants a fairly urgent medical opinion; in a young man it may be due to a type of cancer that occurs peculiarly to this age group. One way to examine the testicle is to form a ring around the organ with the thumb and index finger of the left hand at the root of the scrotum (from where it starts to hang). Gently squeezing on the skin (not the testicle!) the organ can be made more prominent and a swelling made more visible. The right hand is used to identify a swelling different from the otherwise normally smooth surface of the testicle.

Pain and swelling that occur at the back of the testicle maybe due to an infection or inflammation in the epididymis – the first part of the tube that carries sperm from the testicle to the storage sacs (one on either side) that lie beneath the prostate gland. The testicles do not store sperm – they produce them only.

At the time of ejaculation sperm does not come from the testicle but from this sac called the seminal vesicles where they remain until the moment of ejaculation. Secretions added to the sperm in these vesicles provide nutrients while they are in storage; not all of the ejaculation fluid is made up of sperm.

Such an infection of the epididymis may occur without the cause being a sexually transmitted disease (STD) but would, nevertheless, require an antibiotic. The symptoms may mimic those of a bladder infection (i.e. burning on passing urine and passing it more frequently than normal).

Any injury to the testicle followed by pain and swelling should be seen *immediately* by a doctor to exclude a bleed into the organ (haematoma). Pain and swelling that occurs in one testicle following a sudden severe strain, like lifting a heavy weight causing the testicle to twist itself around its 'stalk' (where it is attached to the groin), may compromise its blood supply from vessels that run through the stalk. This is also an emergency; the longer the blood supply is endangered greater is the chance that the testicle may be permanently damaged and, perhaps, lost to surgery.

A single testicle is quite capable of maintaining libido (desire for sex) and fertility – other things being normal e.g. the number and quality of sperm.

A swelling in the scrotum (skin around the testicle) is usually due to accumulation of fluid within the scrotal sac (called a hydrocele). This is not a serious problem as the fluid is harmless, but if the swelling becomes uncomfortably large the hydrocele may need to be drained (with a needle – under local anaesthetic – this is a minor procedure) or a small operation performed to remove the lining of the scrotum that is responsible for making the extra fluid. This does not involve the testicle and will not affect one's sex life. There is little need to put up (sometimes for years!) with a watermelon hanging between the legs simply because of the embarrassment of being examined *down there* or an irrational fear of what is involved in its treatment!

Cyclists are at special risk for traumatising the testicles and epididymis (situated at the bottom and behind the testicles) as they make constant contact with the hard bicycle seat. This becomes more of an issue if the front tapered end of the seat is elevated – making even closer contact with the genitalia. This is independent of the risk posed by the skin-tight apparel that has become fashionable with sports enthusiasts; the heat generated by the exercise is retained between the legs and the testicles. Heat and sperm are unwelcome bedfellows.

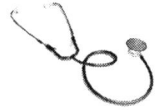

THE THYROID GLAND

The thyroid gland is situated in the lower part of the front of the neck and has the outline of a 'butterfly' in that it has one lobe (wing) on either side of the windpipe (trachea) and a central part that connects the two. If the gland is enlarged (called a goitre) it may become visible as a swelling and moves up and down with swallowing. If it is very big the appearance may be 'unsightly' - justifying removal for cosmetic reasons; goitres are more common in females.

If women can be taught and encouraged to examine their breasts it should not be that difficult to teach them *and men* to feel around the fronts of their necks. With some practice swellings of the thyroid gland can be detected at home. When the gland is not enlarged (i.e. normal) one may not be able to identify it with the fingers.

Firstly, look in the mirror to identify a swelling that moves up and down the neck on swallowing (drink some water). This is discounting the 'Adam's Apple' that also moves with swallowing.

Still in front of the mirror place the middle three fingers together so the tips are in a straight line and slightly bent. Feel on either side, in the narrow groove between the windpipe (trachea) and the muscle, at the lower end of the neck. If no swelling is noted then swallow, with the fingers held in the same position. If a swelling is detected that moves up and down with the motion of swallowing this should be mentioned to the doctor. An ultrasound examination may be necessary and some blood samples taken to test whether the gland is functioning normally.

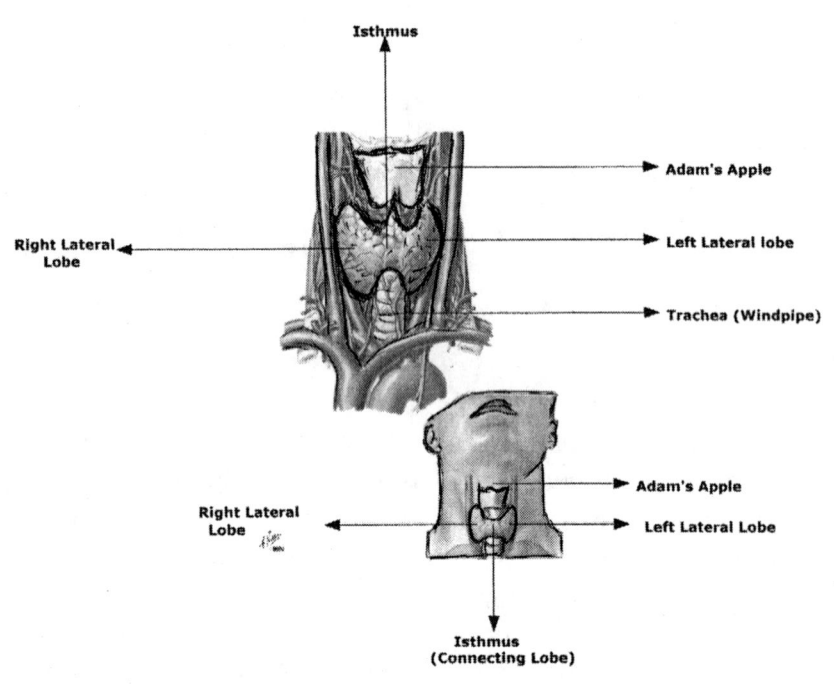

THE THYROID GLAND

Examination of the thyroid gland should be a mandatory part of any doctor's general assessment of a patient. A very small percentage of such swellings (nodules) in the thyroid gland can become malignant.

The hormone produced by the thyroid gland is called thyroxine. Its function may be compared to petrol in a motor car: more petrol and it moves faster, less and the car tends to slow down. How fast or slowly the body functions depends on how much of the hormone this gland makes; too much and the condition is called *hyper*thyroidism, too little – *hypo*thyroidism.

Hyperthyroidism is manifested by a constant feeling of hunger where, after a fair sized meal, the person is ready to eat again – because thyroxine burns up calories. It's like a car that is on the move twenty-four hours a day. This hormone was once used for weight reduction but is no longer advocated because of its possible ill-effects on the heart. Note the weight loss occurs *in spite of the increased food intake.*

Diabetes occurring in a young person who has no insulin (called an insulin dependent diabetic) will also result in weight loss in spite of a good appetite but, in addition, large quantities of urine will be passed and the person will be constantly thirsty.

If the thyroid gland is hyperactive there will be excessive sweating and palpitations i.e. a fast heart rate. The latter maybe regular, i.e. beating rapidly but with a regular rhythm, or irregular where the hearts beats fast and slow in a haphazard manner.

The pulse rate can be measured by using the three middle fingers of the *right* hand (as for feeling the thyroid gland in the neck) placed one behind the other (not side by side) at the *left* wrist just behind the base of the thumb. If one is left handed switch hands. This locates the position of the radial artery. Use the second hand of a watch to count the pulsations in one minute. The normal pulse rate i.e. the number of times the heart beats is about 60 to 80 per minute; persistently more than 100 or less than 60 per minute may be cause for concern. Best time to count is just before nodding off to sleep when the body is most relaxed.

In a hyperthyroid state there may also be a fine tremor (shaking) of the hands – best seen by placing a sheet of paper across the back of the outstretched hands and watching it quiver. Hair loss and menstrual periods that become irregular, and often heavier than usual, may also be noted.

In a certain form of hyperactive thyroid called Graves' disease the eyeballs may become very prominent and appear to be popping out of their sockets. In another condition the gland becomes painful and swollen within a matter of days and the unsuspecting may diagnose a 'sore throat' whereas closer questioning and examination should reveal the pain is *outside* the throat not 'inside' – as occurs in tonsillitis. This condition is called thyroiditis. It usually presents acutely (suddenly) with a feeling of being unwell and feverishness whereas with the other common thyroid problems symptoms appear after weeks or even months.

A hyperactive thyroid left untreated may affect the heart with a fast and often irregular heart beat (called atrial fibrillation) – wearing out the engine with the constant acceleration! This could lead to heart failure or angina (chest pain) - if one is predisposed to the latter.

If the gland is *hypoactive* everything tends to slow down – no petrol! The basal metabolic rate (BMR) slows down accordingly and food that is consumed is not utilised and therefore stored. The result is weight gain – the opposite of what happens with a hyperactive thyroid.

With the lowered BMR cold weather becomes intolerable and the patient wears a jersey in warm weather (cold intolerance), the skin and hair become dry and hair ends tend to split. Left untreated the features of the face become coarse and the heart rate slows down to below 60 beats per minute. The heart may become enlarged and fluid may accumulate around it in the lining (called the pericardium) that surrounds the heart. This is similar to placing the heart within a water filled balloon – making it difficult for the heart to function as a pump. To a large extent these changes are reversible provided the diagnosis is made early and treatment started.

Mental changes occurring in a hypofunctioning thyroid may mimic many of those that occur normally in the elderly – such as forgetfulness and depression. Residents of old age homes should have their thyroid functions routinely checked. All too often these changes are passed off as part of growing old and, furthermore, these may occur subtly over a period of months. The diagnosis should first be considered and then a simple blood test would confirm it. Hypothyroidism and depression may coexist.

Treatment of an underfunctioning thyroid is replacement of the missing hormone in the form of one or two tablets a day – to bring back to life one so easily relegated to the old age heap! A seemingly tired old engine brought back to a new spark within days.

Hyperthyroidism, on the other hand, has everything working at an accelerated pace and is treated initially with medication to slow down the pulse rate to protect the heart and an ' anti-thyroid' drug to bring down the level of this hormone in the blood.

If this has to be used in the long term it is safer and easier to ablate or 'put the gland to sleep' permanently with radioactive iodine. This is quite safe to use and the purpose, as mentioned above, is to medically' destroy' the gland and, thereafter, to replace the 'missing' hormone that the thyroid once made (in overabundance!). How much is required will be determined by blood tests to measure the thyroxine levels - this should be done at least once year.

It is easier to control an underfunctioning thyroid gland than one that is hyperactive. Treatment is usually life-long.

Radioactive iodine is not used if the family is not complete and children are planned, and definitely not before or during a pregnancy. Radioactivity is harmful to the foetus even though the mother would not be affected as the radiation dose is very small.

If a nodule or swelling in the thyroid gland is detected on ultrasound examination to be a cyst (containing fluid) it may be aspirated with a needle or left untreated as this does not become malignant. However, if the nodule is found to be solid it should be removed - as a small percentage of them can become cancerous.

A sensation of discomfort in the throat, difficulty in swallowing food or an unexplained cough that persists for longer than two to three weeks requires a medical opinion. The cause may be that the thyroid gland is enlarging backwards putting pressure upon the windpipe or gullet but other, more worrying, causes like cancer of the throat need to be excluded. A second or third course of antibiotics should not be the order of the day!

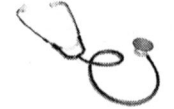

THE PENIS

Circumcision is no longer 'fashionable', neither is it still considered a preventative measure against cancer of the penis. However, religious reasons may prevail.

If the foreskin is too tight (phimosis) and cannot be retracted easily to completely expose the glans (top or head of the organ) this can make cleaning under the foreskin difficult and intercourse awkward. There is also the risk that if it should forcibly be retracted it may not be easy to bring it forward again and, left in this position, will cause the tight band of foreskin to swell and painfully constrict the penis. This will require urgent medical attention. This can happen in children curiously exploring their bodies or during masturbation or sexual intercourse. Being aware of this condition (paraphimosis) and simply pulling the skin back over the glans early will avoid an unnecessary visit to the local emergency unit. However, it will require circumcision at some stage – before it happens again!

Diabetics, who are more prone to infections, should preferably be circumcised. Thrush can lurk and thrive in the warm recesses of the foreskin and the added sugar in the urine will provide nutrition for the yeast (thrush) to flourish.

Premature ejaculation (releasing sperm prematurely) may be given a helping hand if the extra sensitivity of the glans can be reduced. With increased exposure after circumcision the glans becomes 'tougher' as it is no longer protected by the foreskin. This is akin to never going barefoot in the park and attempting this with tender pink feet that have never seen the light of day - let alone the pebbles and stones that will stab at the soles! Sexual prowess is also enhanced after circumcision as the duration of foreplay may be prolonged. Wearing two condoms will have the same effect and this could be a further useful manoeuvre in controlling premature ejaculation. The second condom can be removed at the appropriate moment once its purpose has been served.

Another technique to overcome premature ejaculation is to be seated on the bed or floor and have the female partner sitting behind (the pillion rider on a motorcycle). The man is masturbated until he signals that he is about to ejaculate. The penis is grasped just behind the glans by encircling the organ with the thumb and index finger and gentle but firm pressure applied to the penis to cool things down. Once the urge to ejaculate has subsided masturbation is again started and the procedure repeated until the technique is grasped. During intercourse the man himself can do the squeezing as he will be the best judge of how close he is to ejaculation.

Thinking of the tax man to stave off ejaculation by distracting the 'brain' should be reserved for when more experience has been gained. It carries with it a risk of detracting too much from the matter at hand and backfiring on the pleasure. The tax man may have far-reaching powers!

Circumcision in infancy is usually done without an anaesthetic because the nerve supply to the penis is considered not well developed. Listening to the infant scream in agony is proof enough of how adults abuse children because the latter are believed to have no feelings.

In an older person circumcision can be done under a local or general anaesthetic. Pain after the procedure can be controlled with analgesics. The secret, however, is not to have an erection after the procedure – bearing in mind that the glans will be exposed to the dressing around it and this will stimulate it no end. To avoid this one should be adequately 'sedated' until wound healing is well on its way. Fortunately, this happens fairly quickly (within about three days) as the penis has a very rich blood supply. Initially, contact with underwear will produce frequent and, at inopportune moments, embarrassing erections but these usually subside as the glans quickly becomes desensitised.

The skin over the shaft of the penis and the foreskin (uncircumcised) are at risk of being caught in trouser zips – a point the opposite sex should be aware of. Nothing will dampen the ardour as quickly as an unexpected trip to the emergency unit of the nearest hospital. 'Fractures' of the penis are not uncommon during intercourse and are more prone to occur when the female is on top and her thrusting movements are unchecked. Indulging in fellatio (oral intercourse) in a moving vehicle is more hazardous than using a mobile phone and should be included in the list of things not to do while driving.

A discharge from the penis requires urgent diagnosis. Not every discharge may be due to gonorrhoea (sexually transmitted disease);nevertheless, its presence requires laboratory identification - with a swab sent for culture and sensitivity (to identify the bacteria and the appropriate antibiotic). Sexual activities should be suspended until the cause of the discharge has been established and, if necessary, treated. The other partner should be similarly investigated and treated as required. Infection is usually accompanied by a burning sensation on passing urine and there may be frequency (passing urine very often even though the quantity of urine may be a few drops at a time). These are also the symptoms of a bladder infection (cystitis). It should be noted by both sexes that a female may harbour an infection in the vagina without her having any symptoms to warn her that it exists and, accordingly, prevent its spread to an unsuspecting partner. The spread of HIV infection has this disadvantage thwarting attempts to curb its spread – partners may not be aware they are infective. The same applies to any of the other sexually transmitted diseases – herpes, gonorrhoea, syphilis and chlamydia.

Painful, small, red, pimple-like lesions on the penis (anywhere on it) are most likely due to herpes. Early medical attention should be sought as the antibiotic 'Zovirax' is more effective when used as soon as the lesions appear. The main symptom is burning pain.

The anus and vagina should never be used interchangeably during intercourse as it carries the risk of transmitting bacterial infections from the rectum (where they live normally), hepatitis and HIV.

Intercourse from behind, with the female on all fours, also carries a risk of transmitting infection as the penis can make contact with the anal area. It helps to wash the anal area thoroughly in anticipation of this position – it is the female who is mainly at risk of a bladder infection.

To avoid a similar risk it is safer for the female partner (missionary position – with the female on her back and the male on top) to guide the penis into the vagina - as a 'blind' attempt at entry by the male partner may accidentally make contact with the wrong orifice resulting in contamination of both the penis and the vagina.

Anal intercourse must make the use of a condom and plenty of lubrication mandatory as the lining of the anus is not designed for this purpose and is, therefore, drier than the vagina. Small tears may occur in the anus that can lead to minor bleeding, infection and discomfort. The pain/discomfort in anal intercourse stems from ignorance about how the anal sphincter (valve) functions: the anus can be made to stretch to accommodate a whole adult hand provided it is done very gently (slowly). Introducing a well-greased (preferably gloved) finger into the rectum and holding it in position for two to three minutes will 'loosen' the grip and allow the anus to relax. This happens naturally when the valve has to allow a large piece of firm or hard stool to pass through. The capacity for it to stretch is realised when faecal impaction occurs from long standing constipation and the only way to evacuate the rectum is by introducing the (gloved and greased) hand into the rectum to remove the hard stools. The alternative is to perform the evacuation in theatre under a general anaesthetic!

In the interest of safe sex and the prevention of sexually transmitted diseases, including HIV, condoms are advised to be put on from the moment foreplay begins and *before* any contact is made with the genitalia (private parts) as this poses a risk for both partners.

Oral intercourse (fellatio) also carries the risk of getting or giving an STD. A condom may prevent this and also avoid the ejaculate from 'entering' the mouth – if this should be objectionable to the recipient. There is a risk the teeth could damage the latex.

Introducing the penis in the flaccid state (non-erect/ limp) into rings and other non-yielding orifices or objects in the pursuit of sexual pleasure or experimentation carries with it a risk of serious injury should the penis become engorged and inextricable.

Impotence (penis not erect enough for successful intercourse) can be one of the most devastating disabilities that can beset a man – and a woman. The importance of sex and how the penis functions is often underestimated and ill-understood by both men and women – mainly out of ignorance. Sex is one of the two reasons why the human race and every living being exist. While nature intended for it to be used for procreation - to this basic instinct man has added eroticism and the pursuit of pleasure. Many cultures revere the penis for the important role it plays as an instrument of survival and preservation of the species; small wonder that it should occupy such a prominent position in man's thoughts and actions.

For the penis to become erect blood must first enter the organ and be trapped within it to give it firmness: if blood cannot enter the penis an erection is not possible. The entry of blood can be reduced partially or completely if the artery to the penis is narrowed by hypertension (high blood pressure), diabetes or smoking or all three. These conditions narrow the lumen/diameter of arteries throughout the body (coronary arteries – causing heart attacks, cerebral arteries – leading to strokes, renal arteries – resulting in kidney failure) and the penis is no exception. Perhaps cigarette containers and advertisements should add 'Loss of manhood' and 'gangrene and amputations' to the list of evils that cigarette, cigar, pipe and second-hand smoking causes.

The brain (erotic stimulation) cannot produce an erection without engorgement of blood within the penis. A full bladder on waking can precipitate an erection. An erection may also occur if one is wearing tight pants (jeans) without underwear or while riding a bicycle. If the penis can become erect in this or any other manner (reading, watching erotic material or having successful intercourse outside an impotent relationship) this is proof the organ is functioning normally - and that the cause of the impotence is psychological.

Insufficient production of testosterone (the 'sex hormone') by the body will result in impotence. But prescribing testosterone without first checking the blood levels is a waste of time, expectations and money. It is not a common deficiency but, if proven, will respond to replacement therapy.

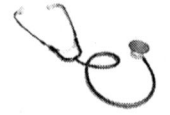

THE THERMOMETER / FEVER

No home should be without a thermometer.

In these days of automation recording the temperature can be done by applying a heat sensitive strip to the forehead. The digital thermometers are more expensive and, often, the battery costs more than the instrument. Then there are the sophisticated ones used in hospitals that record the temperature by placing a probe in the ear canal. These are accurate and give the result within seconds and have the added advantage of disposable ear pieces that eliminate the risk of cross infection between patients. It is impractical for home use.

The old fashioned mercury thermometers while inexpensive have the disadvantages of glass – its risk of injury if bitten and fragility when being shaken down to get the mercury into the bulb. Many a glass thermometer has met an untimely end on the floor before it reached the mouth. They carry the same risk of exchanging bacteria and viruses as the oral digital thermometers. They are not easy to read as the mercury forms a thin silver line that requires a fair bit of swivelling between thumb and index finger to find the upper level. They also have to be sterilised before they may be used again and in today's infective climate this would be unacceptable.

Whatever method is used to check the temperature any level above 37 degrees centigrade constitutes a *fever*.

Whose temperature should be taken? Any person – man, woman or child of any age who in any way feels 'different' from his or her 'normal' self must, as a matter of routine, have the temperature taken and recorded for immediate and future reference. Every patient who is examined by a doctor should ideally have his or her temperature taken at every visit – irrespective of the complaint.

The following symptoms make it necessary to check the temperature.

- headache
- muscle pains
- joint pain
- chest or abdominal pain – any pain in *any* part of the body
- cough
- diarrhoea (watery stools),
- vaginal discharge
- passing urine frequently or a burning sensation on passing it
- confusion, lightheadedness/dizziness,
- not eating and drinking normally
- just a vague feeling of being out-of-sorts

For all *practical* purposes any person with a temperature above 37 degrees centigrade may have an infection somewhere until proven otherwise.

Touching the forehead or any other part of the body and with a learned look pronouncing "Yay" or "Nay" a fever is not acceptable. While it may be easy to do this and be correct when the temperature is very high it is almost impossible to predict when it is only slightly elevated (37.3 or 37.5 degrees centigrade). Such a level would be abnormal and an explanation should be sought.

A temperature of 37.3 degrees centigrade may not be very high at that moment but has the potential to rise at any time – and within 30 minutes become 38 or 39 degrees centigrade. The simple effort of getting to school or work with a fever will drain the person physically and set the recovery process back a few steps.

What does an elevated temperature mean? The problem is no longer 'localised': a runny nose is a local problem involving the lining of the nostrils. However, if an elevated temperature accompanies this then the infection has spread into the body. In order for the temperature to be elevated the infection must trigger a temperature-regulating sensor in the brain - paracetamol and other drugs (antipyretics) that relieve high fevers work by acting on this temperature-regulating centre.

An additional measure to bring down a temperature fairly quickly and easily and without the use of medication is to use a small towel/ face cloth soaked in *warm* water. Wring out the water and swab the face, neck and upper chest and gently blow on the infant or use a newspaper or electric fan to cool the body down. This is a lot more comfortable (and humane!) than near-drowning an ill, and often screaming child, in an icy bath of cold water! The latter is also messy and more time consuming.

Beware the non-steroidal anti-inflammatory drugs advertised for pain and fever. They have the potential for causing problems in the stomach and kidneys. They should not be taken without food – the patient with a fever is unlikely to be eating. Furthermore, these drugs are excreted by the kidneys and therefore rely on an adequate intake of fluid. However, fever, nausea, vomiting and a reluctance to drink will militate against the proper function of the kidneys and increase their risk of damage by these drugs.

An ice cube wrapped in a cloth and placed for a few minutes at a time over the wrist or on the side of the neck, where the arteries are quite close to the skin, is also a simple and effective way to cool down the blood. This 'cooled' blood from the wrist or neck reaches the heart and the brain within seconds. During a fever the heart beats much faster than normal – up to a 120 times in each sixty seconds. This means that within one minute the cooled blood has been carried to the centre for temperature control in the brain 120 times!

Rubbing an ice cube or applying a cold compress to the wrist will do wonders on a hot day! Holding the wrists under a trickle of cold tap water would have the same benefit except that precious water will be wasted down the drain! The radiator in a car plays a similar role in cooling the engine.

If the patient has been vomiting and therefore cannot keep anything in the stomach (medication included) a simple alternative is to use a suppository form of antipyretic and / antiemetic (stop vomiting). Carefully remove the plastic cover surrounding the torpedo-shaped preparation, as it can crumble easily, and introduce it into the rectum.

Many patients of any age are often abhorred by the very idea of a 'foreign' thing being inserted into their backsides: however, it beats getting a rather painful injection.

A suppository takes about 30 minutes to begin working as the rectum is very richly supplied with blood vessels and this makes for rapid absorption of the medication into the body. The procedure is quite safe and no harm will come to the back passage. Smearing a small dab of Vaseline to the opening of the passage will facilitate its entry. Gripping the suppository through a piece of 'cling wrap' will avoid contact with the anal area. The patient should be lying on his or her left side and the upper buttock pulled upwards with one's left hand to expose the anus.

It is important to identify precisely the level of the temperature for two reasons:

a)   If the level approaches 40 degrees centigrade there is a risk of developing a convulsion (seizure), prompting the need to have a lumbar puncture to exclude meningitis (infection of the lining that covers the brain and spinal cord). Better management of the temperature may avoid the procedure. Such a 'febrile (fever) convulsion' may pose a small risk of developing seizures in later life.

b)   The temperature can be recorded at intervals just as is done in hospital and the patient's progress made easier to assess. An accurately recorded temperature chart is of greater value in assessing an illness than the story of a fever determined by placing a hand on the patient's forehead! If this were useful doctors would not need thermometers! After all, their hands have had much more experience!

As mentioned above – and stressed again – no child or student should be sent (forced!) to go to school if the thermometer shows a fever. The same applies to a working person. A person with a fever is unlikely to be faking an illness thereby making the thermometer a more accurate way of ascertaining whether the child/adult should be kept at home.

Any person with an elevated temperature (and that means any level above 37 degrees centigrade) should not be going on a picnic or camp or taking part in any physical exercise regardless of how-ever many months went into the planning or training. Just as there are checks for drugs no athlete should be allowed to participate in any sporting event if their temperatures, taken as a matter of routine, are shown to be above 37 degrees centigrade. This may save unnec-essary sudden deaths in athletes who have trained hard and long and refuse to be denied their moment of glory because of a 'niggling temperature'!

It may be the only clue to a viral infection and there may be no warning symptoms that the virus has affected the heart muscle. Putting the heart through the stress of a marathon is begging for the death penalty. The macho athlete could become the next case on the coroner's autopsy list.

Any person with a fever should be considered medically unfit to operate machinery or drive a motor vehicle – as would have hap-pened had they been drunk!

It should cause no consternation for the temperature level to be requested after an accident enquiry. Do airline pilots have their tem-peratures taken before each flight? Do they have their alcohol lev-els checked before each and every time they take off with the lives of their passengers in their hands? Do long distance truck drivers do this? Do police manning roadblocks check the temperatures of motorists as they do their breaths? Are surgeons checking their own temperatures before they embark on delicate procedures? – A preop-erative surgeon's temperature of 37.3 degrees centigrade could, dur-ing a lengthy operation, become 38 to 40 degrees centigrade! And he or she may imagine the sweating to be due to the difficult case on the table! Such a fever is bound to impair performance.

What could an elevated temperature do to a person? Depending on the level it can vary from a feeling of weakness of the legs, to dizzi-ness, hot and cold shivers (rigors), outright delirium and convulsions.

Temperatures persistently above 43 degrees centigrade are incompatible with life.

During the shivering phase of a fever clothing and blankets should be allowed but once this has subsided (the shaking eases off) most of the clothing, save for underwear, should be removed. Crushed ice may be given to suck upon. Fruit juice, with extra sugar added, can be frozen and then crushed – this would provide much needed calories that are being utilized during the intense bouts of shivering (muscular activity) and also help to lower the temperature.

An effective way to warm up during the rigor (shivering phase) is to stand under a hot shower with the water temperature high enough to be comfortable; a bathtub is less effective because it will not stay constant and cools down fairly quickly. Avoiding the bath tub also saves precious water. Blankets may not be that effective because they do not generate any *additional* heat of their own.

Fever is a defence mechanism whereby the brain, in response to the presence of an intruder in the blood i.e. bacteria , viruses, or certain drugs, sets the 'thermostat' in the temperature-regulating centre at a higher level – similar to the thermostat in a hot water geyser.

Though infection is the main cause of a fever there are others viz.

tumours, inflammatory conditions like gout and other forms of arthritis, drugs as are used in psychiatry and certain forms of strokes may also account for a high temperature.

If a couple wish to ascertain the optimal time in the menstrual cycle to engage in fruitful sexual intercourse recording the woman's daily early morning temperature (while still in bed) can be a guide. Very small but definite elevations may identify the stage when an egg is released from the ovary. By the same observation absence of the temperature elevation at the expected time in the menstrual cycle may imply that the ovary is not shedding the expected egg. This could help identify a reason for an inability to fall pregnant.

Any person with a fever presenting to the doctor should not fail to disclose whether he or she has recently been out of the province or the country even if this information is not requested. Malaria may present just like any other flu-like illness but the diagnosis must first be suspected before the appropriate blood tests to confirm it can be ordered. This could make the difference between life and death! Contact with another ill person may also be relevant. It is not unusual to develop a slight to moderate fever after a vaccination.

Infections like AIDS and other Sexually Transmitted Diseases can only be diagnosed if the history of exposure has been disclosed, as the appropriate blood tests would not ordinarily be requested. A painful, swollen knee joint (any joint) after a history of unprotected intercourse (with an infected partner) may be due to *gonorrhoea* and not *gout!* The former is a sexually transmitted disease and urgently requires antibiotics.

Heat stroke is not common but should be treated as a medical emergency. It usually follows strenuous physical exertion in hot weather conditions or excessive exposure to heat. Factors that make it likely to happen include:- old age, heart disease, alcoholism, recent illness, (especially gastroenteritis) and a generally debilitated state. The underlying problem in this condition is the inability of the body to take the necessary steps to protect itself in the presence of excessive external heat. This is manifested by *high fever and the absence of sweating.* The person may have headache, dizziness, nausea, confusion and convulsions and may end up in a coma. Immediate treatment is aimed at measures to bring down the temperature as quickly as possible while arrangements are being made to get the patient to a hospital.

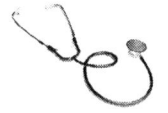

UPPER ABDOMINAL PAIN

The abdomen is the area that lies between the lowest margins of the ribs on either side down to the groin on both sides.

Divide this area into nine equal squares – three across the top, three across the middle (below the top three squares) and three across the bottom (below the middle three squares).

The top right square houses the:

*Right kidney
*Liver
*Gall bladder and
*Part of the large intestine (gut)

The top middle square has the

*Stomach
*Pancreas
*Part of the liver and
*Part of the large intestine

The top left square has the

*Left kidney
*Spleen and
*Part of the large intestine

The middle three squares house the small intestines

The bottom right square has the

*Appendix
*The caecum (beginning of the large intestine)
*Right ovary in a female and the
*Right ureter – the tube that brings urine from the right kidney
to the bladder

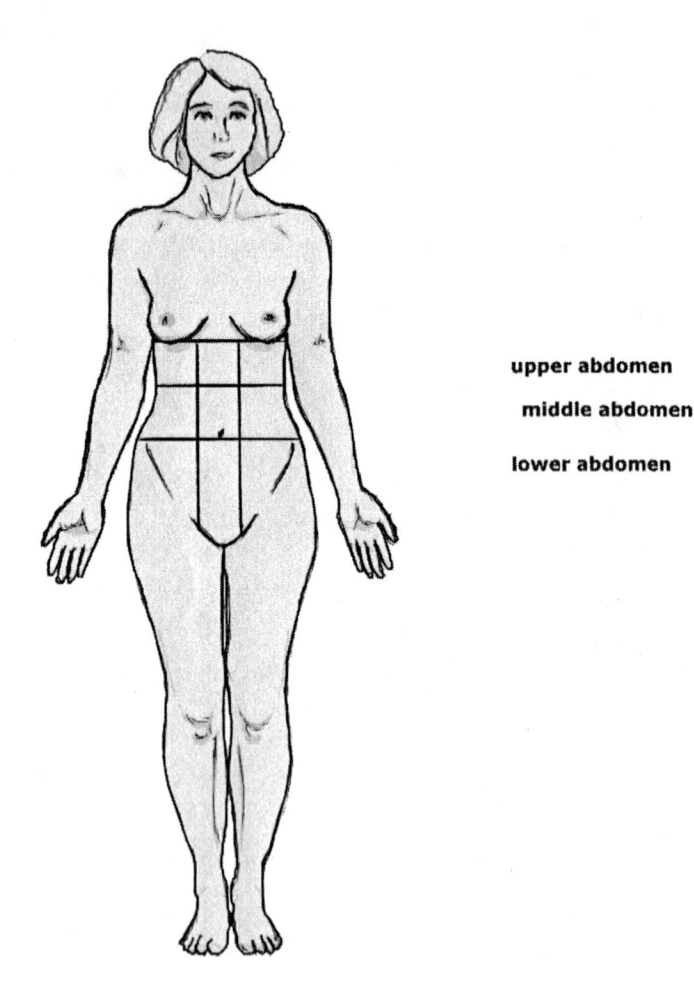

upper abdomen

middle abdomen

lower abdomen

THE NINE QUADRANTS OF THE ABDOMEN

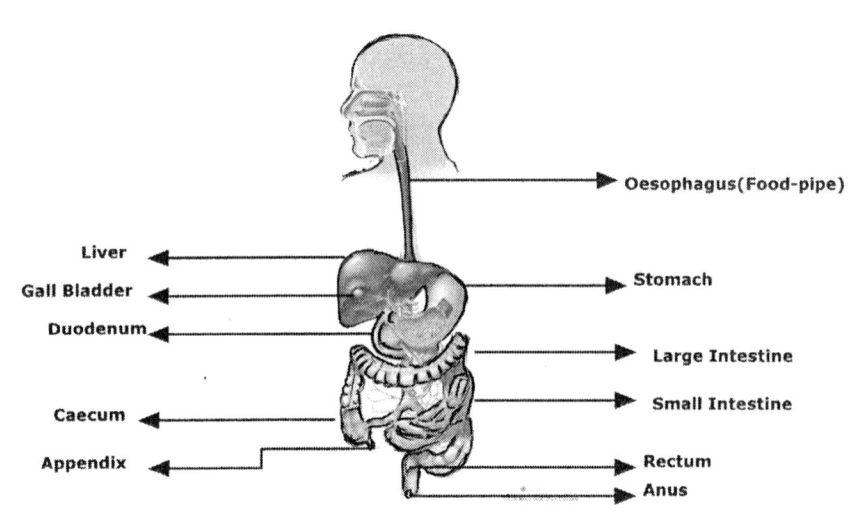

DIGESTIVE ANATOMY

The bottom middle square has the

  *Bladder
  *Uterus in a female

  The bottom left square has the
  *Rectum
  *left ureter as it joins the bladder in the middle square and the
  *left ovary in a female

Nausea as a symptom does not help as it may be caused by a fever, an infection in the stomach, intestine or gall bladder, liver disease, a heart attack, the sight of a bloody car accident or be a side effect of medication.

If nausea is accompanied by a *fever* the most likely culprit is an infection; to determine the source will require additional information.

Pain in the top right square may indicate a problem (infection or stone) in the gall bladder or kidney or abscess in the liver.

The liver makes bile that is carried to the gall bladder through a tube – the bile duct. The gall bladder simply stores the bile until it is required in the gut to digest a fatty meal. If the gall bladder is removed surgically the bile goes directly into the intestine and this new arrangement has no detrimental effects on the patient.

If a gallstone blocks the exit of bile from the gallbladder into the small intestine or a stone blocks the exit of bile from the liver to the gall bladder these obstructions will have serious consequences. The passage of bile may not be impeded under any circumstances. The urine will become dark brown because the excess bile is spilt into the blood and is then carried to the kidneys to appear in the urine. If this blockage is allowed to continue the bile is cut off from the large gut resulting in pale, greyish stools. The excess bile will also appear in the whites (conjunctiva) of the eyes and the skin - making them yellow (jaundiced).

An infection in the liver (hepatitis) usually begins with a few days of feeling unwell, fever and nausea that become progressively worse and may lead to vomiting and the appearance of dark urine and jaundice within five to seven days.

An abscess in the liver may develop more quickly with less nausea but high fevers and increasingly severe pain in the top right square. Pain may also be felt over the tip of the right shoulder. The person with a liver abscess often walks hunched forward - supporting the right side of the abdomen with the right hand. This is to support the liver and prevent gravity from pushing it downward and aggravating the pain. Deep breathing/coughing will also worsen the pain by pushing the diaphragm onto the inflamed liver. Note that pain is not an early sign of hepatitis (see above).

An infection in the kidney (pyelonephritis) may develop within the space of 24 to 48 hours with high fevers and nausea, and there may be vomiting and gradually increasing pain in the right or left upper square (depending on which side is affected – and this almost never does both). The pain characteristically moves down to the groin (or the testicle in a male) on the same side because this organ, in the foetus, lay close to the kidney. During development the testicle on each side travelled down to the respective groin carrying with it the nerve that also supplies the kidney – hence the radiation of pain from the loin to the groin.

Pain from a stone (calculus) in the kidney or the ureter – the tube that connects the kidney to the bladder – starts very suddenly and radiates down to the groin on the same side as the affected kidney as described above. This pain is *distinctive* in that it will not allow the person so afflicted to lie in any one position for long and he or she will toss and turn from one side to another trying to get comfortable. This often gives a clue as to the cause. Pain from a stone is very severe and, invariably, requires an injection for relief.

Early and effective pain relief is stressed as it will save much inconvenience (and suffering) for the patient, the escort/driver and the doctor! Blood in the urine may be visible to the naked eye or it may only be detected by testing the urine at the doctor's rooms. A fever may or may not be present. Nausea and vomiting often accompanies the pain that is matched in severity only by that of a severe heart attack!

If a kidney stone is suspected or there has been a past history of such a stone (and they do recur) pass all urine through an old handkerchief (to act as a strainer) to catch the culprit as the stone could be as small as a grain of sand but have the clout of a horse-kick. This will help prove the diagnosis and identify the type of stone as this information may influence future treatment.

All patients with a suspected kidney stone require an ultrasound (X-ray) examination as soon as possible to identify whether the stone could be obstructing the free flow of urine from the kidney. Such an obstruction can cause the organ to dilate (hydronephrosis) and result in permanent damage and a useless kidney.

An infection or inflammation of the stomach may also be accompanied by nausea and vomiting and a burning pain in the middle of the upper three squares. If this is part of an infection there may be a high temperature. Vomiting may accompany a viral infection (influenza) in children. One, two or three episodes of vomiting within the space of 15 to 30 minutes are usually part of the 'one vomit' – this is an attempt by the body, while it is trying to heal itself, to empty the stomach of its contents. This would allow the inflamed/infected gut to rest and not have to process ingested food.

If a dog is ill from whatever cause it will refuse to eat and neither human nor animal should be forced to eat if either is unwell. In the initial stages of an illness little is lost by simply offering clear fluids in very small quantities +/- 20 ml. at a time at intervals of 10 to 15 minutes to avoid loading the stomach. If this is retained add sugar and some salt to the water (8 teaspoons of sugar and ½ a teaspoon of salt to a litre of boiled water or Fanta - with proportionately less sugar). Ordinary tap water is acceptable – boiling kills bacteria when the quality of the water cannot be guaranteed.

If vomiting persists after the stomach contents have been 'evicted' and small amounts of clear fluids are not retained this requires hospitalisation to prevent dehydration. Beware the very young and the very old as they do not easily tolerate fluid loss from vomiting and / diarrhoea or simply not eating or drinking. The life saving intravenous 'drip' essentially contains sugar, salt and water.

Pain that occurs in the top *middle* square in relation to food i.e. before or after eating may be due to an inflammation in the lining of the stomach (gastritis). Common causes of this are alcohol, aspirin and anti-inflammatory drugs used for arthritis. This inflammation may progress to cause bleeding from the stomach and could lead to the formation of stomach (gastric) ulcers. Stomach ulcers (as different from duodenal ulcers) can become cancerous and require a biopsy and close follow up. It is not the procedure (endoscopy/gastroscopy) that makes the diagnosis but the experience of the person peering down into the stomach.

Pain in the top middle square occurring for the first time in a person past the age of 45 years requires gastroscopy. In this procedure a tube is passed that can visualise the oesophagus (gullet), stomach and the duodenum i.e. first part of the gut after the stomach. A person younger than 45 years experiencing these symptoms for the first time is usually prescribed an antacid to be taken three times daily regularly for about 4 weeks. If the pain disappears the antacids are discontinued and any precipitating or aggravating factors, like alcohol or cigarettes, avoided. If the pain persists or recurs a gastroscopy is recommended – not a prescription for more antacids!

Children often come to medical attention late because mum and/ the doctor think the child is too young to have a peptic ulcer. It is a well-known fact that such an ulcer can also develop within 24 hours of a severely stressful situation such as extensive burns to the skin or a serious motor vehicle accident – these patients are routinely given prophylactic ulcer therapy. The underlying cause of the ulcer in this situation is stress and the outpouring of large doses of adrenaline – the stress hormone.

Pain that wakes a person from sleep needs a doctor's opinion – not 'Jamaica ginger' or 'Rennies'! Beware the pain in the top middle square in a middle-aged or older person who has a normal gastroscope and ultrasound examination (looking for gall stones). Sometimes the lesion (tumour) is lying hidden in the pancreas. This gland lies tucked away below the stomach and adjacent to the duodenum. A CAT Scan is necessary to exclude a cancer – before it is too late! This diagnosis is often missed and should be suspected if the symptoms have been present for several weeks or more and is accompanied by loss of appetite and weight loss.

In the top left square lie the left kidney and ureter – see above. The spleen that lies on this side is usually of little concern to the layperson because it almost never causes a problem on its own – commonly it is part of some other disease and, unless it has increased its size considerably, does not normally cause any warning symptoms. *Symptoms* are what the patient complains of and *signs* are what the doctor finds on examining the patient.

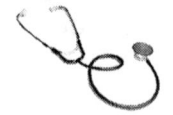

VAGINAL DISCHARGES

Regardless of age any vaginal discharge that has any of the following features warrants a visit to the doctor or clinic:

* Excessive quantity and, as a general rule, having to wear a sanitary pad to cope with the amount
* An unpleasant smell accompanying it
* Any discomfort or pain associated with it (around the vagina or within it [introitus]) – and
* If appropriate, whether there is pain or discomfort during sexual intercourse
* If it is accompanied by a burning sensation during the passage of urine
* If it occurs in the presence of a 'loop' – intrauterine contraceptive device – that has been previously inserted or
* If it persists after a 'womb scrape' (D&C – dilatation and curettage) following a miscarriage.

Though not every discharge is due to a sexually transmitted infection, if the circumstances warrant it this must be excluded with appropriate tests. Any child or young person with a discharge, even if the above criteria do not apply, should have the possibility of a sexually transmitted disease considered - especially if there are people involved in their care and this should include anybody irrespective of whether the person is a friend or relative of whatever age or sex.

Bathing (not that any female of whatever age should be using the bath tub in the first instance!) with bath salts and other 'antiseptics' added to bath water is to be discouraged as these may cause a chemical irritation in the delicate lining of the vagina (vaginitis) and produce a 'discharge'.

The general rule in treating a vaginal discharge requires a swab sent to the laboratory to remove the guesswork in identifying the cause. Using an ointment without the proof of an infection may well 'clear' the discharge with the mistaken assumption that the medication worked! Often the problem will recur if the diagnosis and, therefore the treatment, were incorrect – and the patient lighter in the pocket! The description or appearance of a vaginal discharge, as explained to the doctor or pharmacist, cannot make the diagnosis with any degree of certainty.

Not every discharge is caused by 'thrush'. Advertising that encourages women to buy over-the-counter, expensive medications, often used repeatedly, in the belief that the infection has 'recurred' (when it may not have been present in the first instance!). This serves the interests of the manufacturer and the seller and not those of the patient. Thrush is a 'yeast'/fungus that could be normally present in the vagina but in numbers usually too small to produce symptoms. Yeasts love a dark, warm and moist environment and the vagina meets these requirements admirably.

In a diabetic the environment is made richer with the extra glucose (in the blood and urine) and this makes thrush problematic - especially if the glucose levels are not well controlled. A diagnosis of thrush in any person should make the examination of the blood mandatory to exclude diabetes – another reason for being wary about unsupervised and indiscriminate use of over-the-counter antifungal preparations.

If the pH of the vagina (term used to describe whether it is high in acids or alkalis) is acidic, as may happen during the use of certain antibiotics (e.g. tetracycline) thrush multiplies rapidly - resulting in a vaginal 'infection'. If these antibiotics are prescribed prophylactic use of an antifungal ointment is often recommended.

As an emergency measure (in the middle of the night and with no chemist open!) a vaginal thrush sufferer may obtain temporary relief by using unsweetened yogurt applied within the vagina and the introitus (surrounding area) - as high up the passage as is possible.

Any infection in a sexually active person will also require treatment for the partner: an excellent reason for using a condom. If the penis or vagina does not make contact with the partner's vagina/ anus /mouth the transmission of most infections can be prevented or reduced. Confirming a diagnosis of a vaginal infection from a sexually transmitted disease or infection should, depending on the circumstances, prompt a search for other infections. These usually require blood tests – e.g. confirming an infection with gonorrhoea requires a pus swab taken from the penis/vagina but a blood test is necessary to exclude concomitant infection with the HI virus, syphilis or chlamydia.

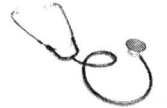

WARTS

Warts are caused by a virus and are therefore infectious and can be passed on by contact with others – as in hand shaking. They commonly occur on the fingers and soles of the feet. They may be painful if situated close to a fingernail or on the sole where, because of the pressure effect of the body weight, they are flattened and may resemble a corn – the latter may also cause pain.

The common practice of continually shaving off the 'tops' of warts will do nothing to get rid of them as their roots go deeper down into the tissue than are visible from the outside. Cutting the surface causes tiny dot-like brown spots; these are due to bleeding. This may help differentiate a wart from a corn – the latter does not bleed.

Painting the wart with a solution called 'Podophyllin' up to 4-5 times a day will eventually 'burn' it out; using it once or twice a day may not be sufficient but helps to earn the comment "It doesn't work!" This solution must be applied carefully so that contact is made only with the wart and not normal skin, as it will burn the latter. To avoid it a small ring of Vaseline may be applied around the wart and the paint applied with the brush kept almost dry to avoid an excess of the solution running off the brush – akin to the way nail polish is applied – by brushing off the excess against the mouth of the bottle.

Another method is cauterising the wart; this is done under local anaesthetic and literally 'burns' off the lesion.

Warts may also be 'destroyed' by the application of liquid nitrogen – called cryotherapy. This may cause some discomfort from the burning sensation that accompanies the application of the nitrogen as it freezes the lesion. Both the above methods obviate the need for compression bandages.

For a large wart more effective treatment would be to have it excised under local anaesthetic. This may not be practical if the wart is situated close to a fingernail. This method requires pressure dressings for about 24 hours to prevent bleeding.

None of the methods guarantees a cure as the cause is a virus and the warts can therefore recur. The ideal time to treat them is when they first appear and the lesions have not had a chance to grow deep into the tissue.

Any wart appearing around the genitalia (private parts) or the back passage needs a professional opinion as syphilis may cause a lesion with a flat top resembling a miniature 'cauliflower'. The wart caused by the virus has a pointed top and may be sexually transmitted, though this is not always the case. A concern about warts in these parts (called condylomata acuminata – meaning 'pointed tops') is that they may, on rare occasions, become cancerous; this complicationdoes not occur when they are situated in other areas of the body.

Warts may be autoinoculated i.e. one can spread them by contact with other parts of the body; walking around barefooted may also infect others. Similarly, the shavings, from misguidedly cutting off the tops with a blade, are also infectious

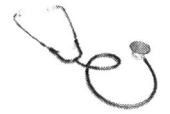

WEIGHT MANAGEMENT

There is nothing magical or mysterious about losing weight. The body cannot produce fat or 'weight' without the intake or increased intake (overeating) of food. To lose weight one must eat less and exercise more. Of the two options exercise is the more important. A person on a hunger strike will not keep his weight.

The ability to lose it is less difficult than maintaining it once it is lost. Almost every 'get thin fast' programme (gimmick) is doomed to fail because any scheme that promises or produces rapid weight loss is pandering to a public that wants the reward (weight loss) without any genuine effort or change in attitudes towards food and health.

15% to 20 % of people will have the motivation to achieve almost any goal, whether it is kicking the smoking habit, exercising, embarking on a new venture or losing weight. Are these the 20% that adorn the advertising that trumpets the successes of 'weight loss programmes'? Do the 80% who do not have this motivation keep the industry in business? This is called the Pareto principle.

What do these 20% have that the others do not? They have the ability to acknowledge that few people have gained success in any field without hard work. Whether it is months of grueling, muscle-straining exercise for a marathon, hours of toiling in the garden to produce 'bowling green' lawns or achieving goal weights – the bottom line is hard work. Not everyone wants to work that hard but that does not stop them from dreaming about the weight they would love to have. These '20 %' do not buy Lotto tickets!

Given the percentage of candidates that will eventually succeed is it small wonder that the unsuspecting public is duped into thinking that anybody can do it? If the majority could lose the excess weight would these schemes remain in business? If preventative medicine was practised successfully it would sound the death knell for much of the medical profession. If heart disease disappeared who will need a 'by-pass operation'? And the attending cardiac surgeon, anaesthetist, nurses, hospitals, and medical aid schemes – the list of people deriving income off the backs of disease is long.

Being overweight and obese (excessively overweight) has a mortality risk all of its own. This risk of dying is independent of any other risk that may be present e.g. high blood pressure, diabetes or coronary artery disease. Tobacco companies are being taken to court for the illnesses and deaths of millions of people who would otherwise be well or alive were it not for the tireless efforts of the manufacturers to ply their products.

When the public wakens to smell the roses (before these are planted on their graves) then the ubiquitous food industry should also be taken to task for the almost continual barrage of 'junk food' that is produced, advertised and sold to a public that laps it up in ignorance of their health risks.

From cool drinks to fried chicken, burgers, fish and chips, margarine, breakfast cereals, chocolates, sweets, sweetened yogurts, cakes, crisps , sugar, eggs, beer, wine, spirits , processed meats, ice cream, fruit juices, coffee, canned foods and ready-to-cook meals - this is a multi-billion dollar concern and will not relinquish easily its grip on the food industry.

The consumer has little chance of escaping the vast network the food industry has created to keep the customer well supplied and well fed. In the name of 'discount' shopping (there is always a sale on!) and bulk-buying the public is cajoled from the cradle to the grave to spend money (which is the basic intention) to buy these products that are guaranteed, one way or another, to help gain weight and cause disease. 'Turnover' is the buzz word in industry whether it is the production of cigarettes, chocolates, cocaine or cars. Never mind that these 'innocent' or ignorant people will, given time, develop cancer, strokes, heart and lung disease. As long as it generates income today who cares about tomorrow?

Obesity has yet to be seriously considered as a disease. Unsuspecting Joe and Jane are unaware that 'food' will lead to their deaths - whereas the consequences of HIV Aids are better known and the end results more dramatic. The media are not averse to the profit to be gained from Aids related topics but may not regard tobacco or obesity and their consequences as deserving of front page newsworthiness.

The busy mother who plonks the young child in front of the television, the nanny or baby sitter who uses the opportunity to keep up with the current episode in their favourite soapie while baby or junior is made to watch the same, the young child who has just returned from school and is now watching its favourite 'children's' programme', the teenager and parents sharing channels between favourite comedies and cartoons and movies – how can the average person escape the well orchestrated advertisement of 'food' that accompanies these programmes? Can one of the secrets to effective weight loss be to ban from television the advertising of all 'food'?

It is difficult to shake off years of "Finish all your food", "Don't waste food" and "God will punish you for being wasteful". Being cajoled and bribed (with promises of sweets and ice cream if they finished all their food) and even punished if they did not comply – is the order of the day. Parents need to be reeducated to desist from these practices and be more streetwise about nutrition and food. These well known one-liners were a product of the post-war era when food was scarce and wastefulness frowned upon.

There are over 2000 separate references on the subject of Omega 3 fatty acids and the health authorities have been publicising its benefits to the foetus to foster the development of the retina and brain. How many medical practitioners routinely prescribe Omega 3? How many gynaecologists are not aware that the multivitamins 'especially designed for the pregnant mother' do not contain Omega 3 (this is an oil and cannot be combined with water soluble vitamins)? To add to the farce they contain so little calcium this would not be sufficient for a cat let alone the 1500mg per day required in pregnancy.

The normal Body Mass Index (BMI) is about 23 for adult women and 25 for men. It has been suggested that the risk of dying from obesity increases 10 to 15% if the BMI is between normal and 30.However, this risk increases 50 to 100% if the BMI is over 30. What is your BMI?

The BMI is calculated by dividing the weight (in kilogrammes) by the height multiplied by itself – i.e. height squared. A calculator would be useful. A male adult weighing 80 kg.and height of 1.5 metres will have a BMI of (80 divided by 1.5 x 1.5) = 32. These are figures used by insurance companies to calculate one's risk to them and their money. What is the risk to your health?

It is generally not realised that feeding (food) and sex (reproduction), in that order, are the only functions required of man and of any living creature on this planet. These are two instincts each organism is born with – created specifically to preserve the species. The newborn infant has the instinct to start feeding almost from birth. The purpose of the feeding and the 'food' is to ensure that the infant reaches reproductive age.

This is the only reason for having that powerful urge called 'hunger' – to ensure the cell/organ/body does not die before it can mature itself to reproductive age when it can perform its second instinctual function – 'reproduction'. Once the latter is achieved (and the newborn independent enough to fend/feed for itself) the parents are no longer required.

The body thereafter begins to age and every cell starts to wind down towards its final demise. The average life span of an adult human should not have been necessary to prolong itself to beyond about the third decade. Have we upset nature's blueprint with 'modern medicine' and the eradication of disease and improved longevity? Small wonder that the animal kingdom still practices as nature intended. However, where man has meddled dogs and cats are dying earlier because of obesity and cardiovascular disease.

Regarding eating and reproduction nothing has been left to chance. The sensation of hunger and the urge to have sex are the most powerful instincts we have. Underestimate these two drives and it is no surprise that so many attempts to lose weight or curb the world's population explosion have met with little success? That 95 % of the American population is estimated to be overweight and the world's population statistic is currently 6.6 billion (2007) are clear signs of the power of food and sex.

There is a special centre in the brain that informs one of hunger and another that signals that it is sated. The stomach distends itself with food supplied to it until it stretches to a predetermined extent (determined by how much it has been accustomed to receive over time). Any attempt to suddenly cut down on the amount it receives on a regular basis, as in 'dieting', is likely to fail as the impulses (messages) from the stomach walls sent to the brain will signal incomplete 'filling' and the hunger pangs will continue. Therefore, to fool the brain the quantity of food taken should be reduced gradually or a bulking agent like fibre used to give the sensation of fullness without the calories.

Food comes in 3 basic forms

- Carbohydrates
- Proteins and
- Fats.

Also essential for the proper functioning of the body are vitamins and minerals. The body cannot manufacture the latter. Vitamins and minerals must be taken on a daily basis as part of the food or, if it cannot be guaranteed that it contains them, as a supplement.

The body cannot store proteins and, therefore, these have to be taken at each meal and everyday. It also cannot store carbohydrates but has found a way to convert carbohydrates to fat to be saved for a rainy day. The original intention was to allow extra food to be stored so that in times of famine the body would draw on these stored fats to supply vital fuel (food) necessary for body functions to be preserved.

This ability has been maintained through time and the body remains an expert at conserving and storing food for energy. Missing a meal sends a signal to the brain that there is threat of a 'famine' and the body goes into 'storage mode'.

'Detoxification' is a much bandied pseudoscientific term used to cleanse the body of toxins that have accumulated in the system. The liver and kidneys have been designed to fulfill this role of detoxifier and are quite capable of performing their function without outside interference (colonic washouts included). However, if a person who has been abusing food and, perhaps, alcohol, checks into a 'health resort' to recover from the overindulgence this may account for the renewed vigour and general well being that follows the expensive weekend.

All three types of foods, vitamins and minerals must be supplied at each meal but the keyword is moderation i.e. eating to live and not living to eat. Carbohydrates are the main source of energy intake. They occur as simple sugars like glucose, fructose and galactose and more complex ones like starch (found in plants) and glycogen (found in animal tissue). Glucose is absorbed quickly into the blood stream pushing up the sugar levels and thereby stimulating the release of insulin. The latter helps to bring down the levels to normal again by carrying glucose from the bloodstream into the cells. Glucose becomes a problem for diabetics whereas fructose, because it is absorbed more slowly, is safer as it does not stimulate the release of insulin as much as glucose does. Complex sugars like pasta and whole wheat bread also take longer to get absorbed into the blood by remaining longer in the intestine, making them better suited for everybody and diabetics in particular.

The lightheadedness that occurs with low blood sugar levels is because brain cells depend, for their energy requirements, on a constant supply of glucose in the blood. Brain cells are unique in that they cannot store glucose (unlike the liver and muscle) and they cannot manufacture glucose as can other cells of the body. In a diabetic, low sugars (that often occur during sleep when one would be unaware) can be a special problem as there is a risk of damaging brain cells and, if allowed to continue to fall, slipping into a coma. The latter can happen within minutes whereas a high blood sugar will take several hours and, depending on other factors, up to 2 – 3 days to push an untreated or poorly controlled diabetic into a coma. In the short term low blood sugars are more dangerous than high ones. Once in a while it is important to check one's sugar level at 3 or 4 o'clock in the morning especially if diabetic medication has been changed.

Protein: Protein means 'of first importance' in Greek. They make up most of the cells and are responsible for breaking down and building up molecules, extracting energy, fighting infections, making enzymes, carrying important hormones and even making genes. There are 22 amino acids that are the building blocks of proteins and must all be present and in their correct sequence before the body can use them. Any product that claims to be a 'protein supplement' must contain all 22 amino acids.

As mentioned above - the body cannot store proteins and therefore must be taken at each meal. The total amount of protein required per day is between 80 to 100 gm. Any amount beyond this is discarded as waste in the urine via the kidneys and not into the gut and out the back passage as is often believed. Of a 300 gm steak eaten in a meal almost 250 gm of it will be passed (pissed) out in the urine as waste products. Furthermore, the kidneys must work (unnecessarily) to get rid of the extra protein, placing it under needless strain. If the kidneys should fail for any reason the first advice given the unlucky patient is to cut down the total protein consumed per day to between 60 to 80 gm. This is the equivalent of a sardine – one sardine for 24 hours is all the protein the body would have needed anyway. Observing this could save the world a lot of food and keep the kidneys healthier for longer. Unfortunately the main source of protein is animal and this carries the additional risk of unhealthy saturated fats (fats that are hard at room temperature). To avoid this fat one could use lentils, beans and Soya as excellent alternatives to animal protein but one would in addition need Vitamin B complex supplementation because the best source of this important vitamin is meat. Vegetarians need to take this vitamin as a supplement. Lean pork has less fat than beef or lamb. Skinless turkey meat has less fat than chicken. Fish (eaten with the skin on) is healthier than all animal meat, provided it is not fried. Fish is a healthier alternative to meat or poultry. Fish-fat is healthy fat and, as in all animals, is stored under the skin. Eating filleted fish with the skin removed is akin to eating the skin of the banana and discarding the fruit! Those engaged in hard manual work and rigorous physical training should take extra protein, as should pregnant women, growing children and patients recovering from illnesses. The body uses protein to promote growth, build muscle and repair tissues. Bodybuilders may take up to 'two dozen raw egg whites' a day to supplement their protein intake. This practice carries the risk of salmonella infection (food poisoning) acquired from the uncooked egg. There are safer and more convenient protein supplements available.

Fats: Fats have become the bane of our health and are the passport to heart attacks, strokes, cancer and obesity. Fat is stored in specialised 'fat cells'. The number of these cells is determined in infancy. If the baby is overweight after birth the total number of these cells increases. This number, once established from a young age, never changes but the size of the cells can increase later and result in obesity. Carbohydrates that have been eaten but not utilised soon after ingestion are converted into fat and stored, along with ingested fats, in certain areas of the body – the breasts, abdomen and thighs in women and the abdomen in men. Carbohydrates are a ready source of energy (hence the 'carbo'-loading long distance runners take in before a marathon). To avoid storage of carbohydrate as fat it should ideally be utilised at the time it is produced. Visible fat is only part of the problem; it is also stored within the abdomen and around the vital organs and, more dangerously, within the arterial walls – causing heart attacks and strokes. Fat (saturated type) is only present in animal sources of food. Vegetables and fruit do not contain this fat. For all the notoriety that fat has earned as a potential 'killer' it is still necessary in our diets for maintaining the integrity of the cell walls and membranes. What are not necessary are the cardiovascular and other problems that accompany the ingestion of animal fat. However, these sterols and lipids that maintain our cell walls can be obtained from supplements that obtain them from plant sources avoiding the need to indulge in saturated animal fats. 'Formula IV' supplies this admirably. Cow's milk is fattier than human breast milk. This is as nature intended. Human milk is quite watery, but with good reason. The human infant does not need as much fat. Cow's milk was designed for the calf and not, as many believe, for human consumption. Cow's milk falls under the category of 'animal fat' and all dairy products are ill advised for humans. Never mind that our mothers insisted – as does the dairy industry – that "Milk is good for you". Full cream milk and its by-products like yoghurt are good sources of calcium but the risk of heart attacks, strokes or cancer in later life from the animal fat in milk makes the prevention of *osteoporosis* pale by comparison. It is safer to use a reliable calcium supplement instead.

The white and low fat cheeses are safer than the yellow ones. Butter is animal fat – this is the equivalent of eating the fat off the lamb chop. There should be little controversy about whether butter or margarine is healthier. The vegetables (sunflower seeds, rapeseed, canola) from which oils are made are not the problem. It is the process of 'hydrogenation' - intended to make the oil solid enough to spread - that causes the health problems of margarines. Hydrogenation is a chemical process that adds hydrogen atoms to unsaturated oil during refinement. Eating butter and working it off almost 'immediately' is used by the body as fuel but margarine causes a whole host of other reactions in the body that have nothing to do with providing fuel.

20 gm. of butter or margarine would be an average spread on two slices of bread –

20 multiplied by 30 (days) = 600 gm. for one month
600 multiplied by 12 (months) = 7200gm for one year

That is a staggering 7.2 kg per year of butter or margarine from using 20 gm. of it on 2 slices of bread each day!

1 gm. of fat contains 9 calories whereas 1 gm of carbohydrate or protein contains only 4 calories each. Simple arithmetic will clarify that in terms of calories – fats (and margarines) contain more than double the calorie content of the other two types of foods.

7200 gm. multiplied by 9 (calories) = 64800 calories for 1 year.

An average office worker uses about 1000 calories per day. 64800 divided by 1000 = 64.8 which means that the 20 gm of butter or margarine each day is the equivalent of the total amount of food that could be eaten in 64.8 days!

Simply cutting out the margarine or butter will save 3 months supply of food! Bread without this spread is often called 'dry bread' and "How can a person eat dry bread?" This is the mischief of television advertising that would have us believe that bread cannot be eaten without a thick spread of butter or margarine. The margarine or oil has often already been added to the bread before it was baked. It may be more cost effective to banish bread altogether - after all carbohydrates can be found in so many other foods besides bread. This would then avoid the need for butter and margarine along with all the other unhealthy fillings that are used to make sandwiches. Television advertising of margarine being spread on everything from bread to the kitchen sink, and with the blessing of the ' Heart Foundation', is responsible for much of the obesity that comes full circle to cause the very cardiovascular disease that is trying to be prevented. Whether it is butter or margarine (or olive oil for that matter) the calorie count is the same for all of them.

The logo 'Don't fool yourself – Speed kills' is used by Departments of Transport to warn motorists of the dangers of fast driving. Many more people die each year from cardiovascular disease, cancer and obesity than from motor vehicle accidents. The logo should rather read: 'Don't fool yourself – Food kills'!

The fat baby will almost certainly grow into a fat adult. Overweight parents invariably have overweight children - so what example can such parents set their offspring? The time to avoid adult obesity starts in infancy. Do not allow the fat cells to increase in number. No amount of 'dieting' will ever change the number of these cells - only the size of each cell can be reduced by weight loss.

Animals store fat under the skin. Therefore the skin of the chicken should always be removed before cooking. Removing it after cooking is shutting the stable door after the horse has fled – the fat has already been absorbed into the meat. Takeaways that serve chicken with the skin intact, battered and *then* deep-fried have gone to extra lengths to make certain the unhealthy fat is well preserved.

On the other hand, the fat in fish is healthy because it contains Omega 3 fatty acids that protect against heart attacks, strokes and helps as an anti-inflammatory in arthritis and Alzheimer's disease. It has also been shown to be beneficial in attention deficit hyperactivity disorder (hyperactivity syndrome). In order to get the benefit of this fatty acid naturally from fish the latter has to be eaten raw – as the Eskimos/Inuits do. Heat from cooking or canning damages the Omega 3 fatty acid. Filleted fish, where the skin is being fed to cats, provides mainly the protein, while the discarded skin keeps the cats' hearts healthy! To derive the benefit of these fatty acids the skin of the fish has to be eaten.

Fish is 'brain food' and for the benefits mentioned above it should be eaten at least 4 – 5 times per week and not just on Fridays! Omega 3 as a supplement supplies more of the fatty acid than one would get from eating fish. This fish oil should be taken during pregnancy and while breast-feeding because it is passed to the infant through the milk. Omega 3 helps the foetus and the infant in the development of the retina (eyes) and brain.

The following guidelines may provide some insight into effective weight management: –

1. Do not allow the infant to become overweight. Watch the clinic weight record card very closely. Fathers should be banned from bringing home 'guilt ridden' luxuries. They cannot make up on Fridays for the time they did not spend with their children during the week by 'bribing' them with chips, sweets, chocolates and fizzy drinks. Weight-for-weight crisp chips have more fat than the average lamb chop! The potato crisp is so thin the oil soaks right through it like blotting paper! Salt sows the seed for the development of high blood pressure. It also teaches from infancy that food 'must' contain salt to taste 'normal'. Ever seen a recipe that did not contain salt as an ingredient or a cooking programme that did not 'throw in some salt for taste'?

Every processed or manufactured food has salt dutifully added to them in the name of *seasoning*. And yet each food has its own taste but this is almost unknown to the average tongue. The brain records the taste of salt in its memory bank from a very early age. Is it any surprise that the boiled potato that does not have any salt added to it is described as 'insipid'? Hypertension is a 'silent killer' and affects a large proportion of the population: salt has been well established as a contributory factor. If one needs to doctor the taste use spices, and any quantity of it, without detriment. Spices do not contain calories and they do not cause hypertension. The common lament that "Food without salt has no taste" implies that the person eating it knows the *taste of salt* in the food but not the taste of the food. Chefs need to be reeducated and 'seasoning' should be banned.

2. Do not readily discuss plans to lose weight with anybody. Sometimes even close family members should be excluded. Those who cannot lose weight themselves and have tried 'everything' will not be overly keen to know that somebody else might succeed. When one is asked by a seemingly innocent "How is the weight loss going?" The unspoken statement may well be "I hope you haven't lost any weight yet because I failed". If both husband and wife are overweight do they support each other or does one partner continually and surreptitiously sabotage the other's attempts at losing weight? Obesity is a disease. Be wary about confiding to the entire workplace about one's 'bleeding piles' or be prepared to continue hearing about them long after they have disappeared. Pneumonia requires a short course of antibiotics whereas hypertension is a life long ailment and accordingly requires lengthy treatment. Obesity is a chronic disease that also requires prolonged treatment. Programmes that promise quick weight loss often fail in the long term leaving the participant more dejected. New Year's resolutions may remain simply that – motivation cannot be instilled on day one and be expected to last for

the rest of the year. It has to be dished out in small regular doses. The best intentions and the most ambitious schemes are doomed to fail if this point is ignored. Stay focused on the goal. Write down the plans and the desired weight where it can be seen e.g. writing the number '75' (if that is the goal weight) on the bathroom mirror, on the television set, the rear view mirror of the car, on the telephone, on your wallet or purse, inside the fridge, on the pantry cupboard and on the inside, where it will stare at you after the door is opened. This reinforcement of one's resolve to improve the weight helps to keep one focused. Any goal or plan that is not written down may remain simply wishful thinking - an architect's plan is drawn on paper!

3. Do not weigh yourself repeatedly after one has embarked on a programme. While the scale is a measurement of one's weight loss it transfers the rewards into the numbers on the face of a machine. The machine begins to control one's life. The person should be in control of one's life and the weight. Furthermore, with exercise fat is converted into protein and this will reflect a weight gain, contrary to expectations, because protein is heavier than fat. The important point is to remain focused and stay doing the right things and *ignore the scale*. The results of one's efforts will eventually show – the scale will not be necessary to verify this. Furthermore, the extra kilogrammes were accumulated over a long period – why should it disappear overnight. Aim to lose only a *single* kilogramme each month. Expecting results overnight and not seeing the desired figures quickly enough will cause dismay and the oft quoted "I tried everything and nothing seems to work!" As already mentioned obesity is a chronic disease – treat it with patience.

4. Make a point of eating all meals on time. Do not allow the work place to sabotage one's plans and do not make excuses if the real problem is that one cannot be bothered to eat timeously. Missing a meal will invariably make one eat more at the next one – partly because one feels deserving of

a bit extra and by then one would be ravenously hungry and ready to eat the proverbial horse.

5. Breakfast is an important start to the day; and point number 4 above will have been ignored. Make the effort to get up earlier or prepare breakfast the night before. It should contain a cereal – preferably oats (the less refined the better – the latter have bigger grains) and bran crushed and sprinkled over the oats. Oats contains soluble fibre and bran - insoluble fibre. If it is inconvenient to cook the oats each day then cook the whole week's supply and store it in the refrigerator whence one can help oneself. 'Weetabix' may be added to oats to increase the fibre content. Most meals fall far short of the daily requirement of the 27 to 35 gm. of fibre per day. The disappearance of fibre from our meals has been responsible for the rise in incidence of heart disease, cancer, raised cholesterol, diabetes, obesity and constipation.

Oats makes the best late night snack if the need for this should arise. It helps one to sleep better, lowers cholesterol – given that the liver makes most of its cholesterol at night, may help in the prevention of certain cancers, prevents constipation and prevents a sudden surge of glucose into the blood thereby avoiding the production of extra insulin to carry glucose into the cells. Adding fruit to oats will provide natural sugar instead of the heavily refined crystals. If one must use a sweetening agent choose fructose.

A slice of wholewheat bread with a helping of tuna or pilchard in tomato sauce – without any margarine or butter – also makes a filling snack. A thin spread of low fat salad-dressing can substitute for butter/ margarine if the latter is considered absolutely necessary. Do not use aspartame or other artificial sweeteners.

A common complaint is the lack of appetite in the morning. Having supper late at night and then retiring will have the food linger on unused in the system and ruin the appetite the following day. Nicotine from smoking on arising will further suppress the appetite. If one is using smoking to dull the appetite and thereby trying to lose weight – do not bother losing weight for health reasons – the cigarettes may kill before the weight does.

A hangover from alcohol abuse the night before will also dull the appetite at breakfast because the liver has not had time to recover from the 'poisoning' effect of the alcohol. In a similar vein, in hepatitis, when the liver is infected with a virus, one of the earliest symptoms is loss of appetite.

If one skips breakfast and the next meal is at 10 am or midday the body has then been without food for between 16 to 18 hours – the last calorie intake being the night before! The liver has only sufficient glucose to last about 3 to 4 hours from the time one arises. Without this ready supply of glucose from the liver the body then has to manufacture glucose to make up the deficit. The school child or employee who does not eat breakfast is not concentrating by 10 am. At a job interview prospective employees who do not regularly eat breakfast (which means ' break the fast') should not be readily employed – their lack of glucose and concentration could cause irritability, lowered productivity, accidents and even loss of life.

Perhaps the traditional tea break at 10 am should be brought forward because the 'tea and sandwiches' taken at this hour may not be available to replenish the liver's depleted glucose stores until after this and closer to 12 noon

School children who do not eat breakfast should be made to understand that this meal is not negotiable – just as wearing shoes or bringing their school books are not negotiable. If necessary the class teacher should be approached – the teacher may have authority far beyond the nagging of the well-intentioned parent. Discourage the sharing of lunches both for school children and for husbands – one's good intentions may be traded for possible junk food. Teachers should have lunch with their protégés.

Educationists need to put aside profit and what is popular on the junk food scene and encourage healthy eating habits from an age when they have our impressionable children under their wings. This may avoid starting the rot then and keeping the 'dieting industry' and pharmaceuticals in business later in life. Educationists and parents should work in collaboration.

Mothers and parents who prepare meals need to be better informed before they undertake this vital task. Imagine if the petrol attendant slipped a bit of oil into one's petrol tank! The garage has a responsibility towards the client and can be sued for such negligence. Parents, grandparents, tuck shop managers, caterers and food manufacturers should pay more attention.

The manufacturers who recklessly flood their crisp chips and other foods with salt should be heavily litigated against for playing such an irresponsible role when it has been shown so clearly that excessive salt contributes to the development of high blood pressure. People from the Transkei and Ciskei – two rural areas in South Africa – in whom hypertension was virtually unheard of 25 to 30 years ago – now swell the hypertension clinics of the hospitals – a classic example of how the introduction of fast foods (fat and salt) have influenced the appearance of disease in previously healthy populations.

Salt and the introduction of fattier food products – battered and deep fried chicken and fish and chips and processed meats are slowly but surely killing those that eat them. If asbestosis and the evils that smoking breeds can be litigated against – then full strength to the rest of the diseased nation.

Cholesterol has been found to be already present *microscopically* in the coronary arteries of three year old children (autopsies performed on cot death victims). It is visible to the *naked eye* (i.e. without magnification) in teenage motor cycle accident victims. This has debunked the idea that cholesterol deposits appeared only around middle age. The seeds of coronary artery disease are being sown from a very early age.

Children should be allowed to sue irresponsible parents and grandparents who believe that eating 'crisp' chips, sweets and chocolates are 'treats'. This encourages the child to believe that these are acceptable forms of 'food'. Placating a difficult child with a 'luxury' helps the future adult to seek refuge in food to overcome boredom and depression and life's other hiccups.

6. Lunch should be the next important meal and still have the advantage of sufficient time during the rest of the afternoon's activities to burn up the ingested calories. Lunch should be partaken as a 'prince'. It should have a balance between all the 3 major foods – as with all the meals.

Having fruit or a salad only for lunch is foolish as it ignores the basics of nutrition – there is no protein in such a meal. Being fed a watery vegetable soup, a sliver of orange and sprig of watercress may appear to suit the ambience of a weekend at a 'hydro' but it is an excellent cost saving ploy to beguile the hapless health fanatic. Restaurants and takeaways cater for a public that expects or demands food that has taste high on their priority disregarding the health hazards of eating such foods. Lunch should be prepared at home. The 'sandwich' is a mistake. Most sandwich fillers are 'unhealthy' and calorie-rich – e.g. processed meats, cheese, peanut butter, jam, butter, margarine, fish paste and sandwich spreads. A lunch box to the rescue! One can select from a helping (half cup = one helping) of baked beans, cottage cheese or yogurt, tuna or other canned fish (half a pilchard) or fresh fish or a chicken drumstick or breast (minus the skin), coleslaw (made with a light salad dressing and not mayonnaise – the latter is made from eggs!) and one or two fruit. A helping of butternut, squash or pumpkin is essential - aim to have at least 2 yellow fruit or vegetables every day (beta-carotene content). For the benefit of antioxidants one should have a daily intake of between 5 and 9 fruit and vegetables with a mixture of colours e.g. red pepper, purple aubergine, yellow squash, carrots, orange, green kiwifruit, red grapes, green ladyfingers / okra (the only vegetable with the highest number of antioxidants), broccoli, brussels sprout, cabbage (the vegetables with flowers in the shape of a cross – cruciferous – beneficial in the prevention of cancer).

7. Supper should be eaten like a 'pauper'. The time-honoured practice of having a 'cooked' meal made by a dutiful wife or concerned mother has been responsible for much of the problems of obesity. After eating this hearty meal, as he considers is his due for working 'so hard during the day', the unsuspecting husband puts up his feet, lets out a belch as he reaches for the newspaper or the remote control – and four hours later is tucking himself into bed. Most of what he has eaten is happily stored away. The body is doing exactly what it has been programmed to do – after years of conditioning – storing the extra energy for a rainy day for it never knows

when its next meal is going to be! The next meal, if he is lucky, is breakfast – more often it is at mid-morning or at lunchtime or, more disastrously, in the evening. But the body does not know this for certain! This extra energy is stored as 'fat'. Any weight loss programme that does not encourage the supper to be drastically reduced in terms of calories taken will not succeed. Supper could be replaced with a well-balanced meal replacement like 'Nutrishake' (GNLD) and, perhaps, a jacket potato (without margarine or butter) and a topping of white chicken or fish and a salsa. One orange (whole – and with the white surrounding the orange eaten – the white contains valuable antioxidants that help to prevent cancer and other diseases) or other fruit could provide dessert.

8. Eat slowly and concentrate on the task at hand i.e. *eating*. Do not eat while reading or watching television. A person watching a horror movie could polish off a whole fried chicken! The stomach needs the brain to guide it to know when to turn off the hunger impulses – it cannot respond to the message if this is being suppressed by 'Dracula'! Popcorn in the cinema will take longer to finish if the film is slow moving or boring. (Many cinemas use coconut oil in their popcorn – this oil carries a higher risk of heart disease than other vegetable oils). Food should be presented to the stomach in a state that makes it easy to digest it. Watching a thriller will make one's heart beat faster and chew and swallow faster sending ill-prepared food to the stomach. The stomach relies on the appearance, smell and taste of food to encourage adequate digestive juices that are vital to the process of digestion. The television should be switched off at meal times or food eaten away from the set if a family sit-down is impractical. The incidence of obesity in adults and children has increased enormously since television was introduced.

Eat only at the table. Teach the brain to associate the table with food and eating; just as one does not shave in the pantry it helps to discipline one's eating habits. Allow the table to stimulate the reflex to feed and not the ice cream parlour in the shopping mall!

9.   On *one day* in the week, more appropriately one day in the weekend, eat whatever takes one's fancy. One day of indulgence cannot cause the damage that six can. Allowing the one day as 'free' allows one some autonomy and does not foster the idea that one can *never* eat ice cream or a favourite chocolate or other 'luxury'. A 'free' weekend day also makes it easier to remember that 'Wednesday' is not the weekend and therefore no chocolate is allowed, instead of trying to remember this from a complicated 'diet sheet' dictating what is to be eaten on which days! Life is difficult enough without having to weigh each banana and chicken breast. Keep the programming simple and doable. People do not wish to be dominated by 'weight loss programmes' to such an extent that life itself becomes 'joyless'. When food is prepared the intention is for it to be eaten or sold and, above all, to be enjoyed. During the weekdays keep the meals simple. Takeaways and fast foods should not even be considered outside of the free weekend day. Children can be taught this discipline from an early age.

The quantity of food prepared at home should be just sufficient for one helping – any extra that is prepared with the intention of labour and time saving later in the week should be removed and stored away out of sight as soon as possible after cooking. It is unfair to have the brain and others in the house know that a second helping is available.

Desserts and sweets do not have to be a regular conclusion to every meal – a fresh fruit salad without cream or ice cream is healthier bearing in mind the stomach does not give a hoot how the food is prepared. Once it passes the mouth it has no choice but to deal with it (digest it); it is the brain that needs to be reeducated. Liquidising the fruit (or vegetables) in a blender is an acceptable form for finicky eaters – provided this is not then stored as this will lose nutrients.

10. Any person who eats food and subsequently vomits to avoid putting on weight that (over) eating will cause should see

a therapist. This condition is called bulimia and requires professional help sooner rather than later. Make the appointment the 'third' time it happens – not after months of secretive vomiting and all pretending that it's nothing! Anorexia nervosa is a serious weight losing condition in which the victim is afraid to eat for fear of putting on weight. Often there are other factors playing a role and food is the common link. Again, professional help should be sought early rather than when the malady has been allowed to become entrenched and therapy made more difficult. Parents and mothers, in particular, who see their daughters as potential 'models' should be held (? criminally) culpable if they should aid and abet this, often life threatening, condition.

11. Criticism does not play a constructive role. Instead it undermines confidence and helps to build a stronger resistance against the problem. Timing is also important. Do not cook a mouth-watering dish and then admonish the obese about 'dieting' when the laden spoon is half way to the open mouth! Do not discuss 'dieting' at the dining table. The bank manager will not entertain your request for a loan in the supermarket.

Do not comment on weight or food related matters in the presence of other people or family members even if there are others who are similarly afflicted. This should be a personal matter and involve only the immediate parties. The doctor does not gather all the new patients with cancer and discuss them en masse; group therapy may be helpful but, only, once the groundwork has been covered. It is often difficult for the affected person to have to cope with other family members or friends who may not always be helpful and can indeed be cruel with their taunts.

12. Avoid eating outside of designated meal times. Ignoring this keeps the stomach active almost throughout the day and accordingly makes it necessary to keep the entire digestive processes working much longer periods. There is little recovery time for the glands and cells that produce the

enzymes. Animals do not eat all of the time. Cows have an especially adapted stomach to cater for this pattern of eating – the ruminant stomach. Try coaxing a trout to bite when it is not feeding time and the amateur angler will soon learn the frustrations of fly-fishing! Eating an ice cream cone in a shopping mall is the equivalent of having dessert when it is not a 'designated' meal time. The message is to the brain and it reads "I'm sorry I don't do that!"

13. If one is invited to a meal it is not compulsory to eat everything in sight – but do avoid talking about one's 'dieting'. The host and hostess may have gone to lengths to prepare food to entertain you, the guest. This is not the time to embark on a weight-loss discussion. Better to accept the proffered food and, once the attention of the host has passed, quietly ask for or find a plate to halve the amount, pleading permission not to waste or that one would have it later. On a special occasion like a birthday or other such function one should regard the time as a 'weekend' and therefore 'free' time to eat as one pleases without feeling guilty. Once a sensible eating habit has inculcated itself into one's brain watching what one eats on these occasions will come naturally and the continual battle "Should I or should I not have the chocolate cake?" becomes easier to deal with. Birthdays do not occur on a daily basis but weekdays do! Watch the weekdays and the weekend will take care of itself! If one has to dine out on a weekday forfeit the free weekend day to make up. There are 52 days in the year that one has as 'free' days and 313 days that make up the time one has to be careful – there being clearly more to lose (gain!) by not being sensible on the latter days. If one should on occasion be indiscreet this should not be a reason to become despondent – acknowledge that this can happen to the best and carry on – Rome was not lost in a day!

14. Do not *force* children to eat! "Finish all your food", "Food should not be wasted", "You should be so fortunate to have food to eat", "I worked hard to cook your meal now eat it all

up like a good boy" and "God will punish you if you waste food" – are well known admonishments mentioned earlier which in present times are designed to cause obesity; these time-honoured comments come from an era when food was scarce and the economy stifled by two world wars, not to forget the ravages of illness and pestilence.

Parents should be more in tune with their children's nutritional needs and serve them accordingly i.e. befitting the age and differing requirements of each individual. However, the parent must first be educated about nutrition. If a child will not eat at meal times, or brings back lunch taken to school, or is overly picky about food, find the reason for this attitude instead of "Eat your food now or else!" or "I'm sick and tired of this nonsense at meal times – now finish your food" or worse still to be sent off to bed as punishment or, criminally, be spanked for not eating as instructed! A child will not deliberately starve itself without reason.

One packet of crisp chips will ruin the appetite, as will juice or chocolates or sweets. Parents glibly teach the young child to eat and enjoy 'luxuries'. Calling these 'junk foods' luxuries is already elevating junk to the level of 'luxury' status. Calling junk food 'food' is another anomaly best avoided. Thirst should be treated with water – not fruit juice. Hunger should be treated with food at the appropriate times.

Setting a routine from a very early age is important. Eating food should not be reduced to the equivalent of sneezing! Any place and anyhow will do. Eating, as mentioned earlier, is as important as sex. It should be respected accordingly. Eating supper in front of the television should become a sacrilege – one would not (normally) have intercourse in the pantry!

Respect for food should not come from a drive-in takeaway just because mum felt it was Friday and she deserved a rest from cooking and dad (and the children) agreed wholeheartedly because dad loves takeaway. Parents who have children must have responsibility for educating them about proper nutrition. Educationists need to value the importance of nutrition with as much emphasis as mathematics and chemistry. Is there a point to producing A grades only to have the chartered accountant, plumber or nurse have their first heart attack when they turn forty? Poor nutrition and obesity in children deserve to be viewed as a form of abuse.

Grandparents should not be party to sabotaging the efforts of the parents to encourage healthier eating habits in their children. The children lose in the end, often with their lives, to diseases like cancer (nitrite preservatives in processed meats), diabetes (obesity and the continual barrage of excessive sugar loads that stimulate the release of insulin), hypertension (excessive salt intake and obesity) and obesity itself (excessive weight gains from overeating and under exercising). Children should be able to sue their parents for 'nutritional negligence' just as not sending them to school incurs a penalty. Does hypertension begin with the first abnormal blood pressure recording? Or is the seed of the problem planted much earlier – when the young inadequate kidneys of innocent children are being bombarded with loads of salt from almost every processed food known to man? Any person who has 'recently' been gaining weight that is not easily explained and having serious difficulties losing it should have blood tests done to exclude hypothyroidism (underfunctioning thyroid gland) and Cushing's disease (overactive pituitary gland in the brain producing excessive cortisol).

Cooking programmes and television chefs should be under few illusions because they advertise food designed to look fabulous and taste great – encouraging the viewer to imagine that food should normally and always be prepared that way. Obesity should be everybody's responsibility. Cocaine is not glamourised on television - food should command the same respect.

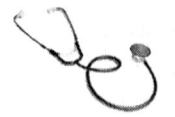

WRIST JOINT

Almost any person, and in particular the elderly, falling on the outstretched arm, will most likely break the bone or bones of the wrist/ lower end of the forearm.

There is often pain and swelling over the wrist or the lower forearm. If pressure applied (gently at first) with the examiner's thumb over the wrist area in a person suspected of such a fracture causes pain – the diagnosis is very likely to be correct.

In a young child bone may not actually break but becomes 'bent' (greenstick fracture). Reluctance in a child to move the joint or adjacent parts should raise suspicion of a fracture. An X-ray is essential for the diagnosis - and this applies to any bone suspected of a fracture. If this cannot be done immediately the joint should be placed in a sling slung from the neck (to support the part), reassure the child and avoid unnecessary movement. In an older person, as an emergency measure, the wrist can be splinted by having the patient grip with the fingers of the affected side one end of a board the width of the forearm and, using a bandage, wrap the board together with the hand, wrist and the forearm into a firmly supportive unit. Any firm cardboard padded with a towel or sanitary pads may suffice until a doctor or emergency unit can be found.

A ganglion is a swelling resembling a knob – situated over the back of the wrist and the adjacent part of the hand. It may become painful when pressure is exerted directly upon it or when pressure is exerted on the wrist joint - as in leaning on the hand while doing a push–up exercise. If one makes a bubble with chewing gum – picture the mouth to be the wrist joint and the bubble to be the lining of the wrist joint that has found a weakness within the joint capsule. Through this weakness the capsule herniates its way to the exterior (through the lips) to form the swelling on the back of the wrist/hand. A ganglion does not become cancerous and if it is not painful can simply be observed. An injection of steroids into the swelling may resolve the problem and, failing this, minor surgery (closing the opening/ defect) will remedy it.

If the thumb is stretched outwards as far as possible away from the index finger a small 'hollow' between two visible tendons will appear at the base of the thumb. This is the hollow in which the customary pinch of snuff is placed from which it is inhaled into the nostrils; this 'snuffbox' has a bone situated within the hollow which may be fractured at the time of a fall on the outstretched hand/arm (scaphoid or boat shaped bone). An initial X-ray may not show up the fracture; the clue that it is present is the continued presence of pain in the 'snuff box' long after the fall. MRI Scans (specialised X-rays) help detect the 'missed' fracture and avoid the risk of negligence liability. If this expensive investigation is not available a follow up X-ray two to three weeks after the fall will identify the fracture – as new bone starts to form at the site of the break the fracture becomes more easily visible.

Carpal tunnel syndrome is another fairly common problem at the wrist joint. All the tendons at the joint are 'held down' in place by a strap akin to the band of a watch. Nerves to the hand pass from the forearm under the strap (ligament). If the band becomes too tight for any reason this compresses the median nerve and produces pins and needles sensation, numbness or a burning pain usually in the 1st (thumb) 2nd, 3rd and half of the 4th (ring) fingers of the affected hand. The pain may travel up the forearm and is characteristically worse at night. Shaking or manipulating the hand/wrist may relieve it. A steroid injection may help for a while but will eventually require referral to a rheumatology department for further tests and possibly minor surgery to release the tight ligament.

I Never Knew That

Both carpal tunnel syndrome and ganglion of the wrist will be aggravated by any position that puts pressure on the joint (press-ups, missionary position during intercourse, handstanding).

It is not often appreciated that within one minute blood from the wrist has circulated to the heart and the rest of the body through every capillary from the brain to the toes up to 70 times in that one minute. It would travel even faster if the heart was beating any faster. The most effective way to cool oneself is to rub an ice cube over the wrist just behind the base of the thumb – where the radial artery is situated ; a useful manoeuvre on a hot day or to bring down a fever.

Karate handchops and boxing will affect the wrist joint at some time and may set the stage for developing osteoarthritis in the joint. The hand and its small joints will suffer a similar fate for they were not designed for such abuse.

ISBN 1425121950

9 781425 121952